C000135042

Basic Clinical Science

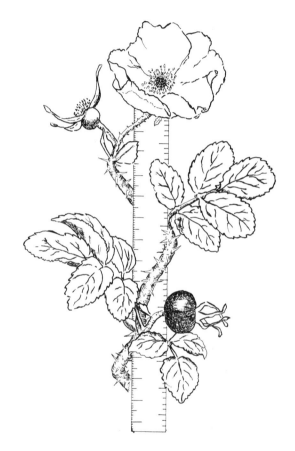

Describing a Rose with a Ruler .....

Hodder & Stoughton
LONDON SYDNEY AUCKLAND TORONTO

British Library Cataloguing in Publication Data
Rowley, N.
Basic clinical science: A complementary medicine
workbook.
I. Title
610

ISBN 0-340-55322-7

First published in Great Britain by
Hodder & Stoughton 1991

© 1991 Dr Nic Rowley

All rights reserved. No part of this publication may be reproduced or transmitted in any form or by any means, electronic or
mechanical, including photocopy, recording, or any information
storage and retrieval system, without permission in writing from
the publisher or under licence from the Copyright Licensing
Agency Limited. Further details of such licences (for repro-
graphic reproduction) may be obtained from the Copyright
Licensing Agency Limited, of 90 Tottenham Court Road, London
W1P 9HE.

Illustrations by Keith Robertson and Kirsten Hartvig.

Cartoons by Keith Robertson.

Designed and typeset by Kirsten Hartvig.

Printed in Great Britain for the educational publishing division of
Hodder & Stoughton Ltd, Mill Road, Dunton Green, Sevenoaks,
Kent by Clays Ltd, St ives plc

Basic Clinical Science

A Workbook for Complementary Medical Practitioners

Nic Rowley, MA, MRCS, LRCP, MBAcA

Lecturer in Orthodox Clinical Science,
the European School of Osteopathy

It is more important to
know what sort of person
has a disease
than to know
what sort of disease
a person has.

Hippocrates

Contents

Preface
 1 Introduction to the Orthodox Approach 3
 2 Inflammation and Tissue Healing 15
 3 Clinical Genetics 35
 4 Basic Immunology 53
 5 Neoplasia 71
 6 Circulatory Disorders 87
 7 Infectious Disease 105
 8 Principles of Orthodox Pharmacology 159
 9 Principles of Epidemiology
    and Overview of the NHS 189
10 Introduction to Clinical Examination 207
11 The Cardiovascular System 237
12 The Respiratory System 267
13 The Gastrointestinal System 295
14 The Endocrine System 337
15 Metabolic Disorders 363
16 Diseases of the Nervous System 377
17 Mental Health 415
18 Joint Disease 437
19 Connective Tissue Disorders 455
20 Bone Disease 463
21 Renal Medicine 475
22 Urology 489
23 Haematology 509
24 Skin Disease 529
25 Eye Disease / ENT 557
26 Gynaecology 589
27 Introduction to Obstetrics 629
28 Emergencies 641
29 The Principles of First Aid 663
30 Dictionary of Differential Diagnosis 677
Further Reading 709
Index 713
Postscript 737

Orthodox and non-orthodox medical traditions have both developed precious insight into the nature of health and disease and apparent contradictions between them are merely reflections of our difficulties in perceiving things as they are (the appearance of a diamond alters with the position of the observer and the nature of the illuminating light). Thus the practitioner of natural medicine should not dismiss the corpus of orthodox knowledge simply because of problems in its *application* in our society any more than the orthodox doctor should dismiss alternative methods and philosophies because of "science's" inability to explain them.

The division of the traditional western medical curriculum into separate disciplines of cell biology, embryology, anatomy, histology, physiology, biochemistry, immunology, bacteriology, chemical pathology, haematology, systematic histopathology, medicine, surgery, obstetrics, gynaecology, psychological medicine, etc etc is largely artificial for in order to grasp the concepts that underlie current orthodox medical practice it is necessary to develop an integrated view of the nature, structure, function and malfunction of the human body.

Nevertheless a fragmented approach to medical education persists because of difficulties in knowing where to start when faced with the huge volume of material now available for study and may account for the fragmented approach to the human condition manifest in some practitioners.

This book is an attempt to provide an intelligible and reasonably comprehensive guide to current orthodox medical practice in a way that is relevant to the needs of students and practitioners of natural therapeutics and, as such, omits much of the hard won detail that illuminates traditional medical textbooks.

Rather than promote the idea that a few months theoretical study of orthodox concepts and techniques is sufficient grounding for the use of such methods in practice, the book aims:

1) to provide the amount of orthodox information necessary for the well informed and safe practice of a natural therapeutic discipline and

2) to facilitate good communication between orthodox and heterodox practitioners and between practitioners and their patients (who often view their complaints from a conventional medical perspective).

Specifically then, the book has the following objectives:

a) To provide a basis for understanding the general pathological processes that underlie orthodox western concepts of disease and treatment.

b) To demonstrate that similar pathological processes can present clinically in a large number of symptomatic guises (depending on the system affected).

c) To introduce the concept that similar symptomatology may have vastly different significance in different groups of patients.

d) To thereby alert the reader to those conditions that would be generally considered to be better dealt with by orthodox medical services at the present time.

e) To provide a good working vocabulary thereby facilitating accurate communication between practitioners and their colleagues and patients.

FORMAT

This book evolved from a series of detailed lecture notes provided for students at the International College of Oriental Medicine, the School of Herbal Medicine and the European School of Osteopathy over the past 5 years. It is an attempt to relieve students of some of the drudgery of note taking during formal lectures, thus allowing them to concentrate more fully on discussion and audio-vis. ¬l presentations. It also attempts to demonstrate that the 'scientific' approach to health and disease, though inherently incomplete, can sometimes be useful in offering patients choices in the management of their ailments.

I have tried to keep jargon to a minimum and to use as few words as possible to explain any given topic, often resorting to abbreviations and sentences in note form. Thus the book will prove more satisfying as a practical reference rather than a textbook to be waded through slavishly from cover to cover.

The open format is supposed to encourage the reader to make notes in the margins referring to actual clinical experience and other, more detailed textbooks.

I have assumed that the reader will have acquired some knowledge of basic anatomy and physiology before embarking on clinical studies but understanding of the text does not depend on this.

Inevitably, the first edition of any textbook will contain textual and factual inaccuracies. I apologize for these and any confusion or inconvenience they may cause. Comments and suggestions from readers on how to improve future editions will be gratefully received.

Acknowledgements

The author humbly acknowledges the help given by the many students, colleagues, teachers and authors who have (knowingly or unknowingly) contributed to this book.

1. Introduction to the Orthodox Approach

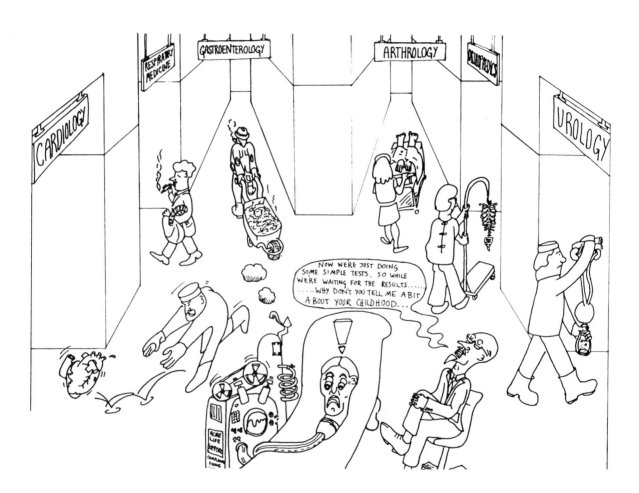

INTRODUCTION TO THE ORTHODOX APPROACH

OVERVIEW

History

Levels of Intervention

The Medical Model

> Pathogenesis
> Diseases as discrete entities
> Differential diagnosis

The Problem Oriented Medical Record

HISTORY

The history of orthodox medicine is a complex and fascinating subject and there are many excellent texts available which detail the development of orthodox western medical practice.

However, it is not always appreciated that institutionalized, technological medicine is a relatively young discipline.

Did you know, for example, that the first successful attempt to formalize nursing practice occurred as recently as 1862 (with the formation of the Manchester and Salford Sanitary Association) and that legislation making trained midwifery care for all mothers a national obligation was not passed until 1936?

And did you know that physicians, surgeons and apothecaries only came together as one (albeit rather disparate) profession in 1853 with the formation of the General Medical Council?

And did you realize that the charitable "voluntary" hospitals, the Poor Law based municipal hospitals, the fever hospitals and the lunatic asylums did not amalgamate into a national hospital service until 1939?

As we shall see in later chapters, many of the most important technical medical "advances" have occurred within the past fifty years. The National Health Service (based on the concept of high quality medical treatment free at the point of need for the whole population) has only been in operation since 1946.

Despite its youth, the growth of the orthodox system since the war has been phenomenal (the NHS is one of the largest employers in Europe) which suggests that conventional medicine must be doing something right. Moreover, the long traditions of some of the non-orthodox therapies have *not* been enough to ensure their position in twentieth century society. Relatively few people feel that the alternative therapy clinic is the first port of call in the face of disease.

Thus, as we review the various aspects of orthodox clinical science, we will try to highlight its strengths as well as its problems since the claims made for non-orthodox approaches to disease are bound to be judged in the light of the *best* of what orthodox medicine has to offer.

LEVELS OF INTERVENTION

Perhaps the highest quality medical intervention is one which prevents the development of disease by **improving the health** of the individual and yet few orthodox practitioners have the time to work in this area.

Nevertheless, a level at which orthodox medicine can claim considerable success is that of physiological support, as seen in intensive care units where the patients are not so much treated as maintained (by high tech means) in broad physiological balance thus allowing the body to mobilize its own healing resources.

Another level of intervention (again one in which the orthodox system is pre-eminent) is the repair of structural damage. Improvements in anaesthetic technique and surgical skill now allow the successful repair of gross tissue damage and many thousands of accident victims would not be alive today without such surgical excellence.

However, the bulk of orthodox medicine is concerned with interventions that either remove diseased tissue, suppress pathological processes or merely provide symptomatic relief with no effect on *underlying* pathology. In other words, much orthodox medical treatment is aimed at relieving effects rather than treating causes.

Of course relieving pain and distress is an important part of all medicine, but in the face of the current tendency for the demand for medical services to increase beyond society's capacity to pay for them, we must surely ask whether the time has come to make a genuine shift in priorities towards primary prevention rather than symptomatic cure.

THE MEDICAL MODEL

The orthodox medical model is really quite simple – learn where all the bits are (anatomy), find out how they work (physiology and biochemistry), observe the sort of things that can go wrong with them (pathology, usually in dead specimens) and then note carefully what sort of symptoms and signs occur in patients who turn out to have the pathologies already studied (clinical medicine). You can then intervene by repairing anatomy (surgery), readjusting physiology (medicine) or removing/suppressing pathology (medicine or surgery).

The "best" cases are those in which it is possible to explain all the symptoms and signs in terms of one pathological diagnosis which can then be treated by a single specific intervention.

The orthodox doctor learns to consider disease in three ways:

1. In terms of pathogenesis (cause).

2. As discrete entities.

3. As part of a differential diagnosis (ie all the possible explanations for a given set of symptoms and signs).

The idea is that when confronted with the clinical problem, the practitioner has these three areas of knowledge whirling in the head rather like drums in a one-armed bandit; hopefully, as more clinical information emerges, the drums will stop and produce three matching pictures thus winning the jackpot of an accurate diagnosis.

We shall now investigate these three concepts in more detail.

1. PATHOGENESIS

A typical orthodox classification of disease:

Conventional medicine divides all disease into 2 broad categories: CONGENITAL (ie present at birth) or ACQUIRED.

Possible causes of **acquired** disease can be listed as follows:
›   Traumatic (injury)
›   Infectious
›   Neoplastic
›   Iatrogenic (drugs, surgery etc. In other words, *caused* by doctors)
›   Metabolic disturbance
›   Endocrine disturbance
›   Multisystem
›   Haematological disturbance
›   Vascular disturbance
›   Immunological disturbance
›   Degenerative change
›   Inflammation of uncertain aetiology
›   Psychogenic
›   Factitious
›   Idiopathic (aka no idea)

Notes:

Infectious disease can be further subdivided into – bacterial, viral, fungal or protozoal (worms, etc.).

Neoplastic disease may be – benign or malignant (primary or secondary).

Multisystem conditions include – rheumatoid and seronegative arthritides, connective tissue disorders, amyloid and sarcoid.

Haematological disturbance can be divided into – red cell disease, white cell disease, proliferative + neoplastic disorders and bleeding disorders.

Vascular disturbance includes – atherosclerosis, embolism and spasmodic problems.

Allergy, hypersensitivity and auto-immune disorders are all examples of immunological disturbance.

2. DISEASES AS DISCRETE ENTITIES

Any disease can be described in detail as a discrete entity (see below). In practice a knowledge of the incidence, affected population, aetiological factors and prognosis are the most useful.

Suggested model for description of a disease:

> › Definition of condition –

> › **Incidence** –

> › **Population** (including age group, sex, occupation) –

> › Geographical distribution –

> › Possible **aetiological factors** (ie possible causes) –

> › Pathogenesis* (including details on transmission and spread of disease) –

> › Gross and microscopical appearances of affected organs or tissues –

> › Major clinical features –

> › Important investigations –

> › Differential diagnosis –

> › Principles of treatment –

> › **Prognosis** –

> › Prevention –

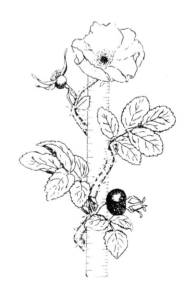

*   Pathogenesis (literally – birth of the pathology) means "how do the pathological changes in the tissues produce the disease in the whole person?".

3. DIFFERENTIAL DIAGNOSIS

As we have already said, rational allopathic treatment of disease is founded on an understanding of specific pathologies that present as recognizable clinical entities, for such understanding carries the potential for the application of specific remedies which remove, reverse or suppress pathological factors.

However, patients present with symptoms and signs and NOT disease labels. Hence the appearance in a surgery or hospital clinic of a "classic" textbook presentation of one of the conditions mentioned in the rest of this book, with a diagnosis confirmed by subsequent investigations (including histological examination of diseased tissue), is surprisingly rare and a matter of considerable interest to the attending physicians.

Thus, although much medical education is aimed at providing the aspiring doctor with a more or less detailed knowledge of myriad "diseases", the clinical emphasis is on the acquisition of a "database" of all the various *possible* causes for any given clinical presentation of symptoms and signs.

For, in a sense, one of the primary duties of a conventional doctor seeing a patient for the first time is to decide what the complaint *could* "be" and then to seek to exclude or confirm the most serious and the most treatable conditions (by physical examination, diagnostic tests, specialist referral, experience of what is common and instinct).

A wide knowledge of "differential diagnosis" reduces the likelihood that something serious (or, worse, something *treatable* and serious) will be misdiagnosed or missed altogether and physicians with encyclopaedic knowledge of differential diagnosis are much admired by their colleagues. However, even a brief survey of the material in the rest of the book illustrates the enormity of the task, for the conditions mentioned represent merely the tip of the orthodox medical iceberg of known pathologies. Thus, for most allopathic physicians, a reasonable approach to the wealth of clinical possibilities contained in the simplest complaints of every patient is facilitated by the realization that **common things are common** and, to a lesser extent, by experience of the fact that **very ill people tend to be very ill** (with some notable exceptions - see chapter 28 for a discussion of "red flag" presentations of importance to practitioners in all disciplines).

Students and practitioners of natural medicine necessarily view their patients in a different (sometimes radically different) perspective from their orthodox colleagues and the differences in the nature of their clinical workload mean (at the present time) that many of the differential diagnoses associated with a given symptom complex will remain "text-book" entities to the majority of natural therapists, making it somewhat illogical to try and commit them to memory.

I have thus included a dictionary of differential diagnosis in chapter 30 listing about 40 common clinical presentations. This is not intended to inculcate a feeling of insecurity about the possible implications of simple complaints and should not stir up worries about the accuracy of alternative diagnostic methods; but neither should it be taken as an exhaustive catalogue to be used without the illumination of clinical experience, for this will lead to oversuspicion of the very rare and possibly disastrous ignorance of the very serious. Rather it is intended as a ready reference to be used when needed and not something to be slavishly (and probably inaccurately) remembered.

» There is never any harm in looking something up since this may lead to greater knowledge for the attendant and better treatment for the patient.

THE PROBLEM ORIENTED MEDICAL RECORD

One of the most useful developments in the recording of patient data has been the widespread acceptance of the **POMR** (Problem Oriented Medical Record) which is a way of recording case notes in terms of the PATIENT'S problems.

A POMR has four parts

1. A database constructed from all the information collected during history taking and examination.

2. A problem list in which all the problems emerging from the database are categorized as **active** (ie needing some action) and **inactive** (ie not causing immediate difficulty but providing a context for the patient's current state).

3. A management plan.

4. A means of recording future progress.

We would suggest that progress notes are recorded under four headings:

S (subjective) for what the patient tells you.

O (objective) for what you observe.

A (assessment) for your assessment of the situation.

P (plan) the management plan resulting from this consultation..

2. Inflammation and Tissue Healing

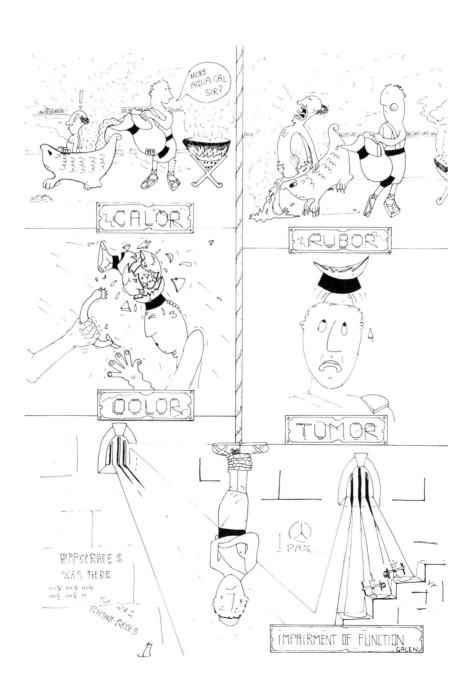

INFLAMMATION AND TISSUE HEALING

OVERVIEW

Introduction

Overview of Inflammation

Sequels to Acute Inflammation

Examples of Inflammatory Conditions

Consequences of Injury

Ulceration

Tissue Healing and Repair

INTRODUCTION

Inflammation is the local reaction of the body to injury. The "cardinal signs" were supposedly first documented by Aulus Aurelius Cornelius CELSUS (53BC – 7AD), a Roman medical writer. They are:

> **HEAT (calor)**
> **REDNESS (rubor)**
> **PAIN (dolor)**
> **SWELLING (tumor)**

> Claudius GALEN (130 – 200AD) who, in his position as Surgeon to the Gladiators at Pergamum, had frequent opportunity to study local reactions of the body to injury, added a fifth cardinal sign –

> **IMPAIRMENT OF FUNCTION**

> In 1927, a scientist called LEWIS performed a series of experiments in which he demonstrated that the cardinal features of acute inflammation were primarily the result of **changes in local vasculature** precipitated by injury and mediated by a combination of chemical factors and local nervous reactions.

You can reproduce his basic observations on yourself:

> "Injure" yourself by drawing a blunt instrument (eg a pen) firmly across the skin of your forearm. Watch what happens.

> Hopefully you observed the following:

> 1) The stroke was marked briefly by a **WHITE LINE** – this was due to a momentary reflex **vasoconstriction.**

> 2) Very soon a dull red line – a **FLUSH** – appeared – this was due to local **capillary** dilatation.

> 3) Shortly after the flush, a brighter red irregular zone – a **FLARE** – surrounded the initial "injury" and was the result of local **arteriolar dilatation.**

> 4) Finally a **WEAL** appeared amongst the redness. This was the result of leakage of protein rich fluid – **inflammatory exudate** – through the dilated vessel walls and into the surrounding tissues.

The **flush, flare and weal** are known collectively as **"Lewis' TRIPLE RESPONSE"**.

The initial injury produced these effects by

1) damaging cells and releasing chemical "mediators";
2) exciting local nervous reflexes termed "axon reflexes";
3) directly affecting blood vessels.

Thus vascular dilatation is responsible for the cardinal signs of redness and heat whilst the leakage of protein rich exudate from dilated blood vessels explains the swelling that accompanies inflammation.

Pain results from a combination of the release of irritant chemicals from locally damaged cells and the pressure caused by the accumulation of protein rich fluid in a confined space.

All animal tissues – internal and external – show features of the inflammatory response when subjected to injury or insult.

In orthodox medicine, therefore, inflammation is a primary manifestation of disease.

OVERVIEW OF THE INFLAMMATORY PROCESS

Inflammation may be:

ACUTE
SUBACUTE
CHRONIC

Causes of inflammation:

PHYSICAL (heat, cold, radiation)
BIOLOGICAL (bacterial toxins, fungi, parasites)
CHEMICAL (poisons and irritants)

The sequence of events in acute inflammation is as follows:

Injury → vascular dilatation → blood flow slows down locally → white cells "fall out" of main stream and "marginate" along the vessel walls → white cells, fluid and protein escape into surrounding tissues as inflammatory exudate causing swelling of affected tissues.

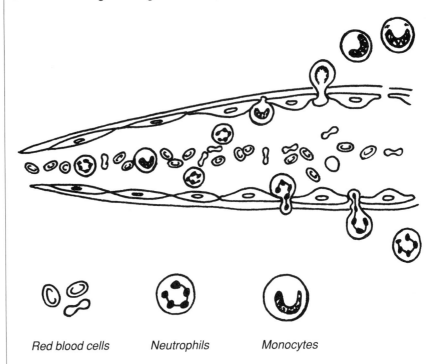

Red blood cells   Neutrophils   Monocytes

Chemical mediators of inflammation include:

HISTAMINE
KININS
COMPLEMENT
IMMUNOGLOBULINS

Constituents of exudate:

WATER
PROTEIN (including fibrinogen)
CELLS (including "polymorphs", macrophages and (later on) lympho-
cytes and plasma cells)

Helpful effects of inflammatory process on local damage:

LOCALIZES injury.
DILUTES irritants with inflammatory exudate.
Allows PHAGOCYTOSIS of bacteria and other foreign particles by white
cells.
Allows NEUTRALIZATION of antigens by antibodies.

SEQUELS TO ACUTE INFLAMMATION

RESOLUTION
ORGANIZATION OF EXUDATE
SUPPURATION
CHRONIC INFLAMMATION

Resolution:

Implies that the inflammatory response has successfully dealt with the injury allowing the situation to "resolve" with little or no damage to the tissues.

The various white cells present combine to break down and "hoover" up any debris and the remaining fluid is take‚ up into local lymphatic vessels.

(**Lobar pneumonia** , a bacterial infection of the alveolar spaces of a lung, is an example of an infection that heals by **resolution**.)

Organization:

Occurs when the acute inflammatory process causes excessive exudation or tissue death and when local conditions are unfavourable for the removal of the debris.

In these circumstances, new capillaries grow into the area and the inflamed tissue is eventually transformed into fibrous tissue (scar tissue). This is achieved by the proliferation of **fibroblasts** (situated around the new capillaries) which manufacture **collagen** – the raw material of scars.

This process is described more fully below (healing by granulation).

Suppuration:

Literally means the formation of **pus** and occurs where pus forming organisms (such as staphylococci) are found – eg on the skin, in an untreated inflamed appendix, etc.

Pus is a thick, creamy, yellow mixture of inflammatory exudate, pus cells (polymorphs), bacteria (dead or alive), cell fragments and globules of fat; an accumulation of pus is termed an **abscess**.

Developing abscesses are ill defined at first but eventually newly vascularized connective tissue proliferates around the edges of the inflamed area and forms a clear boundary. This "demarcation" zone keeps pumping white cells from capillaries into the abscess causing it to swell and then burst, after which healing may take place.

This raises few problems with superficial abscesses but with deeply situated abscesses, discharged pus may have to travel long distances before it escapes to the outside world through the skin. The pathway formed in the tissues by escaping pus is called a **sinus**. A **sinus** is thus defined as a track (lined with granulation tissue) that joins a cavity to the exterior. Sinus formation is a common complication of severe bone infections.

» Note that if an abscess forms on the surface of an organ and discharges its pus in such a way that an abnormal communication is formed between that organ and an *adjacent* organ, the resulting "track" is termed a **fistula**.

A **fistula** is thus defined as an abnormal connection between two surfaces – serous, mucous or cutaneous. (Serous membranes line enclosed body cavities and the outside of viscera. Mucous membranes line all cavities that open to the exterior.)

Chronic Inflammation:

May be a sequel to acute inflammation if the initial irritant, though attenuated by the inflammatory response, still persists. However, chronic inflammatory changes in tissues are, more often than not, a **primary** manifestation of disease and thus do NOT necessarily imply a preceding acute inflammatory phase. **TB, syphilis and rheumatoid arthritis** all produce a chronic inflammatory picture from the outset (though they may be complicated by acute inflammatory episodes).

The microscopic appearance of the affected tissue is different from acutely inflamed tissue with more mononuclear cells present.

EXAMPLES OF INFLAMMATORY CONDITIONS

The suffix "itis" indicates inflammation hence:

Blepharitis	→	Inflammation of the eyelids.
Cholecystitis	→	Inflammation of the gall bladder.
Colitis	→	Inflammation of the colon.
Encephalitis	→	Inflammation of the brain substance.
Endocarditis	→	Inflammation of the heart lining (includes heart valves).
Gastritis	→	Inflammation of the stomach.
Hepatitis	→	Inflammation of the liver.
Meningitis	→	Inflammation of the brain coverings.
Myocarditis	→	Inflammation of the heart muscle.
Otitis externa	→	Inflammation of the external auditory canal.
Otitis media	→	Inflammation of the middle ear.
Rhinitis	→	Inflammation of the mucous membranes lining the nasal cavity.
Salpingitis	→	Inflammation of the Fallopian tubes.

and many, many more.

» It is a good idea to look up the **meaning** of conditions whose name you have not met before as soon as you come across them. You will be surprised how many times a complicated name is merely a Greek or Latin translation of a simple description.

To confuse you:

Pneumonia	→	Inflammation of the lung tissue (alveoli or terminal bronchioles).
Pleurisy	→	Inflammation of the pleura.

CONSEQUENCES OF INJURY

We have seen that the inflammatory response is a local "damage control" strategy employed by the body when faced with tissue injury.

However, if the insult is too great (or long lasting) there may be a variety of **other** consequences ie:

> ›   cell degeneration or death
> ›   tissue death ("necrosis")
> ›   the appearance of "infiltrations"

We will now consider these in turn –

CELL DEGENERATION AND DEATH

Causes of cell degeneration:

Physical agents (heat etc)
Chemical agents
Biological agents
Lack of nutrients and blood

Microscopic signs of degeneration:

Cells swell up.
Fat accumulates inside cells (this sort of "fatty degeneration" is usually found in damaged cell types that have a high metabolic rate in health, eg heart, liver and kidney).
Organelles degenerate.

Mechanisms of cell death:

Self digestion ("autolysis")
Digestion by other cells ("heterolysis")
Shrinkage and fragmentation ("apoptosis")

Nuclear changes in cell death:

Dissolution ("karyolysis")
Fragmentation ("karyorrhexis")
Shrinkage ("pyknosis")

TISSUE DEATH (necrosis)

Necrosis is defined as "death of a **group** of cells in continuity with living cells" and may be caused in the same ways as individual cell death.

The exact appearance of necrotic tissue varies with site and circumstance but there are some common terms that you should have heard of, viz:

Coagulative necrosis:

Caused by inadequate blood supply eg heart muscle in myocardial infarction. The cells die but their outlines remain leaving a "ghost" tissue architecture that can be seen under a microscope.

Colliquative necrosis:

Dead tissue liquefies. Usually only seen in brain tissue which has a high fat content.

Caseous necrosis:

Dead tissue is converted to a granular, amorphous, cheesy mass. After a time, areas of caseation may **calcify**. Caseous necrosis is common in TB.

Gangrene:

Is tissue death + putrefaction and is associated with an abrupt cut off of blood supply in certain vulnerable areas (toes, gut etc). See chapter 6 for more details.

Fat necrosis:

Is death of fat tissue! Dead fat tends to feel hard and is thus a relatively common cause of suspicious feeling breast lumps which may simply be the result of local trauma to the breast (which is very fatty). Fat necrosis may also be followed by calcification.

Fibrinoid necrosis:

Is just a particular sort of tissue damage often seen in the walls of the arterioles of patients with **hypertension**.

INFILTRATIONS

In some chronic diseases, abnormal substances (or normal substances in abnormal amounts) may accumulate in or between diseased cells. The reasons for this are largely obscure.

In the condition known as **secondary amyloidosis**, deposits of a fibrillar protein are laid down in various organs (including spleen, liver, kidney and tongue) to more or less disastrous effect. Amyloidosis may be secondary to several conditions including chronic infection, rheumatoid arthritis and myeloma.

Primary amyloidosis (ie of no obvious cause) also occurs.

ULCERATION

Ulcers are formed when the surface covering of an organ or tissue is lost due to necrosis and replaced with inflammatory tissue.

Ulceration is a complication of many diseases. Tissues most commonly involved are the skin and alimentary tract.

Ulcers may be divided into 2 main categories:

SIMPLE (inflammatory) – which may be acute or chronic
and
MALIGNANT (cancerous)

The differences between simple and malignant ulcers are most noticeable at the **edges**.

Simple ulcer

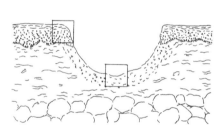

Inflammatory tissue around edge and at the base of the ulcer.

Malignant ulcer

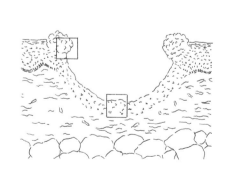

Malignant tissue at edge.

Inflammatory tissue at the base.

TISSUE HEALING AND REPAIR

INTRODUCTION

When cells or tissues have been damaged by trauma or disease, the body attempts to make good the deficit by a variety of mechanisms (some of which can be aided or encouraged by medical or surgical intervention).

These are:

› REGENERATION

› HEALING BY FIRST INTENTION

› HEALING BY GRANULATION (second intention)

» Before considering these in detail, we will explain the phenomenon of **fibrosis** (scarring) which is an integral part of wound healing. All tissue damage results in some degree of scarring (except in those tissues capable of regeneration).

FIBROSIS

Fibrosis is the formation of fibrous tissue (scars).

When tissues are damaged, cells called **fibrocytes** situated around capillaries and in the loose connective tissues are somehow stimulated to enlarge into active cells called **fibroblasts**. These secrete a substance called **tropocollagen** which "condenses" to form a network of **collagen** fibres. Enzyme action over a period of time weaves and remodels the collagen fibres into tough scar tissue.

TISSUE REGENERATION

Regeneration is the replacement of dead cells by new cells.

1) Some tissues regenerate freely:
   surface epithelia, bone marrow, lymphoid tissue.

2) Some tissues regenerate but in doing so do not quite reconstitute normal tissue architecture:
   liver cells, renal tubular epithelium.

3) Some tissues are quite incapable of regeneration under normal circumstances: neurones, renal glomeruli, heart muscle.

WOUND HEALING BY FIRST INTENTION

Healing by first intention occurs in clean wounds whose edges are close together. It results in minimal scarring.

This is the sort of healing that surgical suturing seeks to encourage.

WOUND HEALING BY GRANULATION (second intention)

Healing by granulation occurs in more open wounds particularly if there is significant tissue loss, necrosis or infection.

WOUND HEALING BY GRANULATION

Wound cavity filled with blood clot. Acute inflammation at the junction between healthy and damaged tissue.

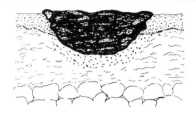

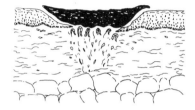

Scab drying out, epithelium starting to regenerate, capillary loops growing into wound bringing fibroblasts.

Clot shed, capillary loops seen as "granulations" of base of wound.

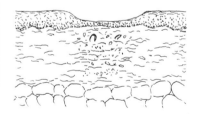

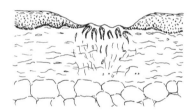

Epithelium covers wound, collagen fibres forming immature scar, capillaries less noticeable.

Mature, avascular scar with full epithelial covering.

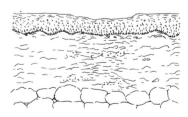

SUMMARY OF WOUND HEALING

Clean incised wounds:

> › Surface glued together by fibrin clot
> › Inflammatory reaction at wound edges
> › Capillary buds join together
> › Fibroblasts align parallel to wound surface and lay down collagen
> › Epithelium covers wound

Wounds with loss of substance:

> › Capillary buds and fibroblasts proliferation in base and at edges
> › Vascular "arcades" build up until gap is filled
> › Fibroblasts lay down collagen from below upwards
> › Epithelium covers surface

FACTORS THAT CAN DELAY WOUND HEALING

Local – Infection
Poor blood supply

General – Vitamin C deficiency
Amino acid deficiencies
Zinc deficiency
Steroid therapy

COMPLICATIONS OF WOUND HEALING

CONTRACTURES
PROUD FLESH
KELOID

Contractures:

Thickening and shortening of collagen bundles in areas of extensive scarring may cause serious cosmetic problems or functional disability.

Burns patients often suffer contractures.

Proud flesh:

> Granulation tissue may form excessively at the base and edges of a wound and prevent proper healing.

Keloid:

> The formation of excessively thick collagen bundles that cause marked swelling at the site of a wound.

» | The condition is more common among blacks and pregnant women.

NOTE:

> Fibrous tissue fills in gaps but cannot perform specialized functions (eg it cannot contract like cardiac muscle fibres).

» | Also don't confuse fibrosis/fibrous tissue with **fibrin** which is involved in blood clotting. Fibrin is the end product of a complex "cascade" of enzyme reactions activated by injury to blood vessels. It forms a matrix upon which a blood clot can be built and thus helps minimize blood loss from a wound. It has no connection with fibroblasts.

3. Clinical Genetics

Sometimes simplicity hides under
complex appearances;
Sometimes it is the simplicity
which is apparent, and which
disguises extremely complicated
realities.

Henri Poincaré

CLINICAL GENETICS

OVERVIEW

Introduction

The genetic code

Mutations

The Transmission of Genetic Defects

Dominant genes
Recessive genetic abnormalities
Sex linked inheritance

Chromosomes and Chromosomal Abnormalities

Disorders Associated with Chromosomal Abnormalities

Autosomal abnormalities
Sex chromosome anomalies
Multifactorial inheritance

Genetic Counselling

INTRODUCTION

Chromosomes were discovered long before DNA and most students are introduced to genetics by way of chromosomes. However, from a functional point of view, chromosomes can be regarded simply as lengths of double stranded DNA, conveniently packaged for cell division. Thus a working knowledge of modern genetics depends on an understanding of the DNA molecule and its ability to transmit genetic information.

THE GENETIC CODE

DNA is made by stringing together chemical entities called nucleotides. Genetic information is encoded by the sequence of nucleotides from which each strand of DNA is made.

There are four types of nucleotide, each containing a different BASE ie Cytosine, Guanine, Thymine or Adenine (C, G, T and A).

The strands of nucleotides that make up DNA molecules are joined together by bonding between bases. Bases always pair off in a particular way ie A binds to T (and vice versa) and C binds to G (and vice versa).

Thus each strand of the DNA molecule will carry a nucleotide sequence **complementary** to its partner eg – "GATCG" would pair with "CTAGC".

DNA molecule

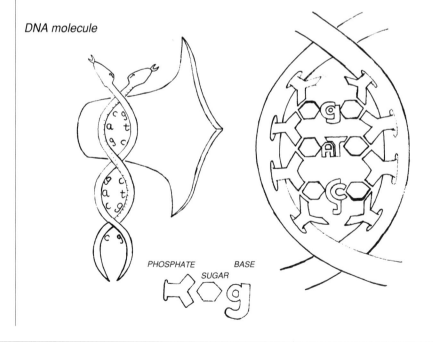

PHOSPHATE   BASE
SUGAR

A sequence of 3 adjacent nucleotides is called a TRIPLET:

A sequence of triplets is called a GENE.

One triplet represents the genetic information necessary for the specification of **one amino acid.** Sequences of triplets (**genes**) thus determine the nature of proteins synthesized by cells.

Although there are 64 **possible** combinations of C, T, A and G within the DNA molecule, the body commonly uses only 20 amino acids to make proteins. This is explained by the discovery that all but 2 amino acids are coded for by a **variety** of triplets. Those triplets that don't appear to code for ANY amino acid probably just provide the "punctuation" marks of the genetic language.

MUTATIONS

Since proteins are just lengths of amino acids strung together in a particular order determined by the order of DNA base triplets, it is fairly easy to see that *mistakes* in nucleotide sequences (known as **mutations**) might produce faulty proteins. If such mutant proteins happen to be important enzymes, bodily function may be compromised to some degree by the genetic error. A variety of environmental factors are known to cause DNA damage and thus mutation, and spontaneous mutation also takes place. However, the frequency of spontaneous mutation is quite low since DNA is a very stable substance that replicates in a very precise way.

The various types of mutation can be considered as misspelt words in the genetic language eg:

Substitution	Hippy Christmas
Deletion	Pubic convenience
Insertion	Public hair
Inversion	Knights in white stain
Nonsense	fhwosapfhs [apologies to fhwosapfhs fans]

>> Note that a **single** nucleotide mistake – sometimes called a "point mutation" – will not *necessarily* cause the production of faulty amino acids since most amino acids are coded for by several triplets (see previous page).

THE TRANSMISSION OF GENETIC DEFECTS

When considering the transmission of genetic defects, it is easier to think in terms of small chunks of DNA (ie chromosomes) rather than the whole DNA molecule. Since chromosomes are easily accessible during cell division, understanding of the transmission of genetic defects depends on an understanding of chromosomes.

Every cell in the body contains a **double set** of chromosomes (one set from each parent) and since chromosomes are just lumps of DNA containing large numbers of genes, it follows that all genes (sequences of triplets) are represented **twice** in every cell. Genes at the same point (locus) on **each** of a pair of chromosomes are called **ALLELES**. When alleles are **identical**, an individual is said to be **homozygous** for the gene in question. Individuals carrying two **different** genes for the same locus are termed **heterozygous** for that gene.

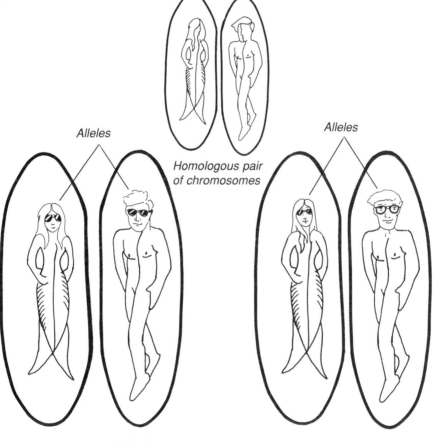

Alleles

Alleles

*Homologous pair
of chromosomes*

Homozygous individual

Heterozygous individual

It is usually only necessary to have **one** normal allele for the production of a normal protein. Thus **heterozygotes** with a defect on only one allele will not usually show any abnormality.

For some loci, however, the amount of protein synthesized by a single normal allele is insufficient for normal functioning and so a harmful mutation of only one gene at such a locus *will* manifest itself as an abnormality. Such aberrant genes are called **dominant genes.**

Harmful mutations which only affect the individual when present in a **double** dose (ie that express themselves only in **homozygous** individuals) are called **recessive genes.**

DOMINANT GENES

Will be transmitted by an affected individual to half his or her offspring.

Dominant genes which don't express themselves in every generation are said to show **incomplete penetrance.**

Note that the degree of abnormality caused by a harmful dominant gene may **vary** from one offspring to another. This is known as **"variable expression".**

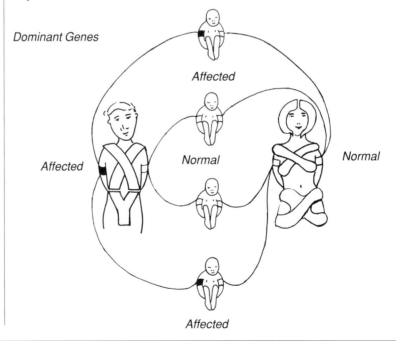

Dominant Genes

Affected

Affected

Normal

Normal

Affected

Common dominantly inherited conditions include:

› Polycystic disease of the kidneys
› Huntington's Chorea
› Polyposis Coli
› Neurofibromatosis

» The overall incidence of dominantly inherited abnormality is about 7 per 1000 live births.

RECESSIVE GENETIC ABNORMALITIES

Are only manifest when the abnormal gene is present in a double dose. Thus the abnormality can only occur in the offspring of a couple who are both "carriers" (heterozygotes).

When carriers mate, 1 in 4 offspring will be affected (homozygotes), 1 in 4 will be genetically normal and 1 in 2 will be carriers (heterozygotes).

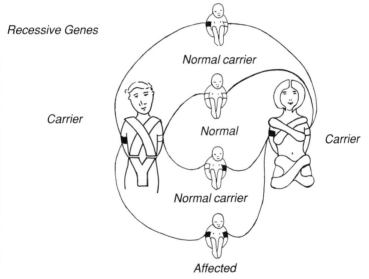

Recessive Genes

Normal carrier

Carrier

Normal

Carrier

Normal carrier

Affected

Common recessive disorders include:

› Cystic fibrosis
› Sickle cell anaemia
› Non-specific severe mental retardation
› Phenylketonuria

The overall incidence of recessive disorders is about 2.5 per 1000 live births.

SEX LINKED INHERITANCE

Genes carried on the sex chromosomes are termed **sex linked**, either Y-linked or X-linked.

X-linked RECESSIVE genes will **only** be manifested in male offspring since males can only have one X-chromosome. If it happens to be an abnormal X-chromosome they will express the disease. By the same token, affected males will pass on the trait to all their daughters but none of their sons.

X-linked recessive traits are only manifest in females who are **homozygous** for the particular gene. Who would manifest **X-linked DOMINANT** traits?*

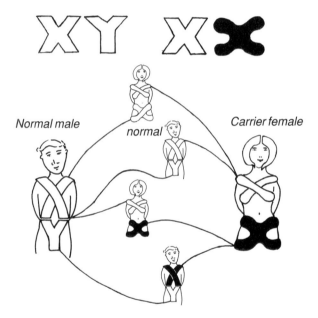

X-linked conditions are all rare and include:

> › Duchenne muscular dystrophy
> › Haemophilia

---

*   Heterozygous females and all males.

TO RECAP

› **The nucleus of EVERY body cell contains a complete set of "chromosomes"** (although the chromosomes are only SEEN as such when cells are in the process of DIVIDING);

› Chromosomes contain strands of **DNA**;

› DNA strands are made up of **nucleotides** linked together;

› The "GENETIC CODE" resides in the **sequences** of nucleotides (arranged in **triplets**) that make up the DNA strands;

› The nucleus "directs" the synthesis of ALL necessary cell **proteins** on the basis of the genetic code contained in its DNA;

› Proteins are made up of very long "polypeptide" chains (that is to say chains of amino acids) which are often coiled and twisted and joined to other polypeptide chains. As well as being important components of most body structures, proteins (as **enzymes**) play critical roles in almost all the body's chemical reactions. In other words you have to have normal proteins for normal functioning;

› Any particular sequence of triplets (in any strand of DNA) that determines the **order** of amino acids in a polypeptide chain is called a **GENE;**

› **Single** gene ("point") mutations can sometimes cause disease.

› **Dominant** genes manifest themselves when present in a single "dose" and are transmitted to half the children of an affected parent.

› **Recessive** genes only express themselves when present in a double dose and thus are only transmitted to children (1 in 4) if both parents are carriers.

CHROMOSOMES AND CHROMOSOMAL ABNORMALITIES

So far we have considered the molecular basis of the human **genetic code**, mentioned the way that cells synthesize proteins on the basis of this code and seen how alterations of a **single gene** on a **single chromosome** can cause disease by causing the production of an abnormal protein.

It should therefore be easy to see that if serious problems can be caused by the mutation of a **tiny** bit of DNA in one **minute** area of **one** chromosome, then serious abnormalities will almost certainly occur if large chunks of chromosomes (containing long strands of DNA and thus **many** genes) get somehow damaged during the course of production of ova and sperms. In fact many of the commonest inherited conditions (such as Down's syndrome) are the result of **chromosomal** abnormality rather than single gene mutation.

Before considering such conditions, it is necessary to briefly consider the structure of chromosomes and the nature and origin of the commonest chromosomal abnormalities.

CHROMOSOMES

In 1956, human beings were shown to have 46 chromosomes, ie 23 pairs, with one of each pair derived from the mother and one from the father.

Of these 23 pairs, 22 pairs were termed **AUTOSOMES** and the members of each "homologous" pair of autosomes look identical under the microscope (though the DNA they carry will, of course, be subtly different).
The remaining pair are called the **SEX CHROMOSOMES** and may be similar or different – ie X and X (female) or X and Y (male) – in type. Each chromosome is itself divided into two identical chromatids joined together at the centromere.

Chromosomes can be individually categorized into three classes (metacentric, sub-metacentric and acrocentric) on the basis of the position of their centromeres.

When stained with chemicals and looked at under a microscope, each chromosome can be seen to have a distinctive pattern of **light and dark banding**.

The last two sentences are unlikely to ever be of any use to you.

CHROMOSOMAL ABNORMALITIES

Chromosomal abnormality may be of **autosomes or sex chromosomes** but, either way, all chromosomal abnormalities are the result of something going wrong with the **meiotic** divisions that are necessary to produce sperms or ova. In simple terms, abnormalities can arise either:

1) Due to **numerical abnormality** ("aneuploidy") involving the loss or gain of one or two chromosomes as the result of **non-disjunction** (non-splitting up) of chromosomes during meiosis.

or

2) Due to **structural** abnormalities of the autosomes (such as translocations, deletions, duplications or inversions of chromosomal material in a way analogous to gene mutation described earlier but on a much bigger scale). In either case, abnormal meiosis produces abnormal gametes. Abnormal gametes produce abnormal babies.
NOTE that translocation of genetic material between chromosomes may **not** result in any abnormality so long as the foetus carries no more or less genetic material than normal in its cells – ie so long as the translocation is **"balanced"**. Problems only arise when some bits of chromosome are **lost** during the exchange, making the translocation **unbalanced**.

Exactly WHY any of these chromosomal abnormalities arise in any given case is largely unknown but we will discuss possible mechanisms later. Before considering some common chromosomal abnormalities in detail it is worth pointing out some of the features common to all of them:

1) All the conditions are **syndromes.**

2) Sufferers are affected to different degrees.

3) As many as 40% of all "spontaneous abortions" (which make up 25% of all RECOGNIZED conceptions) have major **chromosomal** abnormalities.

4) It is possible for a person to have **two or more distinct populations** of cells in their body as a whole (eg half normal and half abnormal) and it is the relative amount of each population which determines the degree of abnormality. This phenomenon is known as **mosaicism.**

Approximately 4 children per 1000 (of those born alive) have chromosomal abnormalities which divide equally between the "autosomal" and the "sex-chromosome" types. Most of these conditions are the result of **numerical abnormalities** of chromosomes.

DISORDERS ASSOCIATED WITH CHROMOSOMAL ABNORMALITIES

AUTOSOMAL ABNORMALITIES

The commonest AUTOSOMAL abnormalities are:
› **Down's Syndrome**
› **Edwards' Syndrome**
› **Patau's Syndrome**

» Many other syndromes have been described but all are rare. However, the **"Cri Du Chat" Syndrome** is also worth knowing about because of its characteristic presentation.

Down's Syndrome:

The commonest autosomal abnormality occurring in 1.5 per 1000 live births. Usually the result of an **extra** chromosome 21 hence the alternative name **"Trisomy 21"**. Can also be caused by translocation. Main features include "floppy" infants with protruding tongue, **characteristic facial appearance** (almond shaped eyes with marked epicanthic folds), round head with low set ears and small ear lobes, broad neck, abnormal palmar creases, short incurving little fingers, **severe mental retardation, heart defects** (20%) **and susceptibility to infection and leukaemia.** These children frequently die young but often have delightful personalities and love music.

Patau's Syndrome:

Trisomy 13. Rarely survive more than a few weeks. Multiple malformations including small head, cleft lip and palate, extra digits, brain damage and heart defects.

Edwards' Syndrome:

Trisomy 18. "Small for dates" as foetus. Death within first few weeks. Low set ears, small mouth, deformed fingers, rocker bottom feet, heart, kidney and brain malformations.

Cri Du Chat:

Partial deletion of the short arm of chromosome 5. Low birth weight, wide set eyes with marked epicanthic folds, small head, severe mental retardation, characteristic cry due to laryngeal abnormality.

SEX CHROMOSOME ANOMALIES

The commonest are: Extra Y = XYY
                         Extra X male = XXY (Klinefelter's syndrome)
                         Extra X female = XXX
                         Missing X = X0 (Turner's syndrome)

The first 3 each occur in 0.5 per 1000 live births. Turner's syndrome occurs in 0.05 per 1000 live births.

XYY	→	Tall males. ? antisocial behaviour.
XXY	→	Tall males with testicular atrophy, gynaecomastia and sparse body hair. Often ↓ IQ.
XXX	→	Female, normal bodies, variable intelligence, sometimes amenorrhoea/infertility.
XO	→	Short females with webbed neck, "cubitus valgus" (forearms bent outwards), poorly developed ovaries, sometimes heart defects. Not all people with such a genetic make up have the syndrome and vice versa.

NOTE:

1) The presence of a Y chromosome makes the person MALE however many X chromosomes they may have.

2) In a normal female only ONE X chromosome is directing cellular processes.

MULTIFACTORIAL INHERITANCE

Some congenital disease patterns are thought to occur only when a **genetic predisposition** coincides with an **environmental influence.** The degree of resulting disability depends on the nature of the interacting factors (including the sex of the individual).

The mode of inheritance of such conditions cannot be coherently explained in terms of our former discussion but it is fairly clear that the more severe the defect is in a given patient, the more likely it is that siblings or offspring will be affected.

» **Various heart defects, spina bifida, cleft lip and palate, congenital dislocation of the hip** and **club foot** are all thought to be inherited in a "multifactorial" manner.

GENETIC COUNSELLING

Involves estimate of **risk**.

» Requires **accurate diagnosis and knowledge** (or estimate) **of mechanism of inheritance.**

» Requires very detailed family history.

» Must put "risk" in perspective. The chance of ANY pregnancy ending with "severe" congenital abnormality is about 1 in 30.

Whilst it is possible to predict the risk of transmission of the autosomal and sex-linked "point" mutations with some accuracy, assessment of the risk in "chromosomal" and "multifactorial" conditions is often very difficult.

Note that the chances of any woman having a child with Down's syndrome (or any of the other *trisomies*) increases with increasing age (over 35 and even more so over 40). However, at least 20% of cases of Down's have their origin in *paternal* non-disjunction so it *may* be that the maternal age effect is due to a breakdown in mechanisms which normally *prevent* the birth of babies with chromosomal abnormalities. A woman who has had an offspring with a "trisomy" has a slightly increased chance of having *another* offspring with a chromosomal abnormality regardless of her age!

The suspicion of foetal abnormality is caused by finding high levels of a substance called 'α-fetoprotein' in the blood of pregnant mothers. Diagnosis can sometimes be confirmed by examining a sample of amniotic fluid. This procedure is known as amniocentesis. Since it involves the insertion of a needle through the abdomen into the uterus, it carries a small risk of direct damage to the foetus and a 1% risk of causing the loss of the pregnancy within a few days of the procedure.

The following table summarizes the risks for some of the commoner genetic diseases:

ABNORMALITY	RISK OF AFFECTED FOETUS
Multifactorial:	
Previous child with spina bifida	1 in 20
Parent with spina bifida	1 in 20
High maternal α-fetoprotein	1 in 10
Chromosomal:	
Previous child with trisomy	about 1 in 100
Parent known to carry translocation	between 1 in 40 and 1 in 10
Mother over 35	about 1 in 20
Autosomal recessive:	
Previously affected child	1 in 4
Both parents known carriers	1 in 4
X-linked recessive:	
(Remember – transmitted through the daughters but expressed in the sons.)	
Previously affected boy + family history	1 in 2 of the sons

» Note that organs and limbs are formed in the foetus in the first three months and thus all drugs are potentially "teratogenic" at this time.

4. Basic Immunology

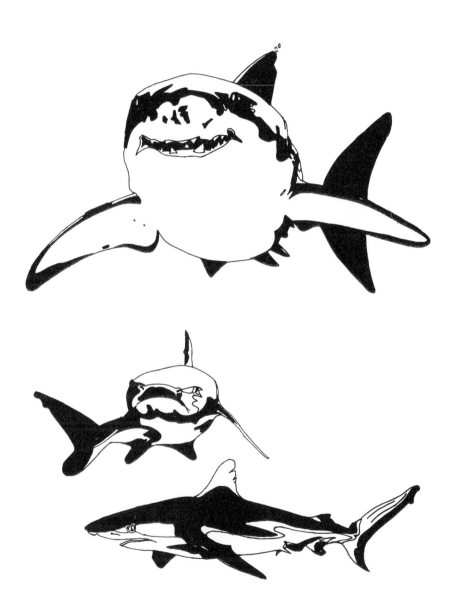

BASIC IMMUNOLOGY

OVERVIEW

Introduction

A Simplified Description of the "Immune Response"

Lymphoid Tissues and Immune Effector Cell Types

Allergy

> Type 1
> Type 2
> Type 3
> Type 4

Auto-immune Diseases

The Principles of Vaccination

> Immunization
> Contraindications to vaccination

Blood Groups

> Rhesus factor

INTRODUCTION

The "immune system" plays an important role in the body's defence against invasion by micro-organisms and other foreign materials. It is also responsible for the destruction of abnormal or mutant cell types that arise within the body from time to time.

However, the effects of immunological reactions are sometimes harmful to normal cells and tissues (a damaging immunological event is termed an ALLERGIC reaction) but there is no fundamental distinction between the mechanisms of "protective" immunity and those of "allergic" reactions. In fact, the concept of "allergy" owes more to the tendency of doctors to distinguish between events they consider "desirable" and "undesirable" than to any particular distinction between protective and allergic immune processes.

OVERVIEW

a) The immune system is similar in some ways to the nervous system in that it recognizes and responds to incoming signals in a way that depends on an **interaction between different cells**.

b) Substances which act as signals to the immune system are termed ANTIGENS and the system responds to the presence of antigens by: 1) producing ANTIBODIES and 2) manufacturing large numbers of LYM-PHOCYTES (particularly T-lymphocytes).

c) A fundamental property of the immune response is that it is **specific** to the antigen which stimulated it. Immune effector cells and antibodies specific to a particular antigen will **not** react with another antigen unless it is **very** similar to the original. Moreover, if the immune system has responded **once** to an antigenic stimulus, it *will* respond *much* more rapidly and abundantly if it is faced with the same antigen on a subsequent occasion.

d) The immune system may "learn" to **tolerate** antigenic signals without responding to them, thereby avoiding potentially damaging responses to harmless antigens (eg one's own body cells).

TO SUMMARIZE

The immune system -

> › Responds to antigenic stimuli
> › Has 2 response modes – humoral (antibody) and cell mediated (T-lymphocytes)
> › Is specific in its responses
> › Has a "memory"
> › Demonstrates tolerance

The ability of the immune system to distinguish self from other seems to be related to the fact that **all** cells carry genetically determined **surface "markers"** which can be recognized as "self" or "not-self" by certain types of antigen sensitive white blood cells.

It is also thought that every human body has a large quota of different **genetically predetermined** antigen sensitive white blood cells (called **T- and B-lymphocytes**) which are found in the lymphoid tissues (lymph nodes, spleen) and circulating in the blood. Such cells are well placed to encounter any foreign antigens that may enter the body.

A SIMPLIFIED DESCRIPTION OF THE "IMMUNE RESPONSE"

If any of the "preprogrammed" lymphocytes mentioned above meets with an antigen in such a way that it *recognizes* the antigen as "foreign"*, it will be stimulated to multiply.
Stimulated T-lymphocytes differentiate as they multiply to produce **4 types** of immune effector cells – **memory, killer, suppressor and helper T-cells**.

Memory cells:

> Are functionally similar to the original undifferentiated antigen sensitive T-lymphocytes and their production allows the immune system to mount a quicker response when faced with the *same* antigen at some later date.

Killer cells:

> Have a direct ability to damage invading antigen carrying cells (such as bacteria).

Suppressor cells:

> Exert a moderating influence on the immune response and stop things getting out of control.

Helper cells:

> Stimulate cells in the lymphoid tissue called **antigen sensitive B-lymphocytes** to divide and differentiate into the so-called **plasma cells** which produce and secrete a variety of high molecular weight substances known as **immunoglobulins** (Ig). These are the **antibodies** mentioned earlier. Antibodies have the property of combining specifically with the antigen molecules that *initially* stimulated their production. They are very important in making bacteria more susceptible to PHAGOCYTOSIS by macrophages and neutrophils (see later) and in the neutralization of bacterial TOXINS.

*   See next page.

Overall then, the immune response to a bacterial infection might go something like this:

› Invading bacterium eaten by macrophage at site of infection or in blood.

› Some bacterial protein is left exposed on the surface of the macrophage.

› Macrophage moves to some lymphoid tissue where it "presents" the dangling bacterial antigen to the resident antigen sensitive T-lymphocytes.

› An appropriate T-cell "looks at" the foreign antigen *and* at the surface "self" markers on the macrophage and "decides" that a response to foreign invasion is called for.

› T-cell multiplies and differentiates into killer, helper, suppressor and memory cells.

› Helper T-cells stimulate resident B-lymphocytes to multiply and differentiate into plasma cells which pass into blood and body fluids and secrete specific ANTIBODIES.

› After a time (depending on whether the stimulating antigen is new or comes from an old adversary) the blood and body fluid levels of antibody and killer T-cells are sufficient for a concerted attack on the "invaders".

› When the fight is over, the body (if still alive) is left with an immunological "memory" of the conflict which will ensure rapid mobilization of resources should it encounter the same challenge in the future.

LYMPHOID TISSUES AND IMMUNE EFFECTOR CELL TYPES

Tissues involved: Spleen, lymph nodes, thymus, bone marrow.
Cells involved: White blood cells and the plasma cells and macrophages derived from them.

1) LYMPHOID TISSUES

Lymph nodes (including tonsils and lymphoid follicles of GI tract)

    i) Formation, storage and removal of lymphocytes.
    ii) Site of ingestion of foreign particles by macrophages.

Typical lymph node

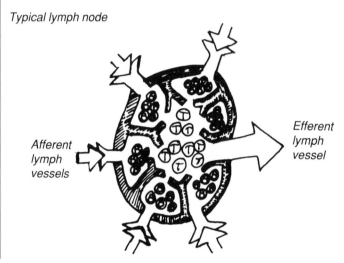

Afferent lymph vessels

Efferent lymph vessel

Spleen

    i) Production of lymphocytes.
    ii) Site of ingestion of foreign matter and worn out red blood cells by macrophages.
    iii) Storage of red blood cells.
    iv) Production of red blood cells in foetus.

Thymus

    i) Production of T-lymphocytes
    ii) Hormone secretion (possibly)

2) IMMUNE EFFECTOR CELL TYPES

WHITE BLOOD CELLS:

Type	% total WBC	Produced in	Function
Neutrophils	50-70%	Bone marrow	Phagocytosis of bacteria, cell debris, antibody "coated" foreign matter etc. Also release various chemicals which can damage bacteria.
Eosinophils	1-4%	Bone marrow	Not well understood. Play some part in controlling inflammatory reactions. Increased numbers in certain allergy states.
Basophils	1%	Bone marrow	Release of histamine and other chemicals involved in inflammation. MAST CELLS are similar but are found scattered throughout connective tissue.
Lymphocytes	20-40%	Bone marrow + lymphoid tissue	T-cells responsible for cell mediated immunity, B-cells for transformation to plasma cells and hence antibody production.
Monocytes	2-8%	Bone marrow	Precursors of tissue MACROPHAGES.

OTHER CELLS:

Type	Produced in	Function
Plasma cells	Lymphoid tissue from B-cells	Production of antibodies.
Macrophages	Formed from monocytes	Phagocytosis of all types of debris and foreign matter, general assistance in immune response.
Mast cells	Derived from basophils	Release of histamine and other chemicals in the tissues.

ALLERGY

Although the immune system is quite good at distinguishing between "self" and "foreign" antigens, it is not much good at discriminating between antigens that are "pathological" (harmful) and those that are not. **Reactions to harmless antigens may cause much tissue damage** and this, in simple terms, forms the basis of the phenomenon of **allergy**.

More formally, allergy may be defined as **a state of altered reactivity of the tissues to antigens which depends upon previous stimulation of the immune system by such antigens.** The term is usually only applied to conditions in which the effects of the immunological reactions in the tissues make a major contribution to the pathology of that condition.

Both types of immune response – humoral and cell mediated – can be involved in allergic reactions. *Antibody* responses tend to occur rapidly on re-exposure to an antigen whilst those mediated by T-cells take longer to develop because of the time taken for cells to accumulate at the "battle ground".

In the jargon of immunology pioneers **Coombs and Gell**, allergy is referred to as **hypersensitivity.** They originally described three types of antibody mediated hypersensitivity reactions and one type of cell mediated hypersensitivity reaction. These are described below.

Type 1

Is termed **anaphylaxis** and is the result of the release of several chemicals (such as histamine) from mast cells and basophils which go about their business with antibody of the **IgE** class sticking to their outer surfaces. If the "free" end of an antibody IgE should happen to latch on to some passing foreign antigen, a mechanism is activated which causes the mast cell (or basophil) to **degranulate** ie release its store of potent chemicals into the blood or tissues.
These chemicals (such as histamine) alter smooth muscle tone and may increase the permeability of blood vessels, so large scale degeneration of many mast cells may produce a variety of unpleasant effects including **bronchospasm, skin rashes, laryngeal oedema and a drop in blood pressure.** A combination of these may even result in death.

Type 1 reactions may be systemic – eg when a drug, a foreign serum or an insect poison enters the blood stream – **or local** – when, for example, pollen grain antigens come into contact with the mucous membranes of the upper respiratory tract and produce **asthma and hayfever.**

For some reason, certain individuals inherit the tendency to develop **local** type 1 hypersensitivity reactions – often referred to as **atopic** reactions. Thus juvenile asthma, eczema, migraine and hayfever often runs in families.

Type 2

Or **cytolytic** ("cell splitting") hypersensitivity reactions occur when certain antibodies of the IgG and IgM classes combine with foreign antigens and trigger off an enzymic system in the blood (the **complement system**) which, as well as destroying invader cells, can destroy red blood cells! Even micro-organisms or drugs long expelled from the body sometimes leave antigenic material stuck to red cell surfaces and these red cells may thus be destroyed by mistake.

Type 2 reactions are thus responsible for **"incompatible" blood transfusions** (including Rhesus incompatibility – see later) and also for **"autoimmune haemolytic anaemias"** caused when certain IgG and IgM antibodies turn against normal red blood cells in the manner just described.

Type 3

Is known as **immune complex hypersensitivity.** It is the result of an excessive build up of "antigen/antibody complexes" in the blood which may cause inflammatory reactions in the tissues. Such accumulations occur when the macrophages are unable to hoover up immune complexes quickly enough and thus are often accompanying infectious disease.

Manifestations of Type 3 reactions include **rashes, glomerulonephritis,** arthritis, **vasculitis and alveolitis.**

Type 4

Delayed, cell-mediated hypersensitivity – is the result of reactions in the tissues between T-cells and antigens causing the release of chemical factors which give rise to inflammation. If such inflammation occurs in the cause of removing some invading micro-organism then we are usually prepared to accept it as a means to an end. If, on the other hand, reactions of this type occur in the skin following *"sensitization"* to substances like industrial and household chemicals then we are apt to feel aggrieved by the resulting eczematous condition.

Delayed hypersensitivity reactions occur in a variety of conditions, some of which will be discussed later.

AUTO-IMMUNE DISEASES

Auto-immune diseases are associated with immune responses against an individual's *own* tissues or organs and the resulting conditions form a spectrum of disease of ever increasing complexity. At one end, "organspecific" antibodies may damage just one "target" organ but at the other, antibodies to various cell components and tissues may produce very involved disease patterns.

Despite enormous research effort, the aetiology of many auto-immune conditions is poorly understood although there are certain important clues suggesting:

1) The possibility of an inborn (inherited) instability of the immune system in some sufferers.

2) The possibility that certain infections (particularly virus infections) and perhaps even vaccinations and other "environmental" factors may cause subtle changes in lymphocyte function and in certain body proteins which eventually lead to a breakdown of the "self" recognition mechanisms of the immune system. This in turn results in "self" *damage* by humoral and cell mediated immune responses.

》　Auto-immune diseases are usually **chronic** and involve the *gradual* destruction of organs or tissues. Several auto-immune conditions will be considered in later chapters. The following table lists some of the more important ones.

Organ specific auto-immune diso. '-rs

> ›　Addison's disease
> ›　Hashimoto's disease
> ›　Idiopathic hypoparathyroidism
> ›　Premature ovarian failure
> ›　Pernicious anaemia
> ›　Alopecia
> ›　Vitiligo

Multisystem disorders in which auto-immune processes are implicated

> ›　Rheumatoid arthritis
> ›　Seronegative arthritides

Connective tissue disorders

› Systemic lupus erythematosus
› Polyarteritis nodosa
› Temporal arteritis
› Polymyalgia rheumatica and the other vasculitides*
› Scleroderma
› Dermatomyositis and polymyositis
› Sjögren's syndrome

*   Pedantic plural of vasculitis.

THE PRINCIPLES OF VACCINATION

People who have experienced and recovered from infectious diseases usually acquire immunity from subsequent re-infections as a result of the priming of the immune system and the persistence of circulating antibodies after the illnesses producing them have subsided. Even "sub-clinical" infections can produce lasting immunity and thus many of us are immune to diseases we never knew we had!

IMMUNIZATION

Describes the process of inducing **artificial** immunity. If the relevant antibody is given **directly** (usually by injection) then the immunization is said to be **passive** and lasts for a relatively short time.

If an antigen (often in the form of a suspension of dead or inactivated micro-organisms) is administered directly as a **vaccine**, an immune response is generated and the immunization is said to be **active.** Active immunization may last for many years.

CONTRAINDICATIONS TO VACCINATION

> › Febrile illnesses, particularly respiratory infections.
> › A history of adverse reaction to a previous dose of the same vaccine.
> › Another live vaccine (eg measles) given 3 weeks or less before.

If live vaccine (measles, mumps, rubella, BCG, polio) add

> › Concurrent treatment with corticosteroids and other immunosuppressants, radiotherapy, cancer chemotherapy.
> › Immune deficiency (leukaemia, lymphomas, AIDS).
> › Pregnancy.

For pertussis vaccine add

> › A history of neonatal cerebral damage or irritation.
> › A history of fits or convulsions.
> › A family history of epilepsy.
> › Suspected neurological disease or defects.

Further details of specific vaccines can be found in the British National Formulary.

The following tables summarize current immunization policies in the UK

DURING THE FIRST YEAR OF LIFE:

Vaccine

Diphtheria/Tetanus/Pertussis (the "triple" vaccine) by injection PLUS oral **polio** vaccine at same time. 3 doses given during year.

Schedule: First dose preferably at 2 months (but often done at 3, 4 or 5). Then 4 week interval before second dose and another 4 weeks before third dose.

Notes: A child's immune system is immature until 6 months and it is arguably slightly illogical to start vaccination before this time. Severe reactions to pertussis vaccine are also less common in children over 6 months of age but on the other hand the most severe complications of pertussis itself occur in infants under 3 months ....

DURING THE SECOND YEAR OF LIFE:

Vaccine

Measles/Mumps/Rubella

Schedule: Since this is a live vaccine, it must NOT be given until at least 3 weeks after polio or other live vaccine.

Notes: The following groups of children are at particular risk of measles infection: children (over 1 year of age) in residential care; children about to enter nursery school; children with serious physical incapacity in whom measles infection may lead to severe illness.

AT SCHOOL ENTRY OR 5 YEARS OF AGE:

Vaccine

Diphtheria/Tetanus booster by injection plus oral **polio booster** (preferably 3 years after initial course).

Notes: If no immunization was given before school entry, a full course of Diphth./Tet. and polio is recommended but NOT pertussis. If no Measles/Mumps/Rubella vaccine in second year, this should also be given.

BETWEEN 10 AND 13 YEARS OF AGE:

Vaccination 1

BCG – TB vaccination.

Notes: Only given to tuberculin test negative children.

Vaccination 2

Rubella vaccine recommended for ALL girls between 11 and 13 years whether or not there is past history of rubella infection (which is notoriously hard to diagnose) unless known to have had Measles/Mumps/Rubella vaccination at an earlier age.

Schedule: Must NOT be given within 3 weeks of BCG.

ON LEAVING SCHOOL (15 OR 19 YEARS):

Vaccine

Polio (oral) and **Tetanus** (injection) boosters.

Notes: Tetanus boosters may then be offered every 5 years and also in cases of contaminated wounds (see later).

Details on immunization schedules for **hepatitis** *and various* **tropical diseases** *can be found near the end of the BNF.*

BLOOD GROUPS

Blood can be classified into four main groups depending on the presence or absence of certain antigens on the red cell membranes (termed A or B "agglutinogens") and the presence or absence of antibodies against these antigens (termed anti-A or anti-B "agglutinins") in the plasma. If a blood transfusion is given in which the recipient's plasma contains antibodies to the antigens on the donor's red cells, the donor red cells may agglutinate (stick together) and finally haemolyze (split apart) in the recipient's body with disastrous results (including shock and kidney failure).

Blood group is genetically determined with inheritance of A and B dominant to O.

> Since an individual may be homozygous or heterozygous for his or her blood group, a child may have a different blood group from either of its parents unless they are both group O (if that makes no sense, we know how you feel).

SUMMARY

A Group O individual's blood:

> › Has no A or B antigens on the red cells.
> › Has anti-A AND anti-B antibodies in the plasma.
> › Can only receive group O blood in transfusion.

A Group A individual's blood:

> › Has A antigens on the red cells.
> › Has anti-B antibodies in the plasma.
> › Can only receive group A and group O blood in transfusion.

A Group B individual's blood:

> › Has B antigens on the red cells.
> › Has anti-A antibodies in the plasma.
> › Can only receive group B and group O blood in transfusion.

A Group AB individual's blood:

> › Has A and B antigens on the red cells.
> › Has no antibodies in plasma and thus can receive all blood groups in transfusion.

RHESUS FACTOR

In addition to the A and B antigens described above there is another red cell surface antigen known as the **RHESUS factor** (so called because Rhesus monkeys carry a similar antigen on their red corpuscles).

84% of the population carry this factor and are termed Rhesus positive. The remaining 16% don't and are thus Rhesus negative!

The practical importance of Rhesus antigens:

is that although there are no naturally occurring rhesus *antibodies* in the plasma, if Rh positive blood is introduced into a Rh negative person then anti-Rh antibodies will be *formed* by the Rh negative person. Thus if a Rh negative woman with a Rh positive partner conceives a Rh positive baby (which is not inevitable) then the woman may form antibodies to her baby's red cells (as long as a few foetal red cells pass across the placenta into the maternal circulation and "set off" the maternal immune system).

The final result may be a stillbirth or a baby with "Haemolytic Disease of the Newborn"(HDN). The risk to the *first* Rh positive pregnancy is fairly small because of the time needed for the immune system to mount an effective response.

HDN can be treated by exchange blood transfusion plus appropriate intensive care. Future pregnancies can be safeguarded by "immuniza-tion" of the Rh negative mother with **anti**-Rhesus factor antibodies soon after the first Rh positive birth.

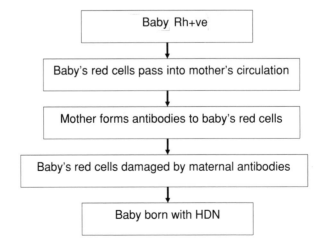

5. Neoplasia

If you don't expect the

unexpected,

you will not find it.

Heraclitus

NEOPLASIA

OVERVIEW

Disorders of Tissue Growth

Carcinogenesis

Carcinogenic agents

Theories of Cancer Causation

Pathological Features of Malignant Disease

Tumour Classification

Staging and grading

The General Clinical Features of Malignant Disease

DISORDERS OF TISSUE GROWTH

There are various "disorders" of cellular and tissue growth described by orthodox pathology, some implying abnormality and others being normal physiological phenomena.

The terms used have quite precise meanings and are worth learning:

> a) to facilitate the understanding of more detailed texts on disease processes and

> b) to make it clear that not all abnormal tissue growth is cancer.

Aplasia:

> Also known as agenesis. Means complete failure of an organ or part to develop eg there are many people who only ever developed one kidney – a fact which is sometimes discovered accidentally during a hospital admission for some unrelated problem.

Hypoplasia:

> Failure of an organ or part to reach full adult size – eg stunted limbs in thalidomide cases.

Atrophy:

> Means a decrease in size of cells or organs which have previously attained full adult size.

> | Cause | Example of effect |
> |---|---|
> | ↓ nutrition | → Starvation (whole body atrophy). |
> | ↓ blood supply | → Kidney atrophy after renal artery blockage. |
> | ↓ endocrine stimulation | → Adrenocortical atrophy in patients on steroids. |
> | ↓ nervous stimulation | → Muscle atrophy after peripheral nerve damage. |
> | Hypersensitivity | → Atrophy of small intestinal mucosa due to wheat exposure in patients with coeliac disease. |

> Pressure, disuse and old age may also lead to tissue atrophy.

Hypertrophy:

Means an increase in the **size** of cells (which may therefore increase the size of an organ). It is caused either by an increased workload (eg high blood pressure where increased peripheral resistance increases the work load on the heart and thus causes hypertrophy of heart muscle cells) or by increased endocrine stimulation (eg uterine muscle cell in pregnancy – a reversible phenomenon).

Hyperplasia:

Means an increase in the **number** of cells in a tissue or organ. It may be the result of increased workload, increased endocrine stimulation or viral infection (eg warts). Hyperplasia is reversible. A good example of physiological hyperplasia is the endocrine stimulated reversible breast growth seen in pregnancy.

Metaplasia:

The ***replacement*** of one adult cell or tissue type with another. It may carry sinister significance eg in smokers, where the normal columnar epithelium of the bronchus is often replaced by stratified squamous epithelium.

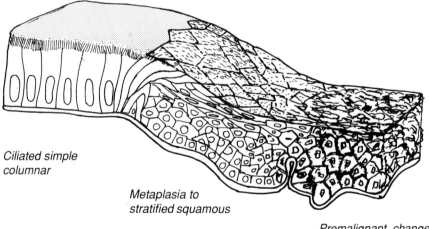

Ciliated simple
columnar

Metaplasia to
stratified squamous

Premalignant change
to cancer in situ

Note, however, that epithelium cannot change to connective tissue or vice versa – the changes take place within the sub-divisions of a particular tissue type.

Neoplasia:

Unlike the above, neoplasia ("new growth", tumour formation) implies a certain degree of **autonomous growth** plus persistence of growth after removal of the initiating stimulus. We will now consider neoplasia and its causes in more detail.

CARCINOGENESIS

Carcinogenesis deals with the facts and theories concerning the cause of tumours.

High tech research into the nature of cancer does not seem to clarify the nature of the essential change which turns a normal cell into a cancer cell. Though we know that many chemicals, radiation and even viruses can produce tumours, it is not known precisely how any of them render cells neoplastic.

CARCINOGENIC AGENTS

Carcinogenic agents are either **exogenous**– that is to say they come from outside the body – or **endogenous**, originating within the body.

Exogenous:

Knowledge of exogenous carcinogenic agents began in the eighteenth century with Sir Percival Pott (the flamboyant barber surgeon and founder of St Bartholomew's Medical School) and his description of the high incidence of cancer of the scrotum in juvenile chimney sweeps.

100 years later the German surgeon (and poet) Volkmann reported the high incidence of skin cancers in people working with mineral oils.

In 1918 it was discovered that painting mice with extracts of coal tar could produce cancers, an effect that could be enhanced by the addition of repeated trauma. It was concluded that certain cyclical hydrocarbons (present in soot and mineral oils) were carcinogenic and also that carcinogenesis may be "multifactorial".

Although skin cancers due to oil and tar are rare today, there are many important examples of modern exogenous carcinogenic agents:

Smoking	→	Carcinoma of the bronchus
Asbestos	→	Malignant tumours of the pleura
Aniline dyes	→	Bladder cancer
X-rays, ionizing radiation and sunlight	→	Various skin cancers and, in the case of ionizing radiation, blood cancers.

Trauma is probably only carcinogenic if it is minor, repeated and of long standing ("it won't get better if you pick it").

There is great variation in the length and intensity of exposure to particular carcinogens needed to bring about neoplastic change; sometimes exposure to "subthreshold" doses of two different carcinogens at the same time may produce cancer where one agent would have been relatively harmless. Furthermore, the combination of certain *non*-carcinogenic factors with a subthreshold dose of a known carcinogen may also cause tumour development. This leads to a concept of carcinogens as **initiators** of irreversible neoplastic change with a host of other "cofactors" acting as **promoters** of tumour growth.

Endogenous:

Knowledge of endogenous carcinogenic factors is largely speculative.

Certain tumours (such as familial polyposis of the colon) are **hereditary** but the fact that some tumours (such as breast cancer) are very common means that their occurrence may *not* have a hereditary component, even if they do occur several times in one family. There is also evidence that some breast carcinomas are related to oestrogen exposure (which would explain the observation that women who have had children – and thus have had periods of relatively low blood oestrogen levels in pregnancy – show a lower incidence of Ca-breast).

Many people take the view that neoplasia can only be considered in relation to the mental, physical and spiritual picture that constitutes the individual. Some would even say that we all have "cancer" all the time, but that in many of us the situation remains in dynamic balance and causes no problem.

On a more mechanical level, it is interesting that the body possesses enzymes which act to chop out erroneous chunks of mutant DNA from aberrant cells. Should the passage of time (or other factors) render these enzymes ineffective, neoplasia would result.

Viruses:

Controversy surrounds the role of viruses in human carcinogenesis since they are exogenous factors that appear to act by disrupting endogenous processes.

Both "DNA" and "RNA" viruses are capable of causing tumours in vertebrates and those that do have been labelled **oncogenic** (which means cancer forming...). Several chicken, rabbit, mouse and cat tumours caused by viruses have been closely studied but the only human tumours

proven to be caused by viruses are warts. As one major pathology textbook states "many of the procedures used to establish the viral nature of tumours are *not applicable to man"* (my italics) but there remains fairly good evidence that Burkitt's lymphoma, nasopharyngeal carcinoma, cervical cancer and liver cell cancer in humans may be virus related.

The **oncogenic theory** of cancer causation is currently generating much interest and can be simplified thus:

After entering the body, oncogenic DNA viruses invade cells in certain tissues and insinuate their own DNA into the host cell nucleus. The result is a population of subtly changed cells.*

In most people (and other animals) "oncogenes" sitting in the nuclei of abnormal cells have no effect. If exposed to carcinogenic agents, however, it is thought that changes might occur that allow the viral "oncogenes" to "express" themselves and transform host cells into full blown cancer cells.

IN SUMMARY

Carcinogenesis may be exogenous or endogenous and in either case more than one factor may be involved (ie carcinogenesis may be multifactorial). Endogenous factors are poorly understood but heredity and infective agents may be involved.

---

*   RNA viruses achieve the same end by slightly different means – they invade cells and then cause production of an enzyme which produces new DNA according to the viral "template". This is then incorporated into the host cell nucleus.

CARCINOGENESIS

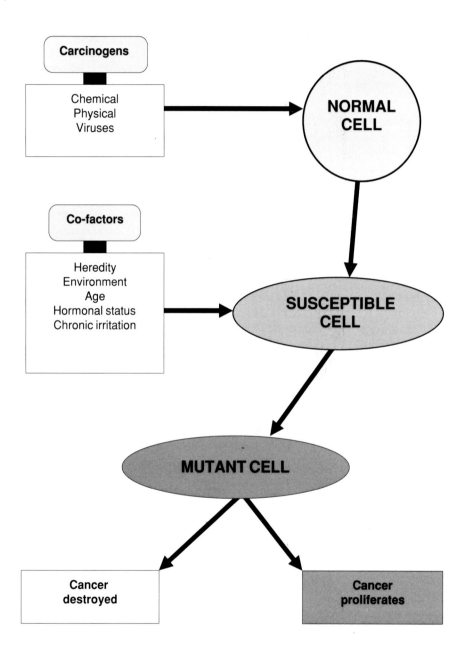

THEORIES OF CANCER CAUSATION

THE MUTATIONAL THEORY – THE EPIGENETIC THEORY

THE MUTATIONAL THEORY:

Proposes that the altered behaviour of the cancer cell arises from mutation, a view supported by the following:

1) Most chemical and physical carcinogens are mutagenic.

2) Chromosomal abnormalities are common features of cancer cells.

3) Oncogenic viruses exert their effects by "forcibly" altering the genetic constitution of the host cells.

THE EPIGENETIC THEORY:

Proposes that cancer cells develop as a result of the reversal of those processes of differentiation which give each cell its character and functional abilities and that such reversal causes the loss of normal cellular homeostatic mechanisms. The need for such a proposal arises from the observation that some inheritable changes in cells occur without mutation – in other words, cells with an apparently normal genetic make up can turn cancerous.

NOTE:

Again it is worth stressing that there is little understanding of the role of the immune system in "protecting" against cancerous change and, so far, experimental studies on the fundamental nature of cancer have contributed little to cancer prevention in man (although they have, of course, extracted a vast toll amongst other species on whom we choose to experiment because they are supposedly like us and yet whom we feel justified in using for experimentation because they are not like us).

PATHOLOGICAL FEATURES OF MALIGNANT DISEASE

A neoplastic tumour is defined as an abnormal mass of tissue which grows faster than normal tissue and in an unco-ordinated fashion. The growth of such tumours continues after the cessation of the initiating stimuli. They thus behave in an autonomous manner.

Neoplastic tumours may be benign or malignant but it is very rare for a benign tumour to become malignant.

Neoplastic tissue seen under a microscope resembles its tissue of origin (the jargon for tissue of origin is "histogenesis") and this forms one basis for classification of tumours (see later).

Since they grow relatively rapidly, neoplastic tumours consist mainly of tumour cells with only sparse amounts of supporting tissue, blood vessels etc.

The rate of growth of neoplastic tumours depends on the life span and rate of proliferation of their component cells.

The overall bulk of a neoplastic growth may be exaggerated by the reaction of the surrounding tissues to its presence.

Neoplastic tumours can become infected, congested, oedematous etc. like any other tissue.

Certain features tend to distinguish malignant neoplasms from benign:

› Malignant tumours grow faster and, if examined microscopically, show a high incidence of abnormal mitoses in their cells.

› Malignant cells look abnormal under the microscope and tend to be poorly "differentiated".

› Malignant tumours tend to undergo ischaemic necrosis as their rapid growth tends to outpace the development of an adequate blood supply.

› In contrast to benign tumours (which mainly cause damage by simple pressure on the surrounding tissues), malignant tumours tend to invade surrounding tissues and then spread via blood vessels, lymphatics or across body cavities to form **metastases.** Virtually no benign tumours metastasize.

TUMOUR CLASSIFICATION

Tumours may be classified according to:

> › their behaviour (benign or malignant).
> › their site (stomach, lung etc).
> › whether primary or secondary.
> › their tissue of origin ("histogenesis").

> **Classification** is important because it has implications for treatment and prognosis.

Nomenclature:

Tissue of origin	Benign type	Malignant type
Germ cells	Dermoid cyst	Teratoma
Surface epithelium	Papilloma	Carcinoma
Glandular epithelium	Adenoma	Adenocarcinoma
Fibrous connective tissue	Fibroma	Fibrosarcoma
Fatty connective tissue	Lipoma	Liposarcoma
Vascular tissues	Angioma	Angiosarcoma

> Note that carcinomas (malignant tumours of epithelium) tend to spread via lymphatics whilst sarcomas (malignant tumours of connective tissue) tend to spread via the bloodstream.

STAGING AND GRADING

> **Staging** refers to the extent of spread of a cancer ie
> › confined to the tissue of origin ("in situ").
> › invading adjacent tissue.
> › distant metastases present.

> **Grading** refers to how much the cancerous cells **look** like the tissue of origin ie a grade 1 tumour would have well "differentiated" cells and a grade 4 would be poorly differentiated. Tumour cells so poorly differentiated as not to resemble any particular tissue are referred to as **anaplastic.**

» The higher the grade and stage, the worse the prognosis and the less likely that conventional treatment will have anything to offer beyond palliation (symptom relief).

THE GENERAL CLINICAL FEATURES OF MALIGNANT DISEASE

1) Mortality league table:

Men	Women
Lung	Breast
Colon/Rectum	Colon/rectum
Prostate	Uterus
Pancreas	Lung
Stomach	Ovary

2) Aetiological pointers in history:

› Chemical → cigarette smoke, exposure to asbestos, exposure to aniline dyes etc.
› Physical → X rays, UV light (incl. strong sunlight), ionizing radiation
› Viral → wart virus, Epstein Barr virus etc.
› Genetic → familial polyposis etc.
› Miscellaneous environmental

3) Danger signals:

› Change in bowel or bladder habit
› Non-healing sores
› Unusual bleeding or discharge, especially from body orifice or nipple
› Newly discovered lumps (esp. breast)
› Problems with swallowing
› Obvious changes in skin moles or warts
› Persistent cough
› Persistent hoarseness
› Loss of weight and appetite

4) Clinical manifestations of neoplastic growth:

Local effects: Expansive growth may cause lumps and obstructions.
Tissue infiltration by tumour may cause pain.
Tissue necrosis may cause bleeding and/or persistent infection.

Metastatic effects:* Swollen lymph glands.
Shortness of breath (lung secondaries).
Jaundice (liver secondaries).
Fractures (bone secondaries).
Epilepsy (brain secondaries).
Skin nodules (skin secondaries).

Systemic effects: Weight loss → cachexia.
Anaemia.
Fever.
Skin conditions.
Polycythaemia and other blood problems.
Thrombophlebitis.
Hormonal and metabolic problems (eg Cushing's syndrome, low blood sugar, high blood calcium).
Gout.
Neuromuscular problems.

» Some of the above are particular features of particular cancers and will be discussed more fully in the relevant chapters.

---

* Malignancy may spread within the body by direct extension, by lymphatic spread, by spread via the bloodstream and by "seeding" across body cavities ("transcoelomic spread").

6. Circulatory Disorders

Big whorls have little whorls

Which feed on their velocity,

And little whorls have lesser whorls

And so on to viscosity.

Lewis F. Richardson

CIRCULATORY DISORDERS

OVERVIEW

Thrombosis

Atheroma

Arteriosclerosis

Clotting Disorders

Oedema

Shock

THROMBOSIS, ATHEROMA & ARTERIOSCLEROSIS

INTRODUCTION

The linked pathological processes of atheroma and thrombosis* together constitute the most serious of all the threats to life and health in the developed world:

1) 160,000 people a year in England and Wales die of heart attacks caused by atheroma and thrombosis in their coronary arteries.

2) 80,000 people a year in England and Wales die of thrombo/embolic strokes.

3) Thrombi in large veins after trauma, serious illness or surgery lead to 20,000 deaths a year from pulmonary embolus.

4) Many amputations are performed each year to mitigate the effects of large artery obstruction.

5) At least 5 men per thousand per year over the age of forty develop angina, caused by partial coronary artery blockage.

THROMBOSIS

A thrombus is a mass formed from blood constituents within a blood vessel (or within the heart) in a living person. **Thrombosis** is the process of thrombus formation.

There are various causes of thrombosis but whatever the *initiating* event, the mechanism of clot formation is the same, ie:

› **Platelets** adhere to the lining (endothelium) of a blood vessel and to each other forming a small projecting mass –

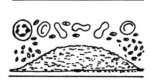

---

*   plus the related phenomenon of embolism.

> The release of chemicals from the platelet mass triggers the **clotting system** locally. The resulting **fibrin strands** add to the growing obstruction –

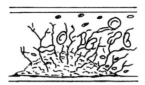

> If the rate of blood flow is slow enough, red cells become tangled up in the platelet/fibrin mass until the blood vessel becomes completely blocked –

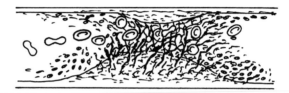

> Blood tends to stagnate behind and in front of the obstruction, causing the formation of more fibrin. The result is a large, fairly solid thrombus that continues to enlarge in both directions, sometimes extending into other vessels

THREE FACTORS MAY INITIATE THROMBOSIS:

> Alterations in blood flow
> Damage to blood vessel lining
> Changes in blood composition

Alteration in blood flow:

Tends to bring platelets into contact with vessel walls.

Slow flow:

May be produced by cardiac failure, enforced bedrest etc. Blood cells "fall out" of the mainstream and accumulate next to the endothelium.

Turbulence:

May occur if vessel walls become deformed (eg in varicose veins or aneurysms); also around venous valves.

Damage to vessel lining:

Leads to platelet adhesion to vessel wall.

Common causes:

› Atheroma (see below)
› Local inflammation

Changes in blood composition:

After operations or trauma, and following childbirth, there may be an increase in concentration of blood clotting factors and platelets and an increase in platelet stickiness.

COMMON SITES OF THROMBOSIS:

Venous:

Systemic vein thrombosis is common because blood flow is slow in veins and there is often turbulence around venous valves. Venous thrombosis frequently arises in the deep veins of the lower limb. Abdominal operations, childbirth, heart disease and varicose veins are all common predisposing conditions (see chapter 11).

Arterial:

The aorta is a common site for arterial thrombosis since it is prone to atheroma and arteriosclerosis (see below). The **coronary arteries, the middle cerebral arteries and the small vessels of the digits (particularly the toes)** are also common sites of thrombosis.

The heart:

Thrombi may form **within the chambers of the heart** as a consequence of heart valve disorders or myocardial infarction.

ATHEROMA AND ARTERIOSCLEROSIS

Atheroma and arteriosclerosis are degenerative conditions that affect ARTERIES and obstruct blood flow.

They are important because they may affect vital organs such as the brain, heart and kidneys. They may also lead to haemorrhage and aneurysm formation. Thrombosis (see above) is the commonest **complication** of atheroma and arteriosclerosis.

ATHEROMA:

Patchy deposition of yellow, fatty, porridgy lumps called **plaques,** just below the arterial intima (the layer nearest the lumen).

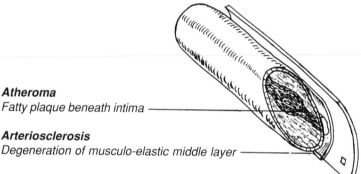

Atheroma
Fatty plaque beneath intima ——————

Arteriosclerosis
Degeneration of musculo-elastic middle layer ——————

ARTERIOSCLEROSIS:

Is also known as "hardening of the arteries" and is characterized by a generalized degeneration of the muscular/elastic tissue of the arterial media (middle layer). Normal tissue is replaced by scar tissue.

In elderly people, nearly all large and medium sized vessels are affected by arteriosclerosis.

Atheroma and arteriosclerosis often occur together. The term **atherosclerosis** is used to describe combined atheroma and arteriosclerosis.

» Atheroma and arteriosclerosis are very much diseases of western "civilization" and are of gradual onset and progression. Thus they may be present for many years before a sudden complication (such as thrombosis) causes dramatic ischaemic damage in a vital organ. It is also important to realize that serious **chronic** ischaemic damage may also result from progressive atheroma (see chapter 11).

Aetiological factors implicated in arterial disease:

> › High calorie, high animal fat, high refined carbohydrate diet
> › Obesity
> › Hereditary peculiarities of lipid metabolism
> › **Smoking**
> › Being male and post-menopausal female
> › Various diseases including **hypertension, diabetes,** underactive thyroid.
> › Sedentary lifestyle

Important sites of atheroma		Possible effects
Cerebral arteries	→	Generalized chronic brain ischaemia and dementia.
Carotid arteries	→	Small emboli may detach and lodge in brain causing strokes.
Coronary arteries	→	Heart attack or chronic ischaemic damage to heart muscle.
Abdominal aorta	→	Atheromatous damage may lead to aneurysm formation. Also, emboli may break off and lodge in leg arteries causing acute ischaemia of limbs.
Renal arteries	→	May cause chronic ischaemic damage to kidneys.
Visceral arteries	→	May lead to chronic ischaemia of bowel (what symptoms do you think this might cause?*).
Lower limb arteries	→	If atheroma *very* severe, chronic ischaemia may lead to symptoms of intermittent claudication (see chapter 11) and eventually to gangrene .....

NOTE:

Ischaemia means lack of blood in a part of the body.

An **aneurysm** is a localized enlargement of the lumen of an artery.

---

*   abdominal cramp related to eating

CLOTTING DISORDERS

INTRODUCTION

When a blood vessel is damaged, liquid blood rushes out until its flow is arrested by a **three stage** process known as **haemostasis**.

The first two stages – **vasoconstriction** and **activation of blood platelets** – are almost instantaneous with activated platelets sticking to the wound edges and to each other to form a "haemostatic" plug.

Activation of the **clotting system*** then generates a chemical called **thrombin** which turns a protein in the blood plasma called fibrinogen into an **insoluble** mesh of **fibrin** which reinforces the platelet plug and turns it into a proper blood clot. This clotting system is triggered off by chemicals released from the platelet plug and by contact of the "clotting factors" with injured blood vessel surfaces.

If blood did not solidify after injury, we would bleed to death. However, after the initial damage has been contained, it is obviously necessary to dismantle blood clots and restore flow through affected vessels. The formation of fibrin, therefore, activates yet another bloodborne enzyme system, the **fibrinolytic system**, which dissolves clots and helps restore the patency of the blood vessels.

Thus you will see that the body's response to haemorrhage depends on a complicated set of interactions between –

› The blood vessel walls
› The platelets
› The clotting system
› The fibrinolytic system

If any of these components is deranged due to hereditary or acquired disorders then the result may be a disease characterized by **abnormal bleeding**.

---

*   A sequence of chemical reactions involving a number of blood coagulation "factors" which normally circulate as inactive substances but which, when activated by vessel damage etc, become powerful enzymes that take part in the chemical reactions leading to fibrin formation.

BLEEDING DISORDERS MAY BE CLASSIFIED AS FOLLOWS:*

Blood vessel abnormalities:

Congenital:	Hereditary haemorrhagic telangiectasia.
Acquired:	Simple easy bruising.
	Bruising associated with old age, steroid therapy and scurvy.
	Vasculitis associated with drug hypersensitivity, infection, rheumatoid arthritis, SLE, Henoch-Schönlein purpura etc.

Platelet disorders:

↓ **platelet production:**	Congenital.
	Vitamin B12 and folate deficiency.
	Blood cancers.
	Severe (aplastic) anaemias related to drugs, chemicals, irradiation etc.
↑ **platelet destruction:**	Immune based "idiopathic thrombocytopenic purpura".
	Disseminated intravascular coagulation syndrome (associated with many severe acute conditions).

Defects in the clotting system:

Congenital:	Haemophilia (factor VIII deficiency).
	Christmas disease (factor IX deficiency).
	von Willebrand's disease.
Acquired:	Liver disease (↓ factor II, V and fibrinogen production).
	Vitamin K deficiency (↓ factor II, VII, IX and X).
	Disseminated intravascular coagulation syndrome.

Bleeding due to overactivity of the fibrinolytic system:

	Is very rare.

* This classification is not comprehensive. Some of the above conditions are discussed in chapter 23; for the rest, consult a standard textbook of medicine.

NOTE 1:

Purpura are small purple bruises that do not blanch on pressure. They are caused by blood leaking into the skin.

Ecchymosis is the jargon word for a big bruise.

Telangiectasia are dilated small superficial blood vessels visible to the naked eye.

NOTE 2:

The case history of a patient with a bleeding disorder often suggests the cause:

Type of bleeding:
> Bleeding from a single site often relates to a local cause (trauma, inflammation etc).
> Bleeding into the skin (bruising and purpura) or mucous membranes suggests platelet or vessel defects.
> Bleeding into joints is characteristic of clotting disorders.

Mode of onset:
> Sudden onset in an adult suggests acquired disorder.
> Surgery: If patient has undergone tooth extraction, tonsillectomy etc without major bleeding problem then unlikely to be severe congenital bleeding disorder.

Chronology:
> Platelet and vessel problems cause bleeding immediately after trauma and eventually respond to first aid measures (ie direct pressure).
> In clotting defects, bleeding occurs up to several hours after trauma, is hard to stop and frequently recurs.

Family history:
> Obviously important – should question about as many family members as possible to detect hereditary disorders.

Drug history:
> Steroids, aspirin and the other NSAIAs may all affect platelet function and cause bleeding.

Other illnesses:
> Liver disease, kidney disease, cancer and auto-immune disorders may all cause acquired bleeding problems.

OEDEMA

Oedema is an accumulation of fluid in the extra-vascular tissues.

Oedema occurs:

> › When the composition ("osmotic pressure") of the blood or the tissue
> fluids is altered.
> › When the pressure ("hydrostatic pressure") inside capillaries rises.
> › When capillary permeability alters for any reason (such as in inflam-
> mation).

> The net effect of these changes is to allow some fluid (and perhaps some
> protein) to leak out of the capillaries causing swelling of the surrounding
> tissues. Oedema may be localized (caused by local pathology) or gener-
> alized (particularly associated with diseases of the heart and kidneys).

LOCAL OEDEMA

INFLAMMATION:

> Causes local oedema and swelling (see chapter 2). **Allergic** oedema is
> a special type of inflammatory oedema in which hypersensitivity (to a bee
> sting or a drug for example) causes rapid (often gross) oedema due to
> histamine release and consequent increased capillary permeability.

VENOUS OBSTRUCTION:

> Is a common cause of local oedema eg deep vein thrombosis affecting
> the lower limb (see chapter 11).

ASCITES:

> Is the accumulation of oedema fluid within the abdominal (peritoneal)
> cavity and is usually associated with cirrhosis of the liver or abdominal
> tumours (see chapter 13).

LYMPHATIC OBSTRUCTION:

> May cause local oedema, eg when an infiltrating breast cancer blocks
> superficial lymphatics (causing the skin of the breast to resemble the skin
> of an orange).

ANGIONEUROTIC OEDEMA:

Is a rare form of allergic oedema of sudden onset and short duration – it may affect the larynx and cause suffocation.

PULMONARY OEDEMA:

Is a most important form of local oedema, associated with serious disease of the heart. Fluid accumulates in the tissue spaces of the lung, and collects in the alveoli. This has a disastrous effect on pulmonary function and gas exchange. The commonest cause is **left heart failure** (see chapter 11) producing increased hydrostatic pressure in the lung capillaries.

Inflammation of lung tissue may also produce pulmonary oedema, eg pneumonia.

GENERALIZED OEDEMA

CARDIAC OEDEMA:

We have just described pulmonary oedema as a consequence of left sided heart failure but it is important to realize that a chronic reduction of left heart output may also have a general effect on body water and sodium homoeostasis because it causes decreased renal blood flow and thus increased aldosterone secretion.

Thus **chronic heart failure can lead to chronic salt and water retention** and if the right heart fails as well, then the resulting peripheral venous congestion (exacerbated by the chronic fluid retention) may lead to **peripheral oedema** where the hydrostatic pressure is greatest, ie around the feet and ankles. This is discussed further in chapter 11.

Note that as the condition of a patient with heart failure deteriorates, fluid may start to gather around the sacrum and in the peritoneal and pleural cavities.

RENAL OEDEMA:

Kidney disease will obviously have an effect on body fluid homoeostasis. Two forms are associated with generalized oedema:

	Acute Nephritis	**Nephrotic Syndrome**
Oedema:	Slight	Marked
Distribution:	Around eyes, ankles	Generalized
Protein in urine:	Moderate	Marked
Plasma osm. press.:	Normal	Decreased
Cause:	Fluid retention	Reduced plasma osmotic pressure

Note that these are syndromes (symptom complexes) and each may have a variety of underlying causes (see chapter 21).

> The message in orthodox medicine is, however:
>
> **If oedema – ? heart or kidney .....**

FAMINE OEDEMA:

In starvation, protein reserves become depleted, In severe cases, the reduction of plasma proteins decreases the osmotic pressure of the blood and causes oedema.

SHOCK

Shock is a condition in which the vital functions of the body are compromised by an acute reduction in effective circulating blood volume.

The causes may be grouped under three headings:

› Hypovolaemic shock (diminished blood volume)
› Cardiogenic shock
› Septic shock

HYPOVOLAEMIC SHOCK:

May be associated with:

Trauma: Severe haemorrhage (internal and external)
              Severe injury (especially fractures and crush injuries)
              Surgery
              Extensive burns
Dehydration: Severe vomiting, diarrhoea, sweating etc

CARDIOGENIC SHOCK:

Results from a sudden fall in cardiac output as seen in acute diseases of the heart such as myocardial infarction.

SEPTIC SHOCK:

Serious bacterial infection may cause shock because of a generalized increase in capillary permeability following the release of bacterial "endo-toxins". It may complicate the other types of shock and is very hard to treat.

NOTE:

Fainting (also known as vaso-vagal attack) is a type of acute self limiting shock mediated by nervous mechanisms.

Anaphylactic shock is an acute reaction caused by hypersensitivity and has been mentioned in chapter 4. It is characterized by acute collapse with bronchoconstriction, skin rash, vomiting and diarrhoea. Subcutaneous injection of adrenaline may be necessary to save life in this condition.

The mechanisms invoked by the body to try and compensate for a relative lack of circulating volume will be described in detail in chapter 11, but an overall picture of shock and its evolution is presented in the following diagram.

The healthy body is extremely good at maintaining blood pressure homoeostasis in the face of small changes in circulating fluid volume.

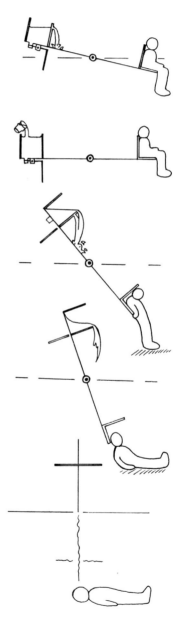

If there is an acute relative decrease in circulating volume –

the body attempts to maintain blood pressure and conserve fluids. Circulation to brain and heart is maintained even at the expense of other organs.

If shock progresses to advanced stage, the patient becomes listless, pale, cold and clammy with blue lips, rapid weak pulse and falling blood pressure.

Eventually tissue hypoxia leads to cell damage exacerbating the fall in blood pressure. Acute hypoxia also leads to changes in the blood, eg disseminated intravascular coagulation. Deranged cell metabolism leads to acidosis.

When systolic blood pressure falls below 50mmHg, serious damage to brain and heart may occur and death often follows.

The OUTCOME of shock:

> **Recovery** (after convalescence)
> **Survival** but with permanent damage to various organs
> **Death**

Early treatment of hypovolaemia, treatment of the initiating cause, youth and good general health all favour recovery.

Delayed treatment, old age, poor general health, pre-existing heart and lung disease and the onset of infection or organ damage tend to favour the progression of shock to the point at which vascular impairment and tissue damage make it irreversible.

7. Infectious Disease

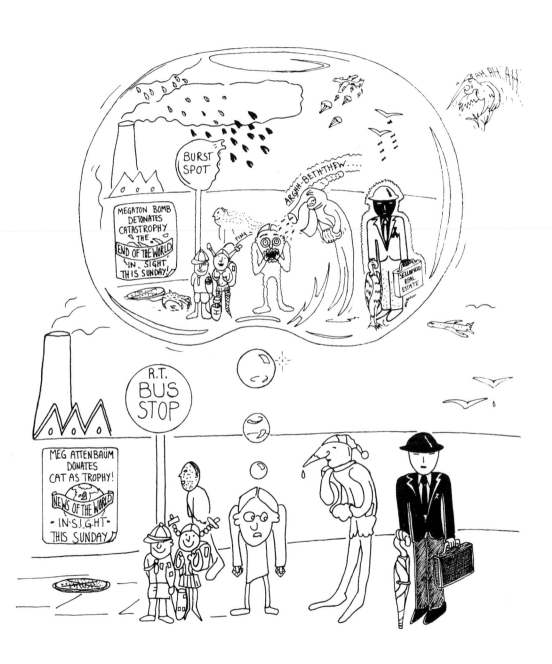

INFECTIOUS DISEASE

OVERVIEW

Introduction

The "they're out to get you" mentality.

General Effects of Infection

– including fever and metabolic changes.

Types of Infective Agent

– including bacteria and viruses.

The Nature of Infection

Commensal growth
Routes of entry of micro-organisms
Host defensive mechanisms
Micro-organism "attack" mechanisms
The course and outcome of infection

Disposal of Micro-organisms by the Body

Opportunistic Infections

The Basic Clinical Features of Some Common Infectious Diseases

Childhood infectious diseases
The herpes family
Staphylococci and streptococci
Diarrheal diseases
Common fungal infections
Sexually transmitted diseases
Tropical diseases

INTRODUCTION

Since Roman times, the idea that diseases are spread by invisible "micro-organisms" has been put forward by people seeking to explain the reason for epidemics.

However, in the absence of positive proof, "germ" theories were widely ignored prior to the late nineteenth century despite some elegant theorizing by philosopher-scientists such as Frascatoro in the sixteenth century and Marcus Plenciz in the eighteenth. Even the microscopic observations of Kircher and van Leeuwenhoek (17th century) and the demonstration of immunization by Edward Jenner (1796) did little to advance the cause. Thus it was not until 1836, when Agostino Bassi published the results of experiments proving that silkworm disease was caused by a parasitic fungus, that the ground was firmly laid for the revolution in medical practice that has resulted from the work of the early giants of microbiology and disease control – Koch, Pasteur, Lister and Ehrlich.

Although it was **Koch** who first showed beyond doubt (in 1876) that an infectious disease (anthrax) was related to "infection" with a **specific** micro-organism, and despite the fact that it was also Koch who discovered the tubercle bacillus (thereby apparently confounding the concept that TB was an emotional or nutritional disorder), history has conferred pride of place in microbiology to the French chemist and son of a tanner, **Louis Pasteur** (1822-1895). His elaboration of the "germ" theory disproved once and for all the idea of "spontaneous generation" and his systematic and meticulous research forms the basis of the current allopathic approach to infection and vaccination.

Some understanding of the history of microbiology is vital to the understanding of orthodox medicine as practised in the West today. You should realize that Pasteur's work is now identified with an unduly narrow interpretation of his findings, for he himself continually stated that he had **not** proved that microbes were the **cause** of infectious disease, merely that they were its **agents**.

Claude Bernard (an experimental physiologist whose holistic approach to the human organism warrants closer study by those who base a part of their practice on his work) and Max von Pettenkofer (a German chemist) suggested that the cause of disease must often be **the bodily "terrain" encountered by microbes** rather than the microbes themselves. Pasteur insisted on his deathbed that Bernard had been right to hold to this view. The fact that much medical research pursues the idea of microbes as concrete causative factors in illness (based on a demeaning interpretation of Pasteur *et al's* work, ie that the microbes are "out to get you") has lead to the development of increasingly toxic drugs, many of which are health hazards in themselves.

This chapter outlines an *orthodox* approach to infection and its agents but we strongly suggest that you refer to appropriate sections in homoeopathic and naturopathic texts in order to broaden your understanding of infectious disease.

GENERAL EFFECTS OF INFECTION

Infection may be defined as the invasion of body tissues by living, multiplying micro-organisms. Such invasion and multiplication may be associated with the manifestations of **disease**.

The general reactions of the body to infection include:

> › **Fever**
> › **Metabolic changes**
> › **Changes in the composition of plasma**

Fever:

Is referred to as "pyrexia" in medical jargon and is a particular feature of **bacterial** infection.

Invading organisms cause the release of **endogenous pyrogens** from white blood cells (especially monocytes) and these chemicals act on the hypothalamus to reset the hypothalamic "metabolic thermostat" to a higher level. The hypothalamus (via local release of prostaglandin E2) signals the vasomotor centre of the brain to reduce heat loss via the skin and this causes the rise in internal temperature that we call fever.

Thus early on in a bacterial infection, the sufferer will look pale and feel cold and shivery and may even experience paroxysmal bouts of shivering known as **rigors**. As fever develops, however, skin vessels dilate and sweating becomes profuse as the body attempts to avoid overheating by facilitating heat loss.

Eventually (hopefully) heat loss exceeds heat production and the body temperature begins to fall towards normal. The mechanisms of fever production and the related metabolic consequences (see below) explain the rise in pulse rate and tendency towards dehydration that are common accompaniments of the febrile state. A body temperature greater than $41°$ centigrade is termed **hyperpyrexia** and is life threatening due to heat damage to brain cells.

Note that fever also occurs in heat stroke and when the body suffers tissue necrosis (crush injuries, myocardial infarction etc).

Metabolic changes:

Tissue breakdown is greatly enhanced by fever, ie:

Fever → increased energy utilization and diminished food intake → breakdown of tissue proteins and fats → weight loss and excretion of excess nitrogenous waste products in the urine (which eventually becomes of small volume and highly concentrated due to dehydration).

Note that tissue breakdown may cause "ketosis"* in children.

Plasma:

In **chronic** infections there is often a rise in plasma levels of γ-globulins and this change is reflected by a rise in the "erythrocyte sedimentation rate" (ESR) (see chapter 23).

---

*   Acetone smell on the breath due to metabolism of fats as a source of energy.

TYPES OF INFECTIVE AGENT

Most micro-organisms are harmless. A few are **pathogenic** (ie capable of producing disease manifestations).

> **Bacteria** and **viruses** are the most important classes of infective agent associated with disease in western societies.
>
> Other important infective agents are:
>
> › Rickettsiae
> › Chlamydiae
> › Protozoa
> › Fungi
> › Worms

BACTERIA

> Are a diverse group of unicellular organisms with "primitive" nuclei containing just one circular molecule of DNA and no nuclear membrane (they are thus known in the jargon as **prokaryotic**). They have no mitochondria and are the only living organisms except plants that possess a rigid cell wall. The cell wall determines the shape of a bacteria and produces characteristic staining patterns when subjected to classical laboratory techniques.
>
> Bacteria reproduce by **binary fission** (up to one division every 30 minutes) and they may also form spores capable of resisting extreme adverse environmental conditions. Different bacteria vary in their oxygen and other nutritional requirements but **pathogenic** bacteria often need a **ready made** supply of organic nutrients for successful growth within a "host".
>
> Local invasion by bacteria causes cell damage and tissue necrosis which in turn evokes a local inflammatory response.

Bacteria may cause cell damage in 3 ways:

> 1) The production of **toxins**.
> 2) **Hypersensitivity** reactions to bacterial proteins.
> 3) **Bacterial spread** via the bloodstream leading to infection of other tissues and organs (and possibly the formation of "septic thrombi").

Note that there are two main types of bacterial toxin:

> **Exotoxins** which are simple proteins secreted by **living** bacteria and which can be neutralized by antibodies.
> **Endotoxins** which are complex chemicals derived from remains of **dead** bacteria that damage capillaries and disrupt blood clotting as well as directly damaging cells. They cannot be neutralized by antibodies.

You should also be familiar with the following terms:

Bacteraemia: The presence of bacteria in the bloodstream.

Septicaemia: The presence of LARGE (potentially overwhelming) numbers of virulent bacteria in the bloodstream.

Pyaemia: The presence of clusters of pus forming organisms in the blood. This may lead to the formation of multiple small abscesses in various organs.

Septic infarction: Is the result of infected emboli (originating from thrombi in deep veins or on heart valves) obstructing the blood supply to organs.

BACTERIAL CLASSIFICATION:

The classification of bacteria is a complex and confusing subject.

They are artificially classified according to certain laboratory characteristics including:

> shape
> staining
> growth characteristics
> biochemical reactions
> antigenicity etc

The major primary classification is according to SHAPE eg:

Spherical   =   "cocci"
Cylindrical =   "bacilli"
Helical   =   "spirochaetes"

Gram positive bacteria:

Are those which stain blue/black when stained by Gram's method*. The Gram positive group contains such important pathogens as the **staphylococci**, the **streptococci** and the anaerobic, spore bearing, rod shaped **clostridia**.

Gram negative bacteria:

Stain pink by Gram's method and the group contains a large number of bowel commensals (the **"coliforms"**) which, though relatively innocuous when confined to the gut, can cause nasty infections if allowed to spread to other sites. Many Gram negative bacteria release endotoxins. **Salmonellae** and **shigellae** (dysentery) stain Gram negative.

Pyogenic bacteria:

May be Gram positive or negative but all share the ability to invade tissues and cause purulent** inflammation. **Staphylococcus aureus, streptococcus pyogenes, meningococcus and gonococcus** are all pyogenic bacteria.

Acid alcohol fast bacilli:

Are organisms which, once stained, resist decoloration by strong mineral acids and alcohol. The "mycobacteria" which cause **TB** and **leprosy** belong to this group.

The following is a simplified classification of important bacterial types.

---

* Gram was a Danish botanist turned medic. who discovered the eponymous staining method when he accidentally spilled some iodine mixture over a bacterial preparation and tried to wash it off using alcohol.

** With pus.

GRAM POSITIVE:

Shape	Oxygen needs	Type	Associated with
Cocci	Aerobic	Staphylococcus	Boils, carbuncles, abscesses etc.
		Streptococcus	Scarlet fever, bacterial endo-carditis, pneumonia.
	Anaerobic	Various	
Bacilli	Aerobic	Bacillus	
		Corynebacterium	Corynebacterium diphtheriae produces powerful exotoxins harmful to heart and nerve tissue and causes the disease diphtheria.
		Listeria	Meningo-encephalitis, infection of womb.
		Lactobacillus	Found in dairy products and as commensals in alimentary canal and vagina. Responsible for souring milk.
		Mycobacterium	Leprosy, TB, etc.
	Anaerobic	Clostridium	Clostridia reproduce by sporing and produce powerful exotoxins. Food poisoning, gas gangrene, tetanus .
		Actinomyces	Actinomycosis.

GRAM NEGATIVE:

Shape	Oxygen needs	Type
Cocci	Aerobes	Neisseria (associated with gonorrhoea and meningitis.)
Bacilli	Aerobes	Pseudomonas
		The **enterobacteria** (including Escherichia, Proteus, Klebsiella, **Salmonella, Shigella**)
		Various other **small** rods (such as Haemophilus, Brucella and **Vibrio**)
	Anaerobes	Includes Campylobacter and Bacteroides.

NOTE:

Legionella pneumophila is a Gram negative rod that thrives in **humid** conditions. It causes Legionnaire's disease.

Spirochaetes are coiled bacteria. The group includes **Leptospira** (aerobic) which causes Weil's disease and **Treponema** (anaerobic) which causes **syphilis**.

CELL WALL DEFICIENT BACTERIA:

Mycoplasma

VIRUSES

Are generally much smaller than bacteria and contain only **one** type of nucleic acid, ie either DNA or RNA. They possess neither mitochondria nor ribosomes and do not have a rigid cell wall. Thus a virus can be thought of simply as an **infectious piece of nucleic acid surrounded by a protective protein coat** (or "capsid").

Viruses can only reproduce **inside other living cells** and they are **not susceptible to antibiotics**. They come in various sizes and may be brick shaped, bullet shaped, icosahedral or helical. An intact virus particle may be referred to as a **virion**.

Most important pathogens:

> › Measles
> › Chickenpox
> › Rubella
> › Mumps
> › Enteroviruses (Polio and Coxsackie) – are viruses that enter the GIT, multiply there, and then (generally) invade the CNS

Mechanism of disease production:

Viruses are **obligatory intracellular parasites**, ie they are entirely dependent on the "host" cells for survival and replication. The life cycle is as follows:

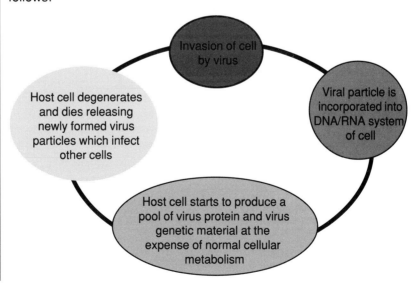

Typical acute viral infection:

Penetration of virus at site of infection → replication of virus within cells locally → cell death + virus liberation → spread to local lymph nodes → further viral replication and release → primary "viraemia"* and spread to lymphoid tissue generally accompanied by malaise, fever, lymphadeno-pathy → secondary viraemia producing specific disease symptoms related to specific target organs or tissues.

Host/virus interaction:

Cells infected by viruses produce **interferon** which stimulates the immune response and produces inflammation. (It also interferes with synthesis of viral protein and hence is an important intracellular defence mechanism.)

Complications of viral infections:

Are often the result of secondary bacterial infection, eg –

›   Pneumonia (especially measles and chickenpox)
›   Otitis media (especially measles)

Also –

›   Post-infective encephalopathy
›   Delayed onset neurological problems
›   Reactivation after long gap (eg shingles many years after chicken pox – also called *latent* infection)

---

*   Viruses in bloodstream.

CLASSIFICATION OF VIRUSES:

Family	Nucleic acid	Shape	Important members
Pox	DNA	brick	Smallpox Vaccinia
Herpes	DNA	icosahedral	Herpes simplex Varicella-zoster Epstein-Barr Cytomegalovirus
Adeno	DNA	icosahedral	
Papova	DNA	icosahedral	Wart viruses
Myxo	RNA	helical	Influenza A Influenza B
Paramyxo	RNA	helical	Para-influenza Respiratory syncytial Measles Mumps
Picorna	RNA	icosahedral	Polio Echo Coxsackie Rhinovirus
Corona	RNA	icosahedral	
Rhabdo	RNA	bullet	Rabies
Reo	RNA	icosahedral	Rotaviruses

Slow viruses are infective agents with incubation periods that may span several years. **Kuru** (a neurological disease found in cannibal tribes) is caused by a slow virus.

Oncogenic viruses have been discussed with neoplasia (chapter 5).

Opportunistic infections are infections occurring in individuals with impaired immunity. The organisms involved are usually non-pathogenic or of low virulence.

RICKETTSIAE

Are similar to bacteria except that they have to infect living cells in order to multiply. They are often transmitted by **insects**.

CHLAMYDIAE

Will also only survive inside living cells. They are between bacteria and viruses in size.

PROTOZOA

Are unicellular microscopic organisms whose cellular organization (such as the configuration of their nuclei and the method of replication) closely resembles the animal cell. They ingest food from their immediate environment and digest it intracellularly and generally have complex life cycles. Protozoa are generally resistant to antibiotics and cause many tropical and sub-tropical diseases.

FUNGI

Relatively few fungi are associated with human disease and those that are generally cause superficial infections. Fungi can be broadly classified into **moulds** which reproduce by sporing and **yeasts** which reproduce by budding.

WORMS

Are **parasites** and a rare cause of disease in the West. They may be classified into **nematodes** (round worms, thread worms), **cestodes** (tapeworms and their cysts) and **trematodes** (flukes).

THE NATURE OF INFECTION

COMMENSALS

Numerous bacteria are **normally** present on the skin and on the linings of the respiratory and alimentary tracts and "swabs" taken from the skin, nose, mouth, hands etc of healthy human beings will produce exuberant bacterial growth in laboratory "cultures".

These **non-pathogenic** bacteria that live upon and within us are termed **commensals** and many are positively beneficial to the human organism (eg certain organisms in the gut produce vitamin B12 and many commensals will **exclude** pathogens from various sites by simple weight of numbers).

ROUTES OF ENTRY OF MICRO-ORGANISMS INTO BODY

Skin and mucous membranes:

Direct contact
Contamination of wounds
"Inoculation" by contaminated needles, insect stings etc

Ingestion:

Contaminated food and water

Inhalation:

Dust
Droplets from coughs and sneezes

HUMAN DEFENCES AGAINST INFECTION

Good health and nutrition.

Physical barriers:

The skin
Nostril hairs

Secretions:

> Tears
> Urine
> Mucous in the respiratory tract
> Saliva
> Sweat

Chemical defences:

> Acid secretions in the stomach and urinary tract
> "Lysozymes" in tears and saliva
> Immunoglobulins (of the IgA class) in tears and intestinal secretions

Inflammation:

> Acute and chronic (limits the spread of infection)

Phagocytosis:

> Follows the acute inflammatory response

Immune responses:

> See chapter 4

Interferon production:

> Interferon is a non-specific anti-viral agent produced by infected cells (see above).

MICRO-ORGANISM ATTACK MECHANISMS

> The invasive capacity of micro-organisms depends on the size of the infecting "dose" and the "virulence" of the organism concerned.

Virulence is:

> › The capacity to resist phagocytosis
> › The capacity to produce enzymes which damage host tissues
> › The capacity to produce **toxins** which compromise or interfere with host functioning at physiological, biochemical and immunological levels.

THE COURSE AND OUTCOME OF INFECTION

The course and outcome of any infection may be affected by various factors that compromise host defence mechanisms eg:

Skin:

Direct damage resulting from wounds, burns or skin disease.

Respiratory tract:

Smoking damages the protective lining of the respiratory tract.

Stomach:

Various abuses (eg alcoholism) may lead to decreased acid production and allow unhelpful organisms to flourish.

Commensals:

Helpful commensals may be destroyed by **antibiotics** thereby allowing pathogenic ones to multiply and take their place.

Immunology:

Drugs, such as steroids, may depress natural immunological defences.

Chronic disease and nutritional deficiency:

May significantly lower "resistance" to infection.

DISPOSAL OF MICRO-ORGANISMS BY THE BODY

The mechanisms involved in the removal of micro-organisms from the tissues are the result of co-operation between 3 systems which all depend on the body's ability to recognize "foreign invaders" as foreign:

1) Once they have been "attracted" to the site of infection by certain chemicals released during the acute inflammatory reaction, the **phagocytes** (macrophages and granulocytes) can **ingest** micro-organisms.

2) Certain **accessory chemical factors** and enzymes (eg the **comple-ment system**) are always present in the blood but are only triggered into activity by the presence of foreign proteins. These chemical factors may either act directly to disrupt micro-organisms or alternatively may help to make micro-organisms more "attractive" and digestible to the phago-cytes.

3) **Specific immune responses** such as antibody and killer T-cell pro-duction are important in destroying infective agents (see chapter 4).

MAIN FEATURES OF SOME COMMON INFECTIOUS DISEASES

Childhood infectious diseases: Bacterial meningitis
Chickenpox
Erysipelas
German measles (rubella)
Impetigo
Measles
Mumps
Whooping cough (pertussis) – see also chapter 12 for discussion of bronchiolitis (RSV), croup and epiglottitis.

The herpes family: Cytomegalovirus
Epstein-Barr (infectious mononucleosis)
Herpes zoster (shingles)
HSV1 – see chapter 13
HSV2 – see under sexually transmitted disease

Staphylococci and streptococci

Diarrhoeal diseases: Campylobacter
Cholera
Dysentery
Typhoid

Common fungal infections: Candida albicans – see chapters 13 and 26
Dermatophyte infection – see chapter 24

Sexually transmitted disease: AIDS
Gonorrhoea
Genital herpes
Infestations
NSU
Syphilis
Congenital syphilis

Tropical diseases: Malaria

Note: We suggest you refer to a pictorial atlas of infectious disease to help you to distinguish between the various rashes associated with the above conditions. This is no substitute for clinical experience, however.

CHILDHOOD INFECTIOUS DISEASES

BACTERIAL MENINGITIS

Infection of the arachnoid and pia mater with one of a variety of bacteria.

Responsible for about 300 deaths per annum in England and Wales. Possible organisms include **meningococcus, pneumococcus, haemophilus influenzae** (children), **E.coli** (newborn) and the **TB bacillus**.

This description refers primarily to **meningococcal meningitis**.

Who gets it:

Anyone! May occur in epidemics in closed communities since meningococcus lives in the nasopharynx and may be spread by droplet infection.

Tuberculous meningitis is commoner in Asian communities.

Aetiology:

Predisposing factors include severe middle ear or sinus infection, skull fracture, pneumonia and other severe infections, overcrowding, immunosuppression, neural tube defects.

Pathology:

Infecting organisms reach meninges via bloodstream or by local spread → organisms spread through sub-arachnoid space → gross inflammatory reaction → pus collects in sulci and around base of brain and CSF becomes cloudy → pus + CSF makes good "culture medium" for further multiplication of micro-organisms → untreated this may lead to cerebral vein thrombosis, cortical infarction and septicaemia.

Septicaemia may lead to circulatory collapse (sometimes associated with haemorrhagic infarction of the adrenal glands) and death.

Clinical features:

Headache, dislike of light, drowsiness and vomiting. Patient has fever. May lie curled up. Characteristic haemorrhagic rash (doesn't blanch on pressure) commonly on buttocks/lower limbs in meningococcal meningitis. Signs of meningeal irritation include neck stiffness and pain on passive extension of knee with flexed hip. As condition worsens, drowsiness, confusion, fits may occur.

Complications:

Cranial nerve palsies, hemiplegia* from brain infarction, hydrocephalus, adrenal infarction, circulatory collapse and death. Survivors may suffer permanent brain damage – mental retardation, epilepsy, hydrocephalus.

Basis of treatment:

Investigations:

Lumbar puncture → CSF sent for microbiological analysis; blood sent for microbiological analysis; chest X-ray, sometimes brain scan.

Management:

Intravenous **benzyl penicillin** or chloramphenicol for at least 10 days (plus life support where necessary) usually resolves bacterial meningitis. Repeated lumbar punctures are taken to monitor effects of treatment. In meningococcal meningitis, a 2 day prophylactic course of rifampicin is recommended for close contacts of patients.

Side effects of treatment:

Penicillin	→	Hypersensitivity reactions
Chloramphenicol	→	Bone marrow damage
Lumbar puncture	→	Headache, secondary infection, risk of coning** and death if ↑ICP (risk largely avoided by performing CT scan before LP)

---

*   Paralysis of one side of body.

** If a lumbar puncture is performed on someone with raised intracranial pressure, having a needle in the sub-arachnoid space of the spinal column can produce an effect rather like that of removing a plug from a bath. The resulting downward "suction" can jam vital parts of the brain against the hard edges of the tentorium cerebelli or foramen magnum resulting in rapid death.

Prognosis:

Overall mortality (despite treatment) about 10% (but about 80% in new-born infants). Always assumed to be potentially fatal without antibacterial chemotherapy. Long term neurological damage is much more common in children than adults.

Early treatment improves prognosis in all age groups.

CHICKENPOX

Viral disease caused by varicella zoster virus.

Epidemiology:

Children mostly affected.
Droplet spread.
More serious in immunosuppressed and pregnant.

Incubation period:

About 2 weeks.
Infectious from 5 days before rash until last crop of vesicles crust.

Clinical features:

Fever, malaise. Also sore throat, headache.

Rash:*   Macules → papules → vesicles → pustules → crusting.
Central distribution, limbs relatively free of spots.
Sometimes scars after healing.

Complications:

› Secondary bacterial infection of spots
› Pneumonitis
› Encephalitis

If immunosuppressed, rash is worse and complications are more likely.

Basis of treatment:

Symptomatic.

* Macules = flat red spots.
Papules = raised red spots.
Vesicles = smooth fluid filled blisters.
Pustules = pus filled blisters.

ERYSIPELAS

Streptococcal skin infection.

Incubation period:

Up to a week.

Clinical features:

Fever, malaise (sudden onset).

May be headache, vomiting.

Raised red rash: Butterfly distribution on face.
                          Lower limbs may also be affected.
                          Blisters may form on facial rash.

Basis of treatment:

Antibiotics.

GERMAN MEASLES (RUBELLA)

A mild viral infectious disease, mainly affecting children and young adults.

Epidemiology:

Incubation period 18-21 days.
Infectious from 7 days before rash appears until 5 days after.
Droplet spread.

Symptoms and signs:

Starts with slight fever, malaise, runny nose and sore throat.
Then flat pink spotty rash on face and neck spreading downwards over rest of body (although rash does *not* appear in all cases).
Often generalized lymph node enlargement (suboccipital/posterior cervical in particular).
Occasional joint pains.

Complications:

Are rare, except for pregnant women infected in the first trimester, whose babies are at risk of developing the **congenital rubella syndrome** (multiple defects especially of eyes, ears and heart).

Basis of treatment:

Symptomatic.

The national measles/mumps/rubella vaccination programme (given to 2 year olds) and rubella only vaccination of 12 year old girls aims to eradicate congenital rubella from the community.*

---

*   See chapter 4 for more information on vaccination programmes.

IMPETIGO

Superficial, highly infectious skin condition caused by streptococci or staphylococci.

Incidence:

Predominantly a disease of childhood.

Clinical features:

Localized smallish blisters (ie a vesicular rash) usually around mouth and nose.
Vesicles burst and crust over.

Basis of treatment:

Local antiseptic preparations to clean skin and remove crusts.
Systemic antibiotics if necessary.

MEASLES

Highly infectious viral disease of young children that is still an important cause of death in the Third World.

Epidemiology:

Infective agent is from paramyxovirus family. Most common in 1-7 year olds. (Rare<6 months since babies protected by transplacental maternal antibodies.) Probably droplet spread. Incubation about 10 days. Infectious for 1-2 days before symptoms to 5 days after appearance of rash.

Clinical features:

Day 1:   Miserable, sore eyes, runny nose, dry cough, fever.
Day 2-3:   As 1, plus Koplik's spots* in mouth.
Day 4:   Koplik's spots fade as dark red flat rash starts behind ears and spreads to trunk then limbs.
Day 6-8:   Rash fades (sometimes leaving shortlived brown staining) and fever subsides.

Complications:

More common: Middle ear infection
                   Bronchitis
                   Pneumonia/pneumonitis (the commonest cause of death)

Less common: Febrile convulsions
                   Post infective encephalitis

Basis of treatment:

Symptomatic + appropriate management of complications. Vaccination now being offered to 2 year olds as component of measles/mumps/rubella vaccine.**

---

* Henry Koplik (1858-1927) – Attending Paediatrician to Mount Sinai Hospital, New York and founder of the American Paediatric Society – who described the small white spots seen in the mouths of children with measles.

** See chapter 4 for more information on vaccination programmes.

MUMPS

Viral infectious disease causing systemic disturbance accompanied by local inflammation of salivary glands, especially parotid glands.

Epidemiology:

Affects children more than infants or adults.
More common in winter/spring.
Incubation period about 18 days.
Only moderately infectious – droplet spread (or oral contact).
Infectious from prodrome until swollen glands go down.

Clinical features:

Malaise, fever, sore throat followed by tender swelling of parotid glands (usually both, sometimes one; may be submandibular gland swelling).

Sufferer starts to feel better after 3 or 4 days but may take 2 weeks for glands to go down.

Complications:

Mumps meningitis is a relatively common cause of viral meningitis.

Other complications (such as encephalomyelitis causing cranial nerve damage) are rare.

Orchitis*/oophoritis** (post puberty) and pancreatitis are rare but important.

Basis of treatment:

Symptomatic/supportive.

---

*   Inflammation of the testes.
**   Inflammation of the ovaries.

WHOOPING COUGH (PERTUSSIS)

A highly infectious bacterial disease of young children, characterized by paroxysmal coughing.

Epidemiology:

Infective agent = bacteria Bordetella pertussis. Occurs in 4 yearly epidemics affecting infants and young children under 7.
Droplet spread.
Incubation period about 10 days.
Infectious from onset of symptoms and for up to 1 month after onset.

Clinical features:

About a week of cold-like symptoms plus fever and dry cough.
Fever diminishes and paroxysmal coughing starts.
Coughing fits end with characteristic "whooop" and may produce transient cyanosis. Often accompanied by vomiting.
Worse at night.
Usually quite well between coughing attacks.
Gradual recovery over 4-6 weeks.

Complications:

Are more likely and more dangerous under 1 year old. Nearly all deaths occur in the under 2's, mostly in babies under 6 months old. Pneumonia, patchy lung collapse and convulsions may all occur. Pneumonia is responsible for most deaths.

Basis of treatment:

Supportive. May need hospital admission if paroxysms very severe. Antibiotics used for secondary infection. Vaccination programme (part of DTP "triple vaccine") aims to eradicate whooping cough. Pertussis vaccine* sometimes provokes encephalopathy (rare).

*   See chapter 4 for more information on vaccination programmes.

THE HERPES FAMILY

CYTOMEGALOVIRUS INFECTION (acquired type)

Background:

CMV is a herpes virus causing "glandular fever" type syndrome in young adults (can also cause congenital problems (especially mental retardation) if transmitted from mother to foetus).

Clinical features:

May be asymptomatic or glandular fever picture with malaise, lymphadenopathy, sore throat and enlarged spleen.

May cause more serious problems in immunosuppressed patients.

Basis of treatment:

Supportive.

EPSTEIN-BARR VIRUS INFECTION

Background:

EBV is the herpes virus apparently responsible for infectious mononucleosis (**glandular fever**).
Affects young adults.
Spread by close contact/kissing.
Can be long incubation period.

Clinical features:

Slow onset.
Tiredness, headache, fever. May be lymphadenopathy.
Occasionally very severe sore throat ("anginose" glandular fever).
Spleen may be enlarged.

Complications:

Relatively common: Tiredness and debility during convalescence

Rare: Blood disorders
         Nerve palsies
         Heart disease
         Pneumonia
         Glomerulonephritis
         Meningo-encephalitis

Basis of treatment:

Supportive.

NOTE:

The EBV is one of the few viruses known to cause tumours in humans –
ie Burkitt's* lymphoma.

---

*   Dennis Burkitt, FRS, formerly senior surgeon, Mulago Hospital, Kampala, Uganda.

HERPES ZOSTER (SHINGLES)

Background:

Herpes zoster is another name for the varicella virus of chickenpox.

Shingles may be thought of as a late complication of chickenpox where the virus, having lain dormant for years in sensory root ganglia, "reactivates" and produces a painful rash following the distribution of a dermatome or sensory part of a cranial nerve.

Often afflicts people who are generally "run down" or immunosuppressed.

Clinical features:

Intercostal nerves and the ophthalmic division of the trigeminal nerve are most commonly affected.
Initially pain/sensitivity of skin plus malaise.
Then vesicular rash which crusts and heals after a week or so.

Complications:

Corneal damage in ophthalmic herpes.
Post herpetic neuralgia (desperately uncomfortable).
Disseminated disease (in immunocompromised).

Basis of treatment:

Pain relief (analgesia) + supportive.

STAPHYLOCOCCI AND STREPTOCOCCI

There are many types of staphylococci and streptococci, but only a few are of medical importance, ie –

> β-**haemolytic streptococci** (groups A, B, C & G) cause sore throat, skin infection, puerperal* sepsis etc.
>
> **Group A** β-**haemolytic streptococci** are well known because of their tendency to cause post infective immunological complications such as –
> › glomerulonephritis (chapter 21)
> › rheumatic fever (chapter 11)
> › Henoch-Schönlein purpura** (chapter 23)
> › erythema nodosum (see below)
>
> Staphylococcus aureus is becoming well known (and feared) for the development of strains resistant to antibiotic therapy (partly in hospitals).
>
> α-**haemolytic streptococci** cause bacterial endocarditis, dental caries etc.
>
> **Faecal streptococci** cause pneumonia and sometimes meningitis.
>
> **Staphylococcus aureus** cause infections of **skin**, lungs, gut, urinary tract, bone and joints.

Note 1:

> **Group A** β-**haemolytic streptococci** are probably responsible for about 1/3 of the sore throats seen in general practice. "Strep. throats" are seen more often in autumn and winter and are commoner in children. Transmission is by droplet spread. The sore throat is accompanied by fever, malaise and headache and the tonsils may look red, swollen and covered in pus.
>
> Occasionally, a strep. throat is rapidly followed by a fine red rash which spreads downwards over the trunk and limbs – **scarlet fever**.

---

*   After childbirth.
** Edward Henoch (1820-1910), professor of paediatrics, Berlin
     Johan Schönlein (1793-1864), teacher of medicine and pathology in Zürich and Berlin

In this condition, the papillae of the tongue may become inflamed and interspersed with white "fur" giving a "strawberry tongue" appearance.

Note 2:

Erythema nodosum is a condition characterized by red, tender, raised, shiny lesions on the shins accompanied by fever, malaise and a raised ESR. As the lesions fade, they go through the same colour changes as a bruise.

Erythema nodosum is an **immunological cross sensitivity reaction** and, although quite commonly seen as a complication of strep. throats, it may also accompany TB, sarcoid, inflammatory bowel disease and adverse drug reactions etc.

DIARRHOEAL DISEASES

CAMPYLOBACTER

Certain types of campylobacter bacilli have recently been recognized as important causes of diarrhoea/acute gastro-enteritis.

Epidemiology:

Campylobacters are normal commensals in a number of animal species and it is thought that they sometimes spread from animals to humans. Raw milk and undercooked chicken may be sources of infection.

Clinical features:

Incubation period is 3-5 days.
Fever, muscle aches and abdominal pain for a couple of days followed by explosive diarrhoea (eventually containing some mucous and even blood).
Vomiting is uncommon.
The abdominal pain tends to be relieved (for a short time) by defecation.

Complications:

› Patients with inflammatory bowel disease may experience a severe exacerbation.
› Reactive arthritis
› Pancreatitis
› Septicaemia

Basis of treatment:

› Supportive
› Encourage fluids
› Antibiotics if prolonged

CHOLERA

Severe epidemic diarrheal disease caused by the toxin produced by the organism Vibrio cholerae.

Epidemiology:

Endemic in parts of Asia.
Faecal-oral spread (usually via contaminated food or drinking water).
Incubation period up to 5 days.

Symptoms and signs:

Rapid onset of vomiting and continuous, copious, watery diarrhoea accompanied by abdominal pain and leg cramps.
The fluid loss can be so severe that shock/acute renal failure may cause death within 24 hours.

Complications:

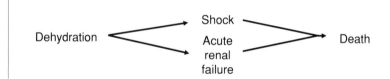

Basis of treatment:

Enthusiastic rehydration (eg with oral glucose/electrolyte solutions).
Clean up water supply.
Ensure good personal hygiene.
Vaccination not very effective.

DYSENTERY

Dysentery is a collective name for a group of conditions characterized by bloody diarrhoea. The two main groups are **amoebic** dysentery and **bacillary** dysentery.

AMOEBIC:

Epidemiology:

Occurs in tropics.
Caused by the organism **Entamoeba histolytica.**
Faecal-oral spread (food/water).

Clinical features:

Fever, abdominal colic and bloody diarrhoea.
May persist for many weeks.
Diagnosis requires examination of fresh faeces sample under microscope.

Complications:

Amoebic hepatitis or liver abscess (may also occur without diarrheal illness).

Basis of treatment:

Metronidazole *(Flagyl).*

BACILLARY:

Epidemiology:

Organisms come from **shigella** group.
Worldwide problem.
Faecal-oral or fly-borne spread compounded by overcrowding, poor hygiene etc.
Faeces may remain infected for some weeks after acute illness.

Clinical features:

Sudden onset with fever, malaise, headache and abdominal pain followed by watery diarrhoea (± blood/mucus). Usually resolves within a week.

Complications:

Arthritis
Haemolysis*
Renal failure

Basis of treatment:

Fluid replacement
General hygiene/public health measures
Antibiotics if severe

* = red blood cells splitting apart.

TYPHOID

Intestinal infection caused by the organism Salmonella typhi. (The salmonella group is huge, containing several organisms responsible for food poisoning associated with contaminated meat and poultry.)

Epidemiology:

Occurs in many parts of the world but now uncommon in Britain thanks to public health measures designed to ensure clean water, safe sewage and good food handling procedures in shops and restaurants. Faecal-oral transmission. Humans may become **asymptomatic carriers,** spreading disease via their faeces or urine. Incubation period about 2 weeks.

Pathogenesis:

Contaminated food/water ingested → organism multiplies in small intestine → spread to mesenteric lymph nodes and then to bloodstream. Gut then re-invaded via liver and biliary system → infection of Peyer's patches*.

Clinical features:

May be asymptomatic – **or**

Week 1 →   Fever, abdominal pain, **constipation,** headache and non-productive **cough** in a patient with recent history of foreign travel.

Week 2 →   Fever, abdominal pain worse, malaise ++, pale face, "rose spots" on trunk (small crops, gone in 1 or 2 days).
May develop diarrhoea.

Week 3 →   Abdominal distension, fever, weakness, sometimes delirium.

Week 4 →   Gradual return to normal.

---

*   Johan Peyer (1653-1712), Swiss professor of logic, rhetoric and medicine – named patches of lymphatic tissue in small intestines.

Complications:

Coma
Gastrointestinal haemorrhage or perforation
Cholecystitis
Myocarditis
Pyelonephritis
Pneumonia
Deep vein thrombosis
Death

Prevention:

Clean water. Good public health system. Vaccines (~ 80% protection for 5 years)

Treatment:

Barrier nursing.
Antibiotics.
Good hydration

NOTE:

Paratyphoid is a milder version of typhoid caused by the organism Salmonella paratyphi.

SEXUALLY TRANSMITTED DISEASES

AIDS

The Acquired Immunodeficiency Syndrome.

Background:

Perhaps should be called Acquired Immunodeficiency Syndrome**s** – a group of clinical presentations apparently related to previous infection with the Human Immunodeficiency Virus.
98% of sufferers have HIV antibodies in their serum (2% don't ....).

Worldwide problem of increasing magnitude (number of cases currently doubling every 11 months) ie:

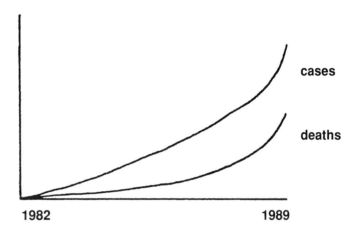

1982   1989

1000 plus deaths in UK at time of writing.

Transmission:

Sexually transmitted and also via blood and blood products.

Risk groups:

Everyone, but classically homosexuals (especially "receptive" partners), IV drug abusers, haemophiliacs, recipients of blood transfusions.

Clinical features:

HIV infection is often asymptomatic. The incubation period may last for years and the progression from primary infection to "seroconversion" to the "antibody positive" state is still poorly understood.

Being antibody positive by no means ensures that you will go on to develop full blown AIDS and anyway, there is little on offer (at the moment) in the way of effective treatment.

There are 4 basic AIDS related states:

1. "Carriers" –
ie "antibody positive" people with serological evidence of previous HIV infection but no symptoms.
It is incredibly difficult to estimate numbers but could be well over 20,000 in UK alone.

2. PGL (or persistent generalized lymphadenopathy) –
Patient fairly well but widespread lymph node enlargement.
May occur BEFORE seroconversion.

3. ARC (AIDS related complex) –
Patients must have 2 UNEXPLAINED clinical features of chronic disease (eg fever, diarrhoea, weight loss, malaise, liver/spleen enlargement, oral thrush) plus abnormal blood test results (anaemia, ESR$\uparrow$, WCC$\downarrow$ etc).

4. FULL BLOWN AIDS –
Two commonest presentations are –
a) Opportunistic lung infection by **Pneumocystis carinii** causing pneumonia (PCP) or b) **Kaposi's sarcoma**[*] – an unusual looking insidious skin malignancy characterized by red plaques on skin and in mouth.

Lymphatic cancers (lymphomas) and other opportunistic infections (especially of the CNS) may also occur in full blown AIDS.

---

[*]   Moricz Kaposi (1837-1902), professor of dermatology in Vienna.

GONORRHOEA

A sexually transmitted disease associated with the gonococcus (Neisseria gonorrhoea) which affects primarily the anterior urethra in the male and the urethra and cervix in the female.

Incidence:

66,000 cases seen per year in the UK.

Incubation period:

1-10 days.

Clinical features:

Male: Mucoid urethral discharge with painful micturition*
          (dysuria).
          Carriers (5%) may have no symptoms.
          May be pharyngitis or proctitis depending on type of
          sexual activity engaged in.

Female: **7% asymptomatic.**
          Clinical picture is not definitive.
          May be slight dysuria or vaginal discharge.

Complications:

Male: Rare if treated.
          Otherwise prostatitis, urethral stricture etc.

Female: Proctitis from vaginal discharge.
          Infection of the Fallopian tubes = **salpingitis**.
          Infertility following bilateral salpingitis.

Babies: "Gonococcal ophthalmia neonatorum" – a purulent dis-
          charge from the eyes of a baby within 21 days of birth due
          to infection during the passage through the birth canal –
          can lead to corneal ulceration and blindness.

---

*   Weeing.

Basis of treatment:

> Penicillin is still effective in about 90% of cases.
> Allergy to penicillin or discovery of a "resistant strain" of gonococcus necessitates the use of newer – often more expensive – antibiotics.
> Patients should refrain from intercourse until tests indicate cure.
> Recent sexual contacts should be traced if possible.

NOTES:

1) Post-gonococcal urethritis is a *non*-specific urethritis which remains after treatment in up to 50% of cases.

2) Gonorrhoea can produce a number of **"systemic"** symptoms, the commonest of which is **arthritis**.

GENITAL HERPES

Sexually transmitted viral infection of genitals caused by HSV-2 (herpes virus type 2).

Incidence:

More common in younger age group with multiple sexual partners.

Incubation period:

4-5 days.

Clinical features:

May be brief prodrome of malaise followed by vesicles on genitals, anus etc + tender inguinal lymphadenopathy.
Vesicles burst leaving painful erosions.
Generally heals after about 10 days.
Tends to recur sporadically.

Complications:

› Neonatal infection (if mother having attack around time of delivery)
› Urinary retention
› Encephalitis/meningitis

» Cervical HSV-2 infection may predispose to cervical cancer.

Basis of treatment:

Antiviral drugs (eg acyclovir) have limited success.
Antibiotics if secondary infection.

GENITAL INFESTATIONS

Pubic lice and scabies.

PUBIC LICE:

= **Pediculosis pubis** = crabs = nits

Live in pubic hair and feed on blood.
Occasionally spread to other hairy areas (but not scalp).
Female lays eggs on hairs.
Transmission by direct contact or contact with infested clothing and bedding.
Bites cause itching/possibly rash (eggs or lice may also be seen).
Easy to treat with special shampoos and lotions.

SCABIES:

Caused by the mite **Sarcoptes scabei**, which burrows under skin to lay eggs.
Burrows show up as exceptionally itchy bumps and may appear anywhere except the head.
Wrists and ankles, genitalia, armpits and skin between toes and fingers are common sites.
Transmission by direct contact.
Treatment involves painting (twice in 24 hours) with benzyl benzoate.
Clothing and bedding should be disinfected.

NSU

Non-specific urethritis

Background:

The expression NSU is used to distinguish between urethritis related to gonorrhoea infections and urethritis from other causes.

The commonest organism implicated in non-specific urethritis is **Chlamydia trachomatis**.

Clinical features:

May be asymptomatic or cause dysuria + urethral discharge.

Complications:

Male: Prostatitis
             Reiter's syndrome*

Female: Pelvic inflammatory disease

Basis of treatment:

Treat both partners.
Antibiotics effective in about 80% of cases.

---

*   Hans Reiter (1881-1969), lecturer at the Institute of Hygiene, Konigberg and later Honorary Professor of Hygiene in Berlin during the 2nd World War. See chapter 18 for description of syndrome.

SYPHILIS

Sexually transmitted disease caused by the organism Treponema pallidum.

Overview:

These days most commonly diagnosed in male homosexuals.
Illness progresses through various stages.
The early forms are associated with superficial infectious lesions.
The late stage causes serious damage to the CVS and nervous system.

Clinical features:

Primary syphilis:

1 month after exposure, hard, well demarcated **painless ulcer** (chancre) appears on penis, vulva or anus (sometimes lip or breast).
May be local lymphadenopathy.
Chancre heals after 4-8 weeks.

Secondary syphilis:

As chancre heals, patient develops widespread, non-itchy red rash (especially trunk, face, palms and soles) plus generalized lymphadenopathy.
May be moist, fleshy, mucocutaneous lesions around anus (anal condylomata lata).

Tertiary syphilis:

Characterized by formation of **gummata** – hard, red, painless, well demarcated patches on skin, mucous membranes or bones.
May not develop for up to 10 years after primary infection.

Eventually (up to 20 years after primary infection) aortic aneurysm or coronary artery damage may develop and the posterior columns of the spinal cord may degenerate ("tabes dorsalis") leading to ↓ position sense in lower limbs, ataxia and incontinence.
Dementia ("general paralysis of the insane") is the final insult.

Basis of treatment:

Penicillin is effective at most stages of the condition.
The earlier the treatment, the better the result.

CONGENITAL SYPHILIS

Epidemiology

Preventable.
Transmitted during or after 4th month via placenta from mother to baby.

May result in:

1) Abortion @ around 28 weeks
2) Stillbirth
3) Live child with signs of congenital syphilis
4) Healthy child that develops congenital syphilis in later years

Clinical features:

Early stage:

Birth – 2 yrs
> rashes
> condylomata lata
> snuffles
> malaise
> lymphadenopathy
> large liver + spleen etc

Late stage:

2-40 yrs = tertiary syphilis
> gummata (on palate)
> inflammation + damage of cornea (keratitis)
> deafness (bilateral VIIIth nerve damage)

Other stigmata:

> peg shaped teeth
> sabre shaped tibia
> facial abnormalities ("saddle" nose)

Treatment:

Early treatment of mother will treat foetus.

TROPICAL DISEASES

MALARIA

Tropical disease caused by parasites of the plasmodium family.

Background:

The most common (and most serious) tropical disease, endemic in most of Asia, Africa, the Middle East and South America.

Pathogenesis:

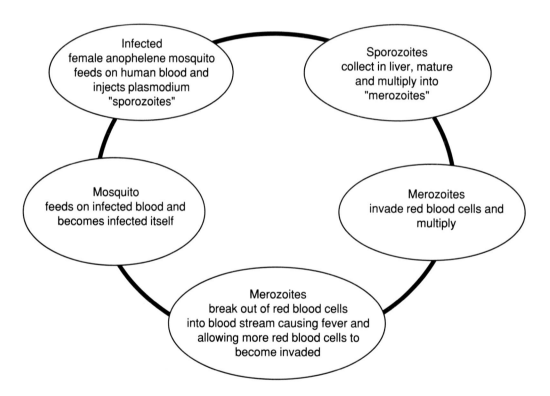

3 members of the plasmodium family (Vivax, Ovale and Malariae) cause a relatively mild disease which tends to recur every few years (if treatment fails to eradicate the parasites from the blood and liver).

The 4th member, Plasmodium falciparum, causes a much more serious and progressive illness that can be rapidly fatal.

Clinical features:

Benign relapsing malaria:

Incubation period 10 days.
Sudden onset fever/sweating/rigors/malaise; spleen usually enlarged.
Symptoms recur every other day or every 3rd day depending on which parasite is involved.

Malignant malaria:

Incubation period 10 days.

Insidious onset of headache, vomiting, malaise, fever, cough and diarrhoea
↓
hepatosplenomegaly + jaundice
↓
haemolysis and anaemia
↓
widespread ischaemic organ damage
↓
renal failure
liver failure
pulmonary oedema
encephalopathy/fits

Basis of treatment:

Drugs derived from quinine (type depends on strain of parasite).

Prevention:

Tablets such as maloprim, fansidar or chloroquinine taken regularly whilst travelling through endemic areas.

Also mosquito nets and avoiding uncovered skin after sunset.

8. Principles of Orthodox Pharmacology

Doctors are people who prescribe
medicines of which they know very little
to cure diseases of which they know less
in human beings of which they
know nothing.

Voltaire

PRINCIPLES OF ORTHODOX PHARMACOLOGY

OVERVIEW

Introduction

Principles of Chemical Medicine

Introduction of New Drugs

Pharmacological Mechanisms and Terminology

Adverse Drug Reactions

Drug Interactions

Common Drug Classes

INTRODUCTION

This chapter is a brief introduction to a huge subject. We strongly suggest that you obtain an up to date copy of the British National Formula (BNF) and that you get into the habit of looking up individual drugs when you come across them in practice.

In the BNF, drugs are classified by "system" for quick reference and are referred to by their generic (chemical) names. Trade names are also given. Most doctors make a point of referring to drugs by their generic names only (to the distress of the drug companies).

You must realize that the decision to withdraw allopathic drug treatment is a serious matter with potentially far reaching consequences and should *never* be undertaken lightly. It would be best managed as a co-operative exercise between the patient and *all* the practitioners involved in his or her care and certainly not without the approval of the original prescriber.

Remember – allopathic drugs are powerful chemicals and their therapeutic manipulation needs considerable skill, due caution and not a little nerve.

PRINCIPLES OF CHEMICAL MEDICINE

At the Congress for Internal Medicine, Wiesbaden in April 1910, a young Prussian biochemist called Paul Ehrlich presented a paper on the discovery of the therapeutic properties of Dioxydiamino-arsenobenzol dihydrochloride which was to revolutionize western medicine. For, by showing that synthetic chemicals could mimic the highly selective anti-bacterial action of endogenous antibodies, he implanted in the public consciousness the idea that it would be possible to produce all manner of chemical "magic bullets" which could free mankind from the scourge of infectious disease – the major health problem of his time. The fact that **salvarsan** (as his arsenical compound came to be known) was active against the organism causing syphilis assured the acceptance of his work amongst the rulers and the powerful of the western world.

It is easy for us to forget how urgent the problem of infection was in the early part of this century and how desperate many doctors were to find some sort of therapeutic intervention to reduce their impotence in the face of great suffering and loss of life. In concert with major changes in social policy and improved standards of public health, the subsequent discoveries of prontosil (Germany 1935) and penicillin (UK 1928-40) had genuine impact on human morbidity and mortality and, together with Banting and Best's discovery of insulin (1921-3) and the improvements in general anaesthesia, the scene was set for the headlong rush to find chemical remedies for all ills in which we are caught up today. (It is interesting to note, however, that whilst up to one quarter of all drug prescriptions contain substances extracted from plant sources, there is very little research to discover *new* drugs amongst the 750,000 species of flowering plants of the earth. It is also important to realize that when the drug industry does research plant material, it extracts individual substances and concentrates them according to the theoretical constructs of biochemistry and physiology rather than looking at the therapeutic activity of the whole plant.)

Much of the rest of this section is concerned with the problems of drug overuse, misuse and commercial exploitation but it is important to take a balanced view of the current uses of chemical medicine.

To start with, we should be clear about why drugs or chemicals may be prescribed in the first place, ie:

›   As prophylaxis – to prevent disease
›   To support physiological processes – "homoeostatic replacement"
›   As treatment for an underlying disease process
    (as understood by orthodox pathology)
›   To suppress disease processes
›   To relieve symptoms
›   To keep a patient happy
›   To stop a doctor from feeling useless

You may care to consider which drugs are used in which category as you come across them in practice.

THE INTRODUCTION OF NEW DRUGS

In the aftermath of the thalidomide disaster, the British Minister of Health established a Committee on Safety of Drugs whose efforts culminated in 1968 with the publication of the Medicines Act that became law in 1971.

The Act provides for the licensing of *all* medicinal products and controls their advertising, supply and retail sale.

Under the Act, every medicine currently on the market when the act became law was given a licence "as of right", but a process of review was instituted with a view to conversion of all licences of right to full product licences by 1990. (There are currently about 10,000 requiring review out of an initial 39,000 licenses of right. Something over 4000 *new* product licences have been issued since 1972. Product licences are valid for 5 years, after which they must be reviewed.)

Note that the Medicines Act does *not* control the *use* which a doctor may make of any licensed product for his/her own patients.

Under the terms of the Act, a Medicines Commission was set up to act as an "independent" advisory body on drug matters to the Ministers of Health and Agriculture (the ultimate licensing authorities). The Minister of Health also set up two powerful sub-committees:

The Committee on Safety of Medicines (CSM) which scrutinizes drugs at three stages in their development – before clinical trials (clinical trial certificate stage), before advertising and marketing (product licence stage) and after marketing

and

The Committee on the Review of Medicines (CRM) which advises on all matters relating to the process of converting licences of right to full product licences.

Both bodies make their assessments on the basis of the following criteria:

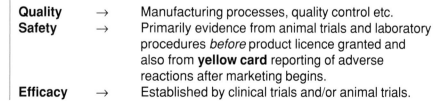

Quality	→	Manufacturing processes, quality control etc.
Safety	→	Primarily evidence from animal trials and laboratory procedures *before* product licence granted and also from **yellow card** reporting of adverse reactions after marketing begins.
Efficacy	→	Established by clinical trials and/or animal trials.

The life story of a new drug from synthesis to sale can be represented as follows:

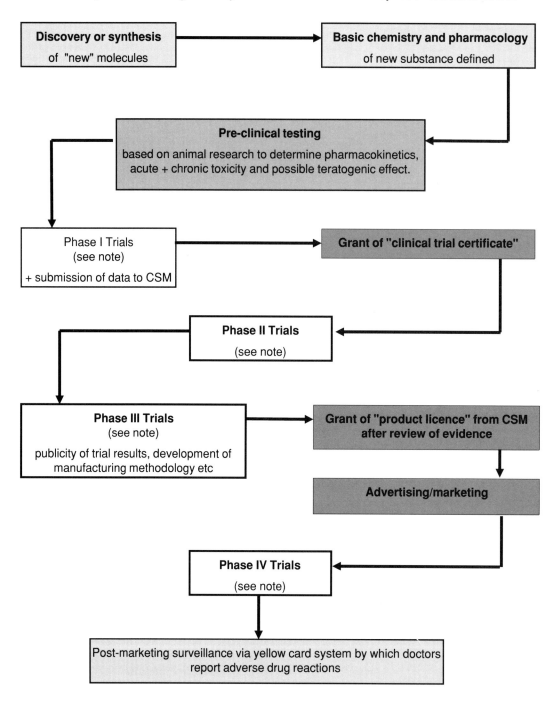

NOTE 1:

Phase I trials are the first limited trials in which drugs are given to humans.

Phase II trials are therapeutic trials by independent (usually hospital) researchers to try and establish appropriate indications and dosage regimes for the subsequent prescribing.

Phase III trials are the formal clinical trials comparing the efficacy of a new drug with another established treatment or placebo.

Phase IV is the general release of the drug for prescription by doctors.

NOTE 2:

Common tests in the pre-clinical testing stage include:

› **LD50** test in which the dose of a drug that will kill 50% of a group of animals is determined -

› **Chronic toxicity** tests in which the chronic toxicity over 3-6 months in at least 2 species (one of which is not a rodent) is measured.

> 3,280,135 experiments were carried out on living animals in 1985:
>
> 76% without any anaesthetic.
>
> 1,699,384 of these were experiments relating to medical, dental and veterinary products/appliances.
>
> 51% of all animal experiments were carried out by commercial concerns.
>
> Between 1985 and 1987 these numbers decreased by 5% which is encouraging but nevertheless
>
> On average, an animal dies in British laboratories every 10 seconds, every day of the year.

The development of a new drug now takes about 10 years and costs over £15 million. ICI produces over 8000 new substances a year for evaluation of which less than 10 go on to pre-clinical evaluation. Only one in twenty of the products reaching the clinical trial stage goes on to full scale evaluation.

Yet despite all this time and money spent on research, and despite the "exhaustive" animal testing, more than 10,000 "yellow cards" are returned each year by GPs and other doctors who suspect that adverse reactions are being caused by supposedly "safe" drugs.....

PHARMACOLOGICAL MECHANISMS AND TERMINOLOGY

Most allopathic drugs operate by influencing physiological processes at the cellular level, eg by altering membrane function, blocking or stimulating receptors, promoting or inhibiting enzyme activity etc. In this way they can regulate organ function, modify immune responses, influence the rate of cell division etc. Some drugs are used as simple mechanical barriers and some act as synthetic replacements for bio-chemicals present in insufficient quantity to maintain normal functioning.

Generally speaking, the life cycle of a chemical medicine is as follows:

Prescription → administration orally, rectally or by injection ("parenteral administration") → absorption from site of administration → distribution to site of action → therapeutic action and side effects → metabolism/inactivation, predominantly in the liver → excretion from body, mostly via the kidneys. Some drugs are excreted via the kidneys "unchanged".

The study of these various phases as they occur in different drugs is the work of clinical pharmacology. As with all branches of orthodox clinical science, a mini language has been developed by pharmacologists to help them describe their observations and the terms used appear so frequently in the medical literature that you should have some understanding of the commoner expressions.

PHARMACOKINETICS:

Is the study of what the patient does to the drug, ie the quantitative study of drug absorption, distribution, metabolism and excretion.

PHARMACODYNAMICS:

Is the study of what the drug does to the patient with particular emphasis on the extent and time course of any effect.
These two aspects are obviously closely inter-related.

HALF LIFE:

Represents the time taken for the concentration of a circulating drug to fall by half once absorption and distribution are complete. Knowing the half life of a drug helps the clinician to estimate the frequency of administration which will maintain a clinical effect. It may also help to predict the rate of elimination following withdrawal of therapy. Some drugs have very long half lives (eg diazepam = 24 hrs+). To confuse matters, some of the **metabolites** of drugs also possess pharmacological activity and thus produce a therapeutic action longer than anticipated. Note that continued administration of any drug eventually produces a "steady state" blood concentration where the amount of drug absorbed is similar to the amount excreted.

VOLUME OF DISTRIBUTION:

After administration, drugs are distributed throughout the plasma, extra-cellular fluid and tissues. When given by injection, this process may be complete within minutes. Volume of distribution is an artificial mathematical representation of the amount of drug in the tissues and fluids at any given time.

CLEARANCE:

Is a complex theoretical concept which expresses the rate of elimination of a drug from the body via all available routes. For most drugs, the rate of elimination from the blood is proportional to the amount present. Drugs which behave like this are said to have **first order kinetics.**

ZERO ORDER KINETICS:

Sounds frightening, but is an important clinical concept. Some drugs such as phenytoin, aspirin and alcohol, are metabolized in the liver by enzymes which may become overloaded (or "saturated") if the dose administered causes the blood level of the drug to reach a certain height. When this happens, elimination from the body ceases to be in proportion to the amount of drug present and subsequent doses may produce rapid and severe toxicity.

Alcohol elimination displays zero order kinetics after a very small amount has been ingested and the fall in blood alcohol levels after a drinking bout occurs by a FIXED amount each hour. Thus the more you drink, the longer the hangover will last ....

BIOAVAILABILITY:

Is defined as **the rate and extent to which a drug is absorbed and becomes available at the site of drug action** and is an important concept because many things can happen to a drug on its journey from the pill box to the toilet which may diminish its effectiveness.

Thus when taken by mouth, a drug must dissolve in the intestinal contents before absorption can take place and this process depends on the physi-co-chemical nature of the drug formulation. Drugs that are fat soluble tend to be absorbed more quickly. The absorption of some drugs is inhibited by the presence of food in the gut. After absorption through the gut wall into the bloodstream, a drug is immediately carried to the liver via the portal system where it may undergo extensive metabolism (the "first pass effect"). This means that only a small amount of unchanged drug reaches the systemic circulation. If first pass metabolism is extensive, it may be better to give the drug by injection directly into the systemic circulation thus avoiding the first pass effect; dissolving tablets under the tongue achieves the same end..

EFFICACY:

Is the ability of a drug to produce a therapeutic effect. It is expressed in terms of the maximal effect obtainable with that drug; eg morphine has greater analgesic efficacy than paracetamol.

POTENCY:

Is a measure of **how much** drug is needed to produce a given effect. In other words, 20 mg of a potent drug may produce the same effect as 500 mg of a less potent drug, but that doesn't mean that it is more effective.

POTENTIATION:

Occurs when the clinical effect of two or more drugs in combination is greater than the sum of their individual effects. This may apply to efficacy OR toxicity and is often the result of one drug altering the metabolism or excretion of another.

SYNERGISM:

Is said to occur when one drug enhances the effect of another without altering itself.

BLOOD/BRAIN BARRIER:

Drugs which are administered for their effects on the CNS have to cross the blood/brain barrier into the CSF and extracellular fluid surrounding brain cells before they can act. Only lipid soluble drugs can rapidly penetrate the BBB and, for such drugs, the rate of onset of therapeutic action simply depends on the route of administration.

Note that lipid soluble drugs are more likely to produce CNS side effects (eg the anti-hypertensive lipid soluble drug propranolol often causes sleep disturbance).

ADVERSE DRUG REACTIONS

INTRODUCTION

Up to 20% of hospital in-patients suffer an adverse drug reaction.

5% of hospital admissions are precipitated by drug reactions.

At a conservative estimate, 3000 deaths per year are directly attributable to drug treatment in the UK alone.

The very old, the very young and people with liver and kidney disease are most susceptible to adverse drug reactions.

The drugs most commonly implicated in adverse reactions are:

> antibiotics
> anticoagulants
> aspirin
> digitalis
> diuretics
> insulin
> steroids

The drugs most commonly implicated as a cause of death include:

> amitriptyline
> aspirin
> chlorpromazine
> halothane
> indomethacin
> isoprenaline
> oral contraceptives
> phenylbutazone
> steroids

Drug reactions may be classified into two types:

Predictable reactions are reactions that can be predicted from the known pharmacology of the drug eg effects on receptors other than the "target" receptor or exaggeration of the desired therapeutic effect. Such adverse effects are directly related to the amount of drug administered and are, in theory, avoidable.

Unpredictable reactions are unrelated to the *known* pharmacology and are not "dose dependent". They thus carry a higher risk of death. Drug allergies are common unpredictable reactions.

Any drug may cause both types of reaction.

Since most adverse drug reactions are **predictable**, it follows that factors that alter drug levels in the body (or render the body more sensitive to drug action) may predispose to adverse effects.

MECHANISMS OF ADVERSE DRUG REACTIONS

>> Pharmacokinetic mechanisms, pharmacodynamic mechanisms, and unpredictable genetic and immunological mechanisms may all contribute to adverse reactions:

PHARMACOKINETIC:

Absorption:

Any changes in stomach acidity, gut motility or gut lining* may decrease or increase drug absorption.

Liver metabolism:

The liver converts fat soluble drugs (which are easy to absorb through the gut) to water soluble waste (which is easy to eliminate via the kidneys). Some people inherit certain liver enzymes of unusually low activity and may thus be highly sensitive to large doses of certain drugs (eg **sulphonamide** antibiotics). Moreover, old age and liver disease also reduce the drug metabolizing capacity of the liver which increases the chances of toxicity.

Plasma proteins:

A proportion of drugs are transported in the bloodstream bound to plasma proteins (usually albumin) and are only pharmacologically active when free of these bonds. Thus, in diseases which reduce plasma albumin concentration, the activity of certain drugs alters markedly.

---

*   Caused by disease or other drugs.

Tissue distribution:

Disease and ageing may alter the volume of distribution of drugs; old people (whose total body water is diminished) are vulnerable to toxic effects of drugs at much lower doses than young adults. Some drugs also bind to body tissues irreversibly with unfortunate effects (eg tetracycline incorporates itself into growing bones and teeth). Obese people may accumulate fat soluble drugs in their fat tissue and may thus require higher doses to achieve therapeutic effect.

Kidney excretion:

Damage to glomeruli and tubules will slow down the excretion of water soluble drugs making them more toxic.

PHARMACODYNAMIC:

Any condition which affects the pharmacokinetics of a drug may also alter patient **sensitivity** to a drug.

GENETIC AND IMMUNOLOGICAL:

Many unpredictable reactions (including drug hypersensitivity) have a genetic or immunological basis.

IMPORTANT ADVERSE DRUG REACTIONS

Heart arrhythmias may be caused by:

> beta-blockers
> carbamazepine
> digoxin
> diuretics
> L-dopa
> lithium
> phenothiazines
> phenytoin
> salbutamol
> tricyclic antidepressants

Heart failure may be caused by:

> anti-arrhythmics
> beta-blockers
> verapamil

Nausea and vomiting may be caused by:

> antibiotics
> bromocriptine
> digoxin
> L-dopa
> oestrogens
> opiates
> theophylline

Diarrhoea may be caused by:

> antibiotics
> laxatives
> magnesium salts

Constipation may be caused by:

> aluminium
> anticholinergic drugs (including tricyclic antidepressants)
> hydroxide
> iron
> opiates

Peptic ulcer may be caused by:

> aspirin
> NSAIAs
> steroids

Pancreatitis may be caused by:

> opiates
> sulphonamides
> thiazide diuretics

Jaundice may be caused by:

> chlorpromazine
> erythromycin
> oral contraceptives

Gallstones may be caused by:

> clofibrate

Hepatitis may be caused by:

> anti-TB drugs
> halothane
> NSAIAs
> paracetamol o/d
> sulphonamides

Kidney damage may be caused by:

> aminoglycosides
> captopril
> cephaloridine
> gold
> penicillamine
> phenacetin

Any drug can cause skin rashes.

DRUG INTERACTIONS

Drug interactions are of two main types:

Pharmacokinetic – in which one drug alters the nature of the other and **Pharmacodynamic** – in which the interaction results from effects at the site of drug action.

For every drug there is a range of blood concentration within which the drug will exert its maximum therapeutic effect – the so called **"therapeutic range"**. Above the upper limit the drug will become toxic, below it will exert no useful effect.

A number of common drugs have **very narrow therapeutic ranges** and their action is consequently frequently compromised by the presence of another drug.

› anti-hypertensive drugs
› digoxin
› lithium (and some other drugs altering brain function)
› oral contraceptives
› oral hypoglycaemic drugs for diabetes
› phenytoin
› warfarin

all have narrow therapeutic ranges.

Some drugs (see below) have the unusual power to increase the activity of enzyme systems in the liver thereby increasing the rate of breakdown of drugs normally eliminated via that system. This phenomenon is called **enzyme induction** and has two important clinical consequences:

1) If an enzyme inducing drug is administered at the same time as a non-inducer, the therapeutic effect of the non-inducer may be seriously diminished and

2) If the dosage of the non-inducer is increased to compensate and then the inducer is withdrawn, the patient may rapidly develop signs of toxicity due to the non-inducer.

>> Enzyme induction may take several days to develop.

The following common drugs are enzyme inducers:

> › carbamazepine
> › chlorpromazine
> › griseofulvin
> › phenytoin
> › rifampicin
> › spironolactone

Enzyme inducers will DECREASE activity of:

> › **oral contraceptives** → may result in unwanted pregnancy.
> › **steroids** → will reduce the anti-inflammatory and adaptive effect of steroid therapy.
> › **tolbutamide** → may result in hyperglycaemia.
> › **warfarin** → may result in thrombosis.

Some drugs are liver enzyme **inhibitors** and present precisely the opposite set of problems when combined with non-inhibitors.

The enzyme inhibitor CIMETIDINE will INCREASE activity of:

> › diazepam
> › labetalol
> › propranolol
> › theophylline
> › warfarin

» Drugs which alter brain function tend to be additive in their effect and are potentiated by alcohol.

» **Aspirin** may **potentiate** the action of warfarin and phenytoin by displacing them from their protein carriers.

COMMON DRUG CLASSES

ANALGESICS

Are used to relieve pain. **Non-narcotic** analgesics such as aspirin and paracetamol are unrelated to opium and are mostly used for musculo-skeletal disorders.

Narcotic analgesics form a large class of drugs (all related to opium) and are used in the control of severe pain.

ANTIBACTERIALS

Are "antibiotics" used in the treatment of bacterial infectious disease. They may be **bactericidal**, which means that they actually kill micro-organisms, or **bacteriostatic** which means that they simply inhibit bacterial multiplication. Antibiotics related to penicillin exert their action by interfering with bacterial cell wall synthesis. Many other antibiotics act by interfering with bacterial metabolism.

Aminoglycosides:

Are potent bactericidal antibiotics used particularly for the treatment of "Gram negative" infections. Side effects (which include deafness) are dose related and may be very serious in cases of kidney damage.

Broad spectrum antibiotics:

Are therapeutically active against a wide range of micro-organisms.

Cephalosporins:

Are expensive cousins of the penicillins and tend to have broad spectrum activity.

Macrolides:

Have a similar spectrum of action to the penicillins and are thus used as alternative medication in cases of penicillin hypersensitivity. **Erythromycin** is the best known macrolide.

Penicillins:

Are bactericidal and act by interfering with cell wall synthesis. They often cause allergic skin rashes.

Penicillinase resistant penicillins:

Resist the enzymes produced by certain "penicillin resistant" bacteria and are thus not inactivated by such organisms.

Sulphonamides:

Are an older class of antibiotic that declined in popularity as more active and less toxic compounds came on the market. Combinations of sulphonamide and trimethoprim* (eg Septrin) have much greater activity than the sulphonamides alone and remain very popular. Trimethoprim is also used on its own.

Tetracyclines:

Are an older class of antibiotic whose use is limited these days by bacterial resistance and the fact that they are deposited in growing bones and teeth (causing discolouration).

>> **There are a number of other important antibiotics (such as chloramphenicol) that do not fall into any particular class.**

ANTICHOLINERGICS

Many drugs have an "anticholinergic" effect which means that they tend to interfere with the activity of the parasympathetic nervous system. All drugs with anticholinergic properties have the following possible side effects:

› Dry mouth from ↓ salivation
› Blurred vision and photophobia from dilated pupil and paralysed accommodation
› Constipation
› Urinary retention

---

* A chemical that disrupts bacterial metabolism.

ANTICOAGULANTS

Prevent thrombus formation (or slow down the propagation of existing thrombi). They do this by interfering with the clotting "cascade" reactions. **Warfarin,** a common anticoagulant, "antagonizes" the action of vitamin K.

ANTIDEPRESSANTS

Are used to relieve the symptoms of severe depression. **Tricyclic antidepressants** (so called because of their chemical structure) form the largest group.

Monoamine oxidase inhibitors (which interfere with the metabolism of neurotransmitters) are also used as antidepressants.

ANTI-EMETICS

Are drugs used to relieve symptoms of nausea and vomiting. Most are related to major tranquillizers.

ANTI-EPILEPTICS

Or "anti-convulsants" are used to prevent fits. Their mode of action is not well understood.

ANTIHISTAMINES

Inhibit the action of histamines by blocking histamine receptors on cells. They thus inhibit the action of one of the most potent chemical "mediators" of the allergic response.

ANTIPSYCHOTICS

Are also known as **neuroleptics** or **major tranquillizers**. They are supposed to tranquillize without impairing consciousness and are thus used in the management of mania and schizophrenia.

Some people who have experienced these drugs describe them as chemical strait-jackets.

ANXIOLYTICS

Are certain members of the benzodiazepine **group** of drugs that are supposed to relieve the symptoms of anxiety.

Diazepam (Valium) is the archetypal benzodiazepine anxiolytic.

BARBITURATES

Are old fashioned very potent hypnotics used for intractable insomnia (and occasionally for epilepsy).

Very short acting barbiturates are used to **induce** anaesthesia.

BETA-BLOCKERS

Should really be referred to as beta adrenoreceptor blocking drugs. They act by blocking adrenaline receptors in the heart, peripheral blood vessels, bronchi, pancreas and liver.

They are used in the treatment of hypertension, angina, myocardial infarction, arrhythmias, hyperthyroidism, anxiety and stage fright.

BRONCHODILATORS

Are substances which relax bronchial smooth muscle and thus relieve symptoms and improve respiratory performance in conditions such as asthma and chronic bronchitis. **Sympathomimetics** such as salbutamol are widely used as bronchodilators.

Xanthines form another popular group of bronchodilators. They work by interfering with the chemical messengers within smooth muscle cells and thus inhibit contraction.

CARDIAC GLYCOSIDES

Are a group of drugs used in the treatment of heart failure and disturbances of cardiac rhythm. They improve the muscular "performance" of the heart and slow down the rate of conduction through the A-V node.

Digoxin is the best known cardiac glycoside. It is a close relation of the cardiac glycosides found in the common foxglove *(Digitalis purpurea)*.

CYTOTOXIC DRUGS

Damage dividing cells and are thus used in the chemotherapeutic treatment of cancer.

DEMULCENTS

Are supposed to soothe dry, irritating coughs.

DOPADECARBOXYLASE INHIBITORS

Are drugs given in conjunction with dopaminergic drugs (see below) to avoid their complete metabolism before reaching the brain.

DOPAMINERGIC DRUGS

Are used in the treatment of **Parkinsonism** and act by replenishing supplies of the neurotransmitter **dopamine** in the basal ganglia region of the brain. They thus help reduce rigidity. **Anticholinergic** drugs are also used to relieve tremor in Parkinsonism.

EXPECTORANTS

Are claimed to promote expulsion of bronchial secretions.

HYPNOTICS and SEDATIVES

Are used in the relief of insomnia and control of agitation. **Benzodiazepines** are the most commonly used **group** of sedatives.

IMMUNOSUPPRESSANTS

Depress the immune response.

LITHIUM SALTS

Are drugs with an unexplained mood-regulating action of use in controlling manic disorders.

Side effects include gastrointestinal disturbance, tremors, weight gain, oedema, goitre and hypothyroidism. In overdose they can produce vomiting, diarrhoea, lack of co-ordination, fits, coma and occasionally death.

LOOP DIURETICS

Are very potent diuretics which inhibit water reabsorption from the ascending limbs of the loops of Henle.

MAST CELL STABILIZERS

Stop tissue mast cells degranulating as part of the allergic response and thus can help avoid bronchial smooth muscle constriction in allergic asthma.

NSAIAs

Are non-steroidal anti-inflammatory agents. Widely used in the symptomatic relief of arthritic disorders.

OXYTOCICS

Can be used to induce or augment labour because of their stimulant action on smooth muscle. By the same token, they can be used to stop bleeding due to incomplete abortion, post-partum haemorrhage etc.

POTASSIUM SPARING DIURETICS

Are weak diuretics that cause the retention of potassium.

They are thus used in combination with thiazide and loop diuretics which cause potassium loss!

PROSTAGLANDINS

Crop up everywhere as endogenous chemical mediators and are used as drugs for the induction of therapeutic abortion (and occasionally labour).

SALICYLATES

Includes aspirin and aspirin like compounds.

STEROIDS

Are a subclass of lipids with a characteristic chemical structure based on four interconnected "carbon rings".

Common types:

› Hydrocortisone
› Prednisolone
› Betamethasone
› Dexamethasone

» Steroids are also available in drops (eyes, ears) and inhaler form (asthma).

Skin preparations:

› 1% Hydrocortisone cream (Mild)
› 0.05% Clobetasone (Eumovate – Fairly potent)
› 0.1% Betamethasone (Betnovate – Potent)
› Hydrocortisone butyrate ("Locoid" – similar strength to betamethasone)
› 0.05% Clobetasol (Dermovate – VERY potent)

Indications for steroids include:

› Asthma
› Connective tissue/auto-immune disease
› Addison's disease
› Surgery transplant
› Malignancy

Side effects:

› Fluid retention →may lead to heart failure
› Slow wound healing
› Appetite stimulation →weight gain
› Reduced resistance to infection
› Masks fever response in infection
› High blood pressure
› High blood sugar
› Skin atrophy
› Peptic ulceration
› Depression →psychosis
› Necrosis of the head of the femur

> › Softening of bones (osteoporosis)
> › Cataract
> › Buffalo hump
> › Myopathies (ie muscle disease)
> › Cardiomyopathies (ie heart muscle disease)

Interactions with other drugs:

Steroids may antagonize action of anti-epileptic drugs (phenytoin and barbiturates). They can be dangerous if used in presence of:

> › TB
> › Herpes
> › Pregnancy
> › Psoriasis
> › Peptic ulcers

» Steroid eye drops may be catastrophic in glaucoma.

» The side effects of topical steroid therapy are much less severe than systematic steroid therapy in the short term.

**Abrupt withdrawal of systemic steroid therapy may be fatal.
The pituitary/adrenal axis will be deranged for at least 2 weeks after cessation of treatment.**

A schedule for prednisolone withdrawal:

If on 40mg/24hrs then: Reduce to 30mg/24hrs for week 1.
15mg/24hrs for week 2.
10mg/24hrs for week 3.
7.5mg/24hrs for week 4.
5mg/24hrs for weeks 5 + 6.

and THEN stop IF ALL IS WELL!

» **IMPORTANT:** This schedule is **not** to be taken as a recommendation for the withdrawal of steroid therapy in any particular case!

SULPHONYLUREAS AND BIGUANIDES

Are oral hypoglycaemic agents and are thus used to lower the blood glucose in certain patients with Type II diabetes.

SYMPATHOMIMETICS

Are drugs which mimic the effect of sympathetic stimulation and are thus useful as cardiac stimulants in cardiogenic shock.

THIAZIDE DIURETICS

Are relatively mild diuretics which act by altering the properties of renal distal convoluted tubules.

VASODILATORS

Cause blood vessels to dilate. This can prove advantageous in heart disease since

1) if the coronary vessels are dilated the blood supply to the heart improves and

2) if systemic vessels are dilated the amount of blood returning to the heart is "off-loaded" to a certain extent thereby reducing the workload on the heart.

Vasodilators are therefore used in the treatment of angina and heart failure.

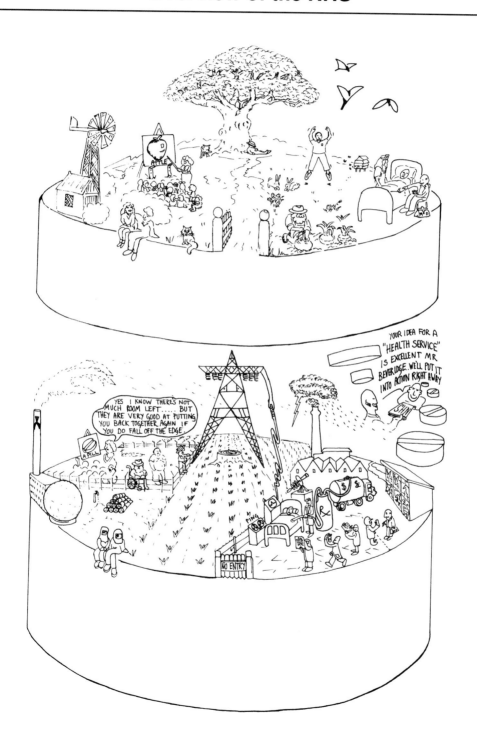

PRINCIPLES OF EPIDEMIOLOGY
AND OVERVIEW OF THE NHS

OVERVIEW

Epidemiology:

Epidemiological methods
Clinical trials
Common terms in epidemiology

The NHS:

History
Structure
Funding
Social services

EPIDEMIOLOGY

INTRODUCTION

Epidemiology is the study of health and disease in the community.

By studying the characteristics of populations, the epidemiologist tries to formulate hypotheses to explain the **cause** of illness. The tools of the trade are careful, systematic observation and statistical analysis.

By collecting data on the natural history of all types of disease, the epidemiologist can try to devise effective **prevention** programmes and can help in the planning of health services. He or she also has the expertise to help colleagues in their assessment of new treatments. Within the National Health Service, epidemiology is the basic skill of practitioners of public health medicine. They have the responsibility of assessing the health needs and health status of the population as a basis for planning and resource allocation.

Much of what is good in orthodox medicine comes from epidemiological study, because epidemiology is primarily concerned with improving the **health** of the community and the **prevention** of disease by identifying avoidable risk factors. (The classic example is that of John Snow, the nineteenth century London physician, who noticed that the cholera out-break in Golden Square in 1854 could be traced to the water drawn from one particular public water pump. By chaining the handle to the pump, he stopped the outbreak.)

But you don't need to be a specialist in public health medicine to study the health of the population under your care; every practitioner can be an epidemiologist -

To quote William Pickles, a country GP working in the first part of this century -

".......personal knowledge and love of the country in which we live fit even the most commonplace of us for epidemiological research."

EPIDEMIOLOGICAL METHODS

1. DESCRIPTIVE STUDIES/SURVEYS:

Before epidemiologists can investigate *specific* hypotheses on disease causation, they need to find out certain basic facts about the population in their district, region or country.

In other words, they need to make **descriptive** studies ("cross sectional surveys") in which the incidence and prevalence of diseases are related to basic variables such as:

Time:	? long term changes ? cyclical changes ? epidemic

Place

and

Person:	age sex race marital status occupation etc

Having collected this data, they may see certain patterns which suggest links between population variables and disease.

They may then decide to test out their ideas by planning **analytic studies**.

2. ANALYTIC STUDIES (case control/cohort studies):

Analytic studies are used to test the validity of hypotheses linking specific aetiological factors with specific diseases.

They may look at the pattern of past events using retrospective (case control) studies or they may follow the fortunes of a group of patients for several years in prospective (cohort) studies.

If their hypotheses hold good for a large enough section of the population (statistically speaking), epidemiologists will suggest that a specific link between disease cause and disease effect has been made.

The next step (to the orthodox doctor) is to try and devise treatments or prevention strategies which will relieve the community from the burden of a particular disease, but coming up with a treatment is only the first step – the problem is to prove that it works! The only way to do this (from the orthodox perspective) is to perform a "clinical trial" (intervention study).

3. INTERVENTION STUDIES (ie clinical trials):

A clinical trial is an experiment designed to evaluate the effects of various treatments or preventive measures on a particular disease.

For many years the biggest "problem" in the design of clinical trials has been the tendency for the placebo effect to alter the results.

The first systematic investigation of the "placebo" effect was undertaken by William Evans and Clifford Hoyle at the London Hospital in the early 1930s and involved comparing the effects of thirteen different drugs with the effects of placebo sodium bicarbonate. After three years work they concluded that (statistically) placebos gave better results than the majority of chemical remedies tested. However, rather than stimulate interest in the role of the mind in disease and healing, these observations indirectly spawned an entirely new approach to clinical experimentation which we now refer to as the **controlled randomized double blind cross over trial**.

Controlled – Means that the new treatment is compared with an existing standard treatment or a placebo. Thus controlled trials have a "treatment group" of patients receiving the new drug and a "control group" of patients on standard therapy or placebo. If the intervention is a preventive measure, such as reducing smoking in middle aged men at risk of ischaemic heart disease, the control group would be middle aged men who have *not* stopped smoking.

Randomized – Means that patients are allocated to the treatment or the control group in an entirely random fashion irrespective of the nature of their presentation.

Double blind – Means that neither the patient nor the attending practitioner knows whether the patient is taking new drug or standard drug (or placebo) until the trial is complete. This is supposed to eliminate the influence of the hopes and expectations of the doctors on their perception of clinical result.

Cross over – Means that half way through the trial patients will be swapped from treatment to placebo to eliminate possible "bias" from "placebo reactors".

The design of clinical trials:

It is often hard to reconcile the unbiased assessment of a treatment's value with the need to ensure that each patient's care does not suffer as a result of the experiment.

Before starting a clinical trial, a **study protocol** must be produced which describes all aspects of the design, organization, data and intended evaluation methods of the study.

The **type of patient** eligible for inclusion in the trial must be precisely defined and any exclusions specified. The source of all patients must be recorded.

Treatments need to be **defined** in considerable detail, including dose schedules (where appropriate), duration and any extra patient care offered.

Trials involving comparison between more than two treatments are clumsy and usually avoided.

Clinical trials are usually comparative studies of a "treatment group" of patients on the new therapy and a "control group" of patients on standard therapy (or no therapy). Treatment and control groups should (as far as possible) be recruited in the same place at the same time.

Random allocation of patients between treatment and control groups is necessary to avoid systematic differences between the groups. (If, for example, patients with the better prognoses were all put in the treatment group, then the results would appear more impressive .....) The researcher should have no involvement in allocation of patients between groups.

Written, informed consent should be obtained from each patient entering the trial.

Double blind, cross over design (using placebo if necessary) should be considered as a way of avoiding biased evaluation. If used, the protocol must allow for the double blind code to be broken in the event of any adverse reaction to treatment.

Methods of **response evaluation** should be defined in advance and strictly adhered to. Special training of those involved in patient assessment may be necessary to reduce **observer variation**. Any **adverse** reactions must be recorded.

Data should be recorded on specially designed, standard forms and **not** on case notes.

It is important to have sufficient patients in a trial to reach what is known as a statistically significant result ; that is to say, a result which reflects a genuine difference between treatments rather than a chance difference.

Poor design and inappropriate statistical analysis tend to produce **Type 1** errors (false positives), ie one treatment will be pronounced better than another when no real difference exists. Studies with insufficient patient numbers produce **Type 2** errors (false negatives) ie two treatments will be pronounced equally effective when an important difference does, in fact, exist. Proposed methods of statistical analysis should be defined at the outset of the trial.

Violations of the study protocol must be honestly reported – in particular, any patient **withdrawals** must be documented.

The progress of the trial must be carefully monitored in case the treatment differences are so large that the trial has to be stopped because it would be unethical to withhold the more effective treatment or allow the more dangerous one to continue.

Nevertheless:

> There are well documented examples of "suggestion" influencing results **despite** the elaborate precautions that are supposed to eliminate bias –
> Successive trials on the same drug using virtually identical research protocols often produce conflicting results –
> A large number of papers published in medical journals contain statistical errors, many of a serious nature –
> An enormous amount of clinical research is undertaken in pursuit of career advancement –
> The relationship between researchers and drug companies is often "cosy" to say the least .....
> The orthodox profession regards the controlled randomized double blind cross over trial as almost perfect. If it was abandoned, much of the current clinical research edifice would crumble.

COMMON TERMS IN EPIDEMIOLOGY

Prevalence –

The number of people in a particular group who have a particular condition at a particular time divided by the **total** number of people in the group. Analogous to a "snap shot" of the situation.

Incidence –

The number of people who develop a particular disease in a given population **over a defined period of time** divided by the total number at risk. Analogous to a "movie" of the situation.

Sensitivity –

A sensitive test is one that correctly identifies a high proportion of the people who actually have the disease being tested for with very few **false negatives**. Increasing the sensitivity of a test will increase the number of false positives (people told that they have the disease who actually *don't* have it) but will ensure that **few** cases are **missed**.

Specificity –

A specific test is one that correctly identifies a high proportion of those who do *not* have the disease under investigation with very few **false positives**. Increasing the specificity of a test will increase the number of false negatives (people told they are free of a disease when they do, in fact, have it!) but will avoid the unnecessary treatment of disease free patients.

Crosssectional –

A cross sectional survey is one in which data is collected from a *defined population* at a certain point in time. It attempts to discover if people with a particular disease are more likely to have certain attributes than those who do not (although it cannot, in itself, prove a causal association). Cross sectional surveys are also called prevalence surveys.

Retrospective –

Retrospective studies are also called case control studies. They investigate the attributes of people *known* to have a particular disease to see if their past histories suggest a likely cause.

Prospective –

Prospective studies are also called "cohort" studies. They follow the life stories of a large group of people to see if the *development* of a particular disease could be related to personal characteristics, lifestyle or exposure to possible harmful agents.

Secular trends –

These are changes in disease incidence occurring over periods of many years. Note that it is often difficult in practice to determine whether observed trends are due to *real* changes in disease incidence or to changes in nomenclature, diagnostic criteria or the efficiency with which disease data is collected.

Inference of causality –

Epidemiological research suggests *associations* between diseases and suspected causes. Such associations do not necessarily confirm that suspected causes *actually* cause disease.

It is always possible that an association may have appeared by chance. It is also possible that an *apparent* association could be caused by faulty or biased research methods.

Cost effectiveness –

A health strategy is said to be cost effective if –
i) It genuinely fulfils its objectives.
ii) It is, pound for pound, more effective than other health strategies already known to achieve the same result.

Cost benefit analysis –

An attempt to quantify all possible costs and benefits of a health strategy and to place these in context of the needs of society as a whole.

Marginal analysis –

A technique used by health planners to determine whether **increasing** the money spent on a given health programme actually produces "worthwhile" improvement in the health of the community. The "law of diminishing returns" means that, beyond a certain level of investment and improvement, large amounts spent will only produce small gains.

THE NHS

HEALTH AND SOCIAL SERVICES

Health and social services in this country are provided by five "agencies":

› The National Health Service

› The social services and environmental health departments of local authorities

› The voluntary services

› The private medical sector

› Various occupational health services

THE NATIONAL HEALTH SERVICE

History:

Before 1946, public health services, hospitals, family doctors, district nurses and midwives had limited formal association, since they had all developed independently over the previous 100 years. Despite Lloyd George's NHS Act* (1911), access to medical treatment largely depended on having the money to pay for it and so the report by William Beveridge (1942) suggesting the need for a comprehensive national medical service providing treatment for all, free at the point of need, was a revolutionary document. It formed the basis for the NHS Act (made law on 6th November, 1946).

Unfortunately, when formulating his plans, Beveridge assumed that once people had free access to "modern" medical care the health of the population would improve and thus the cost of providing care would go down.

---

*   which did not cover the retired, women or children.

Moreover he had no real way of knowing how much the cost of medical manpower and technology would rise over the following years. Thus, from the beginning, the NHS has been underfunded.

Despite this (and thanks to the dedication and selflessness of countless NHS staff over the past 40 years or so) the NHS provides a remarkable service to patients, unique in character but, sadly, now under great strain because of increasing demand and limited resources.

The reforms arising from the Government White Paper (1989) **"Working for Patients"** are supposed to redress this imbalance by creating what is called an "internal market". From April 1st, 1991,* District Health Authorities are to act as purchasers ("procurers") of health services for their resident population, by placing contracts with "provider units" (hospitals and community services). Providers will aim to supply services of the highest quality and at the most competitive prices.

Some provider units have become **Self Governing Trusts**, not managed by District Health Authorities, and some GPs have been given their own budgets with which to purchase services for their patients.

The implications of these reforms are complex and it remains to be seen whether they represent an improvement to the "average citizen". The structure outlined opposite shows the relationships between the various bodies concerned with health care provision but functions and responsibilities are still under review and there may be further changes. Note also that arrangements in Wales and Northern Ireland are different from the English and Scottish model and from each other.

---

*   April fools' day.

Structure of the NHS (April 1991) –:

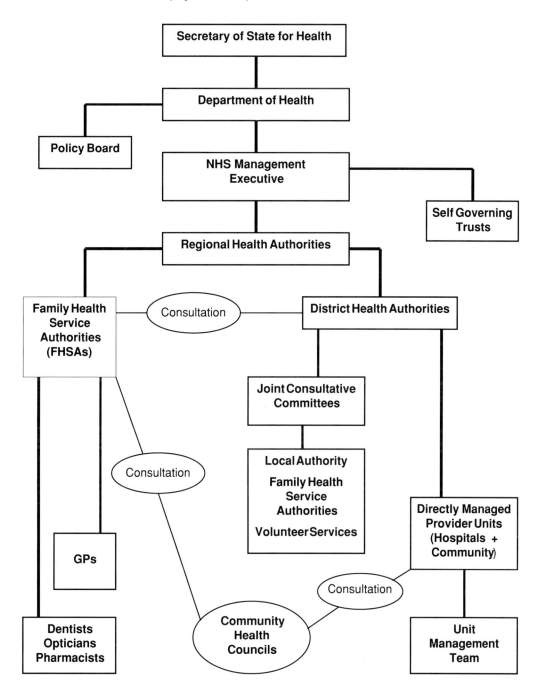

NOTE:

What used to be known as District General Hospitals (Acute Hospitals) are now referred to as "directly managed provider units".

They provide the "specialties" to which GPs refer ie –

› General Medicine
› General Surgery
› Orthopaedics
› ENT
› O + G
› Ophthalmology
› Paediatrics

They may also provide the rest of the region with the "super specialties" to which only consultants refer ie –

› Radiotherapy
› Cardiology
› Cardiac Surgery
› Neurology
› Neurosurgery

FUNDING

Although the following figures relate to 1988, they illustrate some general features of health care budgeting that are still relevant today.

BUDGET ALLOCATION 1988:

23bn to health + social services

18.35bn to health = 6% GNP = 12% government exp.

63% on hospitals
9.4% drugs
6.2% GPs
6.2% community health
4% administration
3.9% dentists
7% miscellaneous (including ambulance)

At district level, 70% of money goes towards WAGES.

Money obtained as follows:

88% income tax/local taxes
6% national insurance
5% charges for services
1% miscellaneous

12% total government expenditure compares with:

12% on defence
11.3% on the arts
25% on social security payments

This puts the UK 9th in the league of per capita health expenditure @£375/head.

The US spends most.

Consultation rates:

> 100 million GP consultations
> 51.5 million hospital out-patient appointments
> 7.46 million in-patients dealt with
>
> per year

Use of resources:

> 6% maternity
> 5% mental handicap
> 3% children
> 11% mentally ill
> 13% elderly
> 62% everything else

SOCIAL SERVICES

These are provided by local authorities and are funded by a combination of local taxes and government money.

The services provided comprise domiciliary, day and residential care and thus include:

> › Residential care for the old, the disabled, the mentally ill and children
> › Day centres
> › Social workers
> › Home help, meals on wheels etc (sometimes provided by the voluntary sector)

NOTES:

a) The private sector looks after the equivalent of 8% of the NHS patient load for 1% of the cost.

b) The occupational health services (for prisons, the armed forces etc) are independent specialties and negotiate their budgets independently with the relevant funding body.

CONCLUSION

The effectiveness of any health service is reflected by the extent to which it meets the demands of its population and the NHS unquestionably tries hard to meet the needs of its clients.

Despite these efforts however, cash constraints on the one hand and waste on the other conspire to limit the number of people who could really benefit from treatment actually receiving it.

The following diagram illustrates the problem –

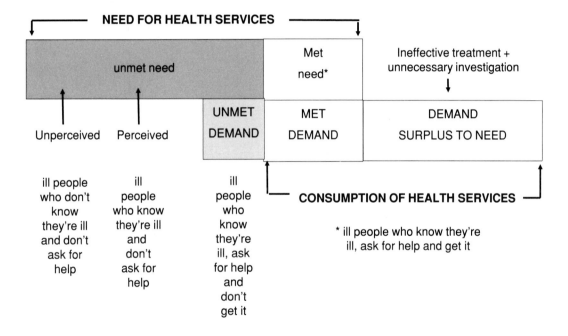

10. Introduction to Clinical Examination

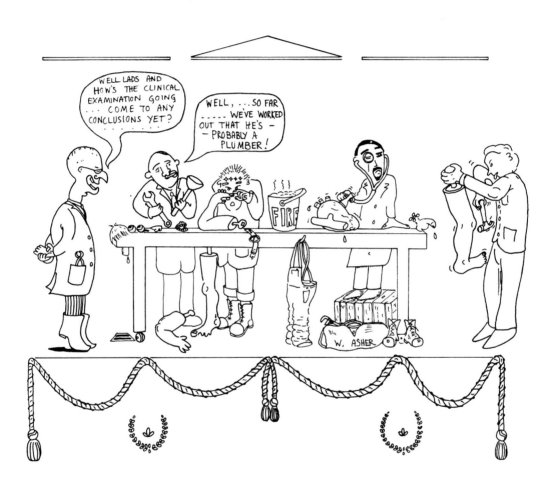

INTRODUCTION TO CLINICAL EXAMINATION

OVERVIEW

Orthodox History Taking and Clinical Examination

The orthodox approach
An integrated approach to basic physical examination
Sequence for a quick "screening" examination

Clinical Assessment System by System

Introduction
The cardiovascular system
The respiratory system
The gastro-intestinal system
The nervous system

Appendices

   i) Dermatomes and myotomes
  ii) Reflexes
 iii) Cutaneous nerve roots
 iv) Joint movement – normal ranges
  v) Pointers in endocrine disease
 vi) Examination of the breast
vii) Blood pressure measurement
viii) Heart sounds

ORTHODOX HISTORY TAKING AND CLINICAL EXAMINATION

There are many excellent texts describing orthodox techniques for gathering clinical information and it would be inappropriate to duplicate that detailed information here. This
chapter is thus an attempt to provide a simple framework on which to hang the more
detailed knowledge that is accumulated through clinical experience.

> Eliciting clinical signs in the orthodox manner is a subtle art and, like all
> art, takes a lifetime (at least) to master. The student and practitioner of
> natural medicine often has little use for the techniques described in
> orthodox texts on clinical methods and would be ill advised to invoke them
> on a casual basis. However, **simply listening to what the patient has
> to say and observing him or her closely will usually provide all the
> information necessary to formulate an appropriate orthodox dif-
> ferential diagnosis.**

THE ORTHODOX APPROACH

- › History taking
- › Clinical examination
- › Formulation of a differential diagnosis
- › Basic investigations (such as blood count, chest X-ray and urine
  analysis)
- › Special investigations
- › Confirmation of diagnosis
- › Treatment
- › Follow up

The history should elucidate:

- › What has happened
- › To what kind of person
- › Why help is being sought now
- › How the illness affects the patient (and their family)
- › Details of the patient's physical and social environment

It should also –

- › Establish the practitioner/patient relationship
- › Provide major clues towards a likely diagnosis

AN INTEGRATED APPROACH TO BASIC PHYSICAL EXAMINATION

The following sequence is not comprehensive and should be altered and adapted to suit the clinical circumstances and the personal style of the practitioner. Whatever sequence is adopted should be practised until it becomes second nature.

It is vitally important to examine as many "normals" as possible because the range of normality is very wide indeed. If an obvious abnormality is detected in the course of a basic routine examination, the system (or systems) concerned should then be thoroughly examined according to textbook protocols.

Above all –

> › be kind and gentle
> › always explain what you are doing
> › try not to examine with cold hands
> › don't subject patients to unnecessary changes of posture
> › always be mindful of modesty but remember that examining a part without adequate exposure may be worse than not examining it at all

» You are examining the patient for their benefit and not to prove that you can perform the exercise in a technically correct manner. Be adaptable. Improvise if necessary. If you aren't certain whether you have detected something or not, take your time and **find out.** On the other hand, first impressions are often the most accurate (before the mind gets in the way!)

» Don't sit on the fence – believe what you perceive and act accordingly. That is, after all, the best you can do.

» Apart from making a note of blood pressure, temperature and heart rate, don't break the flow of the examination by making notes as you go. Complete the examination, let your impressions sink in and then write up your findings in a systematic way (suggested methods for recording data are included in this section). The order of **actual** examination is NOT the same as the accepted formal order for writing up an examination.

» As always – **look, feel, percuss, auscultate.**

SUGGESTED SEQUENCE FOR A QUICK "SCREENING" EXAMINATION

Is the patient well or unwell, alert or drowsy, oriented or disoriented?

Explain what you are going to do.

Place patient in comfortable position, reclining at 45˚.

Examine the hands.

Put thermometer in mouth.

Take radial pulses.

Take blood pressure.

Remove thermometer.

Feel carotid pulses.

Observe face.

Examine conjunctivae and sclerae.

Examine lips, mouth, teeth and fauces (including sticking out tongue and saying ahhh).

Observe neck for swellings – ask patient to swallow.

Feel for cervical lymph nodes and enlarged thyroid from behind.

Consider examining breasts.

Palpate axillae for lymph nodes.

Observe JVP.

Palpate trachea.

Observe chest.

Palpate apex beat.

Feel praecordium for thrills and parasternal heaves.

Auscultate heart in all four areas and, in each area, listen *in order* for the heart sounds, for added sounds and for murmurs.

Thus start listening at the apex with the bell of the stethoscope and the patient inclined to the left – if murmur heard, listen around into axilla.

Then sit patient forwards and listen with diaphragm at LSE, pulmonary and aortic areas and then over carotid arteries (for bruits). Listen once more at LSE with patient holding breath in expiration for aortic murmurs.

With patient still sitting forward, observe back (including spinal configuration) and assess chest expansion.

Percuss and auscultate back of chest.

Look for sacral oedema.

Lie patient back; percuss clavicles, front and sides of chest.

Auscultate front and sides of chest.

Remove pillows, lie patient flat and expose abdomen.

Observe abdomen carefully.

Systematic superficial and then deep palpation of abdomen **observing patient's face.**

Palpate for abdominal organomegaly.

Percuss abdomen.

Auscultate abdomen for bowel sounds and abdominal aortic bruits.

Feel femoral pulses and listen for femoral bruits.

Observe inguinal region and ask patient to cough.

Feel for inguinal hernias asking patient to cough (If hernia suspected, must examine inguinal region with patient standing).

Briefly examine genitalia in male.

Sit patient up to 45° again.

Observe legs.

Assess leg pulses.

Assess ankle oedema.

Perform brief neurological assessment:

Ultra-quick: Assess leg tone
                Straight leg raising against opposition
                Knee and ankle jerks + plantar reflexes
                Tuning fork on external malleoli
                Ask patient to put arms out in front and close eyes
                Observe for tremor or downward drift of one arm
                Press down on arms to assess power
                Ask patient to keep eyes closed and put one finger
                (which you touch) on nose (theirs)
                Test biceps, supinator and triceps jerks
                Observe eyes for squints, examine pupils, look at fundi
                Watch patient walk

More thorough: A more detailed assessment of the **cranial nerves**
                followed by an assessment of **motor function** (inspect
                for wasting, tremor, fasciculation; palpate muscle tone;
                test power of major muscle groups; test reflexes),
                sensory function (touch, pin prick, vibration and
                position sense) and **co-ordination** can be performed
                very quickly and is worth practising.

》   Note that anyone who can stand on one leg and hop on the spot is unlikely
to have a gross neurological abnormality!

CLINICAL ASSESSMENT SYSTEM BY SYSTEM

INTRODUCTION

Neither the notes that follow nor the popular books on clinical examination are any substitute for clinical experience; practise wherever and whenever you can and remember that the more "normal" people you examine, the more likely you are to to notice pathology when it DOES crop up. The aim is to develop a style and system of your own – there really is no RIGHT way to examine a patient!

Remember:

Look – Feel – Percuss – Auscultate.

Always be mindful of your patient's comfort and dignity.

Develop a consistent approach so that you can be sure of making a thorough and reliable clinical assessment.

Clinical signs only achieve significance in relation to the patient's history and general physical state. Remember that a little common sense can go a long way and that you are probably quite good at determining whether someone is really ill or not .....

THE CARDIOVASCULAR SYSTEM

IMPORTANT POINTS IN THE HISTORY:

? Does the patient smoke

? Past history of rheumatic fever or kidney disease

? Family history of heart trouble, high blood pressure etc

? Chest pain –

Pain of **ischaemic heart disease** is severe, constricting, central chest pain **radiating** to neck, jaw and left arm.

» If this sort of pain is precipitated by **exercise** and **relieved by rest** suspect **angina**.

In **myocardial infarction**, the pain may be more severe, may come on at rest and may last for hours.

? Short of breath –

Shortness of breath **on exertion** (of a type which would *not* render a healthy person breathless) may result from a degree of left ventricular failure – often associated with angina.

>> Waking up in the middle of the night gasping for breath ("paroxysmal nocturnal dyspnoea") and breathlessness when lying flat ("orthopnoea") are features of quite severe **left heart failure**.

? Palpitations –

Try and elucidate rate, rhythm, mode of onset and precipitating, aggravating or alleviating factors. Check current medication.

? Ankle swelling –

Especially at end of day. Common symptom in **right heart failure.**

? Fainting ("syncope") –

May be due to cardiovascular pathology.

>> Coughing up blood, particularly in form of red frothy sputum, may be related to valvular heart disease and, in any case, is an important symptom meriting full investigation.

? Symptoms of occlusive vascular disease –

1) **Intermittent claudication** – cramp like pain in the calf, leg or buttock precipitated by exercise and **relieved by rest**.

2) **Rest pain** – suggests advanced pathology – boring, gnawing severe pain often worse at night and relieved by hanging foot over edge of bed.

>> Note that many patients with occlusive vascular disease have symptoms relating to other parts of the circulatory system such as angina, history of strokes etc. Nearly all of them **smoke**.

GENERAL OBSERVATIONS:

? Highly coloured cheeks (malar flush) –

| Sometimes accompanies mitral valve disease.

? Clubbing –

| In relation to heart disease suggests **infective endocarditis** or **"cyanotic" heart disease**.

? Central cyanosis (blue tongue/lips) –

| Suggests the presence of unsaturated blood in the systemic circulation.

? Obvious dyspnoea (eg as patient undresses) –

| May suggest degree of left ventricular failure.

? Swelling of ankles or around sacrum –

| May suggest right heart failure (which may or may not be associated with left heart failure).

? Xanthomata – (xantho = yellow)

| Eg yellow deposits around eyes (= xanthelasma) – may be normal or suggest hyperlipidaemia; deposits in tendons (especially Achilles tendon) or reddish/yellowish lumps around elbows may suggest hypercholestero-laemia; small yellow deposits with red haloes on buttocks and extensor surfaces may also suggest hypercholesterolaemia.

? Jugular venous pulse grossly elevated when patient sitting –

| Suggests right heart failure.

? Any abnormal pulsations anywhere on body

? Varicose veins

SEQUENCE OF CLINICAL EXAMINATION:

- › Observe general state
- › Look at hands
- › Assess radial pulse
- › Take BP
- › Assess carotid pulse if necessary
- › Look at face again, especially colour of sclerae, tongue and mucous membranes
- › Assess JVP (includes pressing on liver – beware tenderness)
- › Observe then palpate praecordium
- › Listen to "4 areas" with bell and diaphragm for normal heart sounds, added sounds and murmurs. Remember that certain abnormalities are heard best with the patient in a particular position.
- › Sit patient forward and listen to lung bases
- › Assess sacrum for oedema, then lay patient back
- › Assess calves for oedema and other vascular problems
- › Assess peripheral pulses if indicated
- › Assess fundi

Recording your findings:

Clinical notes are written up in a standard way and should not be completed until you have FINISHED your examination.

The information is not necessarily recorded in the same order as your examination is conducted.

- › General observations (colour, hands etc)
- › Pulse – rate, regularity, character
- › Peripheral pulses (if palpated)
- › Blood pressure
- › JVP/peripheral oedema
- › Apex beat – position, character
- › Thrills, heaves etc
- › Heart sounds, added sounds, murmurs (eg I + II + 0)

THE RESPIRATORY SYSTEM

IMPORTANT POINTS IN HISTORY:

? Smoker

? Breathless

? Cough -

> Dry or sputum; if sputum, what colour? (green suggests acute infection, clear in winter suggests chronic bronchitis)

? Cough up blood (haemoptysis) –

> If so, merits further investigation – causes include Ca bronchus, pulmonary embolism, TB, bronchiectasis, valvular heart disease.

? Swollen ankles –

> May suggest right heart failure.

GENERAL OBSERVATIONS:

? Clubbing –

> Not explainable by chronic bronchitis unless congenital. Should alert to possibility of Ca bronchus, chronic lung infection, cirrhosis of the liver or even inflammatory bowel disease.

? Evidence of respiratory failure –

> a) CENTRAL cyanosis (blue tongue) suggests a reduction of oxygenation of blood = **hypoxia**.
>
> b) Drowsiness + warm hands, coarse tremor and bounding pulse suggests too much CO_2 in blood = **hypercapnia**.

? Increased respiratory rate or abnormal breathing pattern

? Dyspnoea

? Wheezing

? Using "accessory muscles of respiration" –

ie sternomastoids, strap muscles and platysma.

? Chest asymmetrical or deformed –

"Barrel" or hyperinflated chest suggests chronic obstructive airways disease.

SEQUENCE OF CLINICAL EXAMINATION:

> Patient undressed to waist
> Observe general state
> Look at chest shape
> Look at hands
> Arrange patient to face away from you
> Observe spine
> Palpate for cervical/supraclavicular lymphadenopathy
> Assess chest expansion
> Assess tactile vocal fremitus – upper/middle/lower zones – compare sides
> Percuss upper/middle/lower zones comparing sides
> Auscultate upper/middle/lower zones and assess breath sounds and added sounds
> Assess vocal resonance and whispering pectorilioquy, IF INDICATED
> Turn patient to face you
> Palpate trachea in suprasternal notch and assess the crico-sternal distance
> Palpate apex beat
> Assess chest expansion
> Assess TVF upper/middle/lower zones – comparing sides
> Percuss upper/middle/lower zones – comparing sides
> Auscultate upper/middle/lower zones

Recording your findings:

> › General observations – cyanosis, clubbing, lymphadenopathy, dysp-
>   noea
> › Respiratory rate
> › Trachea
> › Crico-sternal distance
> › Expansion (compare sides)
> › TVF (compare sides)
> › Percussion node (PN)
> › Breath sounds (BS)/added sounds (wheezes, crackles)

THE GASTRO-INTESTINAL SYSTEM

IMPORTANT POINTS IN HISTORY:

? General well-being

? Appetite

? Weight

? Nausea

? Vomiting –

> ? Blood – bright red or coffee grounds?
> Old food may suggest pyloric stenosis

? Problems swallowing –

> Solids suggests mechanical obstruction (tumour etc.).
> Liquids suggests neurological or psychological cause.

? Bowel habit -

> If diarrhoea – ? blood, mucus or pus.
> If pale, bulky, offensive and floating, suggests malabsorption.
> If tarry with peculiar smell suggests melaena (digested blood).
> Bright red blood coating stool suggests haemorrhoids.
> Blood mixed with stool suggests cancer or inflammatory bowel disease.
> Recent change in bowel habit may be due to cancer (in right age group).

Dark urine, pale stools and yellow sclerae suggest JAUNDICE:

> If found, ask about: Alcohol
>   Drugs
>   Recent blood transfusions
>   Recent foreign travel

GENERAL OBSERVATIONS:

Clubbing
White nails
Red palms.
Yellow sclerae
Spider naevi (more than 6)

all suggest chronic liver disease.

A flapping tremor
Sickly breath smell
Confusion

in addition would suggest **liver failure**.

A hard lump behind the left sternoclavicular joint may be related to a stomach cancer.

White nails, a smooth tongue and angular stomatitis together with pallor of mucous membranes may imply anaemia.

Look at the abdomen for nodules, scars, swellings – think flatus, faeces, foetus, fat, fluid! – abnormal movements or pulsations, hernias, dilated veins.

SEQUENCE OF CLINICAL EXAMINATION:

> General inspection
> Examine hands
> Look at eyes and mouth
> Place patient flat with arms at sides and abdomen adequately exposed
> Observe abdomen
> Systematically palpate the 9 abdominal areas, first superficially then deeply
> Palpate for liver (and percuss if in doubt about size)
> Palpate for spleen
> Palpate for kidneys
> Briefly percuss the 9 abdominal areas (and elicit shifting dullness if indicated)
> Listen for bowel sounds
> Briefly examine hernial orifices (first lying, then standing if necessary) and external genitalia
> Perform rectal examination if indicated

Recording your findings:

Hands:

Mouth:

Colour:

Stigmata of chronic liver disease:

Abdomen: ? soft

                             ? tenderness/guarding

                             ? rigidity

                             ? masses/organ enlargement

                             ? bowel sounds

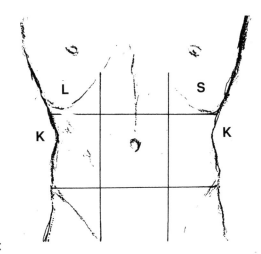

Hernial orifices:

External genitalia:

PR:

L = liver
S = spleen
K = kidney

THE NERVOUS SYSTEM

SEQUENCE OF EXAMINATION:

General assessment including consciousness, orientation and memory.

Arms out in front/close eyes: look for tremor or drift of one arm.

Arms still out in front, ask for piano playing movements.

Finger to nose/heel to shin tests of co-ordination.

Ask for rapid alternating movement of hands.

Cranial nerves II – XII: Visual acuity
Peripheral visual fields
Check pupils for size, symmetry and reactivity to light & accommodation
Eye movements
Look for nystagmus
Check fundi
Trigeminal sensation including corneal reflex
Trigeminal motor function (eg opening mouth)
Raise eyebrows, screw up eyes, show teeth (VII nerve)
Check hearing, including Weber and Rinne
Say AH
Check gag, swallow and cough
Look at tongue, protrude tongue
Test sternomastoid/trapezius

Observe upper limbs for wasting/fasciculation.

Assess upper limb tone.

Assess upper limb power.

Observe lower limbs for wasting/fasciculation.

Assess lower limb tone.

Assess lower limb power.

Elicit tendon jerks and plantar responses.

Test vibration/position sense in feet.

If indicated, perform more complete sensory testing, including light touch/pinprick.

Perform Romberg test.

Watch patient walk.

Recording your findings:

Higher functions:

C N II – XII:

P E R L A*   Fundi:

Tone/Power/Co-ordination Upper Limbs:

Tone/Power/Co-ordination Lower Limbs:

Reflexes**:   B   S   T   K   A   Plantar

              Left: +/–   +/–   +/–   +/–   +/–   ↑or ↓

              Right: +/–   +/–   +/–   +/–   +/–   ↑or ↓

Sensory:

---

*   Pupils Equal and Reacting to Light and Accommodation
**   Biceps, Supinator, Triceps, Knee, Ankle

APPENDICES

Appendices 1 to 8 contain miscellaneous information relating to orthodox clinical examination which you may find useful.

DERMATOMES

The area of skin supplied by a **single spinal nerve** (and thus by a **single segment of the spinal cord**) is called a **dermatome**.

On the trunk there is considerable overlap between adjacent dermatomes and thus dermatome charts are always over-simplifications.

The rather strange arrangement of dermatomes in the limbs results from changes that take place as the limbs grow outward from the body wall during embryological development.

The following represents a MINIMUM basic knowledge of dermatome "levels":

C4	Tip of shoulder
C5	Lateral aspect of elbow
C6	Thumb
C7	Middle finger
C8	Little finger
T3	Axilla
T8	Costal margin
T10	Umbilicus
T12	Pubis
L3	Knee
L5	Big toe
S1	Little toe

CUTANEOUS SENSORY INNERVATION (DERMATOMES)

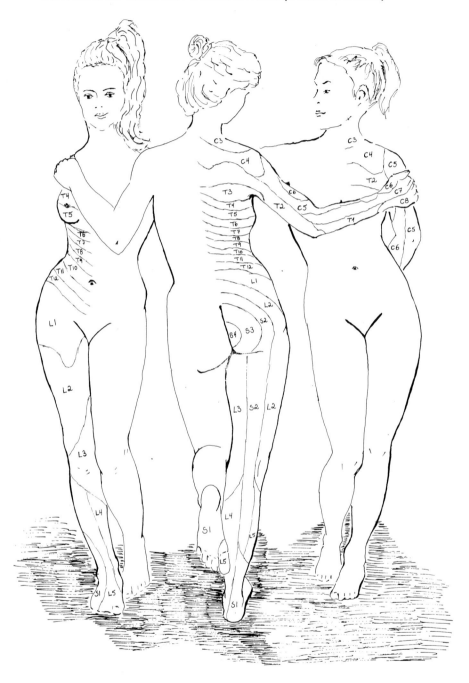

MYOTOMES

Skeletal **muscle** also receives a segmental innervation, but most muscles are innervated by 2, 3 or 4 spinal nerves. Thus the concept of **myotomes** (muscles supplied by particular combinations of spinal nerves) is clinically useful in localizing lesions in the **motor** (efferent) nervous system to *approximate* levels in the spinal cord.

The following table lists the muscles tested routinely in clinical examination together with their segmental and specific innervation:

Shoulder abduction:	Deltoid	C5 (axillary nerve)
Elbow flexion:	Biceps	C5/6 (musculocutaneous nerve)
Wrist extension:	Long extensors	C6/7(radial/post. interosseous n.)
Hand grip:	Intrinsic hand muscles	C8/T1 (ulnar/median nerves)
Hip flexion:	Iliopsoas	L2/3 (femoral nerve)
Knee extension:	Quadriceps	L3/4 (femoral nerve)
Foot dorsiflex:	Tibialis anterior	L4/5 (deep peroneal nerve)
Knee flexion:	Hamstrings	L5/S1 (sciatic nerve)
Foot plantarflex:	Gastrocnemius/Soleus	S1/2 (post. tibial nerve)

TENDON REFLEXES

Biceps	C5/6
Supinator	C6
Triceps	C7/8
Abdominal	T6-12
Patellar tendon	L3/4
Achilles tendon	S1/2
Plantar reflex	L5/S2

JOINT MOVEMENT – NORMAL RANGES

SHOULDER:

180°   ABDUCTION

60°   EXTERNAL ROTATION

90°   INTERNAL ROTATION

ELBOW:

150°   FLEXION

90°   SUPINATION

80°   PRONATION

WRIST:

75°   FLEXION

70°   EXTENSION

HIP:

115°   FLEXION [30° EXTENSION]

50°   ABDUCTION

45°   INTERNAL AND EXTERNAL ROTATION

KNEE:

135°   FLEXION [+ 5° HYPEREXTENSION]

ANKLE:

30°   DORSIFLEXION

50°   PLANTAR FLEXION

POINTERS IN ENDOCRINE DISEASE

THYROID:

Is there a lump in the neck which moves on swallowing?

Warm hands, perspiration, tremor, palpitations, exophthalmos and a preference for cold weather may suggest **thyrotoxicosis**.

Dry hair and skin, puffy face, croaky voice, tiredness and preference for warm weather may suggest **hypothyroidism**.

PITUITARY:

Lack of skin pigmentation, thin skin, decreased secondary sexual hair, delayed puberty and short stature may all be caused by ↓ pituitary function.
Bitemporal hemianopia suggests pituitary tumour.

ADRENAL CORTEX:

Increased skin pigmentation, postural hypotension and decreased body hair (in female) suggests ↓ adrenocortical function.

↑ adrenocortical activity produces Cushing's syndrome: Truncal obesity with round, red, hairy face. Thin, bruised skin with pink stretch marks. Proximal muscle weakness and high blood pressure. Can be caused by exogenous prescribed steroids.

PARATHYROID:

People with hyperparathyroidism (and thus possibly ↑ blood calcium levels) classically complain of bones, stones, psychological moans and abdominal groans.
May also have thirst and polyuria.

EXAMINATION OF THE BREAST

Briefly **inspect** for asymmetry, obvious lumps, retracted nipples and changes in skin texture.

Systematically palpate each quadrant of each breast with the flat of the hand, noting any lumps or tenderness.

If lump found, consider palpating for axillary and supraclavicular lymph nodes and for liver enlargement.

There are 4 major symptoms of breast disease:

> › lumps
> › nipple retraction
> › nipple discharge
> › pain

Here are some questions to ask yourself in each case:

LUMPS:

Who first noticed the lump – ? history of previous lumps or relationship to periods – is it single or multiple – is it vague or well defined – are the edges and surface smooth or irregular – is it mobile or "tethered" to underlying tissue.

NIPPLE RETRACTION:

Long standing or recent – unilateral or bilateral – linear or circumferential – retraction or erosion.

NIPPLE DISCHARGE:

? physiological – ? unilateral or bilateral – ? scanty or profuse – ? spontaneous or only if squeezed – ? colour – ? exudate from eczema rather than discharge.

PAIN:

? actually originating in breast – ? cyclical or spasmodic – ? unilateral or bilateral.

Remember that men occasionally have breast cancer and that breast cancer is a relatively common disease.

With any lump anywhere, note:

> › site
> › size
> › shape
> › fixed or mobile
> › consistency
> › tenderness
> › pulsation
> › transillumination

BLOOD PRESSURE MEASUREMENT

General principles:

A fabric cuff containing an inflatable rubber bag attached to a pressure measurement gauge is wrapped around the upper arm and inflated until the flow of blood through the brachial artery is entirely obstructed.

The pressure in the cuff is then reduced until the pressure in the artery ABOVE the cuff is JUST enough to open the artery momentarily and force some blood through. This can be heard as a knocking sound through a stethoscope placed over the brachial artery.

The measured pressure at which knocking sounds are **first** heard must equal the **systolic** pressure (the MAXIMUM pressure generated by the heart in the cardiac cycle).

If the pressure in the cuff is decreased further, a point will be reached where the knocking sounds disappear (or suddenly go very quiet). The measurement at this moment represents **diastolic** pressure (the lowest level to which the BP drops during the cardiac cycle). Blood flow through a normal unobstructed artery **can't be** heard through a stethoscope, so when the sounds disappear, the pressure in the artery must be just enough to overcome the pressure from the cuff throughout the cardiac cycle.

Basic sequence:

The technique of blood pressure measurement must be learnt in a practical setting and should be practised as often as possible.

The following sequence is simply an aide-memoire:

›   Choose correct sized cuff for size of patient
›   "Unplug" cuff tubing from machine
›   Wrap cuff firmly around upper arm leaving antecubital fossa unob-structed by cuff or tubing
›   Reconnect tubing
›   Fiddle with pressure release valve so that you know which way to turn the knob
›   Palpate radial pulse and pump up cuff until pulse just disappears (this gives you a rough idea of the systolic pressure and avoids the need to pump the cuff up so much that you hurt the patient!)

› Place diaphragm of stethoscope over brachial artery in antecubital fossa supporting patient's arm STRAIGHT with your fingers under their elbow and your thumb holding stethoscope in place
› Pump up cuff to just above systolic pressure
› Release pressure fairly slowly noting SYSTOLIC PRESSURE (sounds appear) and DIASTOLIC PRESSURE (sounds disappear)

NOTES:

1) Don't keep cuff inflated for longer than absolutely necessary. Emergency (!) release of pressure can be achieved by disconnecting tubing.

2) Mercury manometers are generally regarded as more reliable than machines with dials. Nevertheless, no BP machine is accurate to within more than 5mm of mercury (so a measurement of 163/84 is nonsensical!)

3) If using a mercury column, remember to have the machine at the same level as your eye (or vice versa) to avoid optical errors.

4) Small cuffs on big people cause you to over-estimate blood pressure (and vice versa).

HEART SOUNDS

When healthy heart valves open, they make no sound.

When they close, the opposition of the valve **cusps** produce vibrations that may be heard through a stethoscope.

The first sound:

Is low pitched and slightly prolonged.
It is caused by closure of the mitral and tricuspid valves.
The two components may sometimes be distinguished separately on auscultation.
The carotid pulsation occurs just *after* the first sound.

The second sound:

Is shorter and higher pitched than the first sound.
It is caused by the closure of the pulmonary and aortic valves just after the end of systole.
The splitting of the two components may be made more obvious by listening during inspiration (when venous return to the right side of the heart is increased by the negative intrathoracic pressure).

» A **third** (rapid ventricular filling) and/or **fourth** (atrial contraction squirting blood into the ventricles) sound may also be heard in certain conditions (eg heart failure).

11. The Cardiovascular System

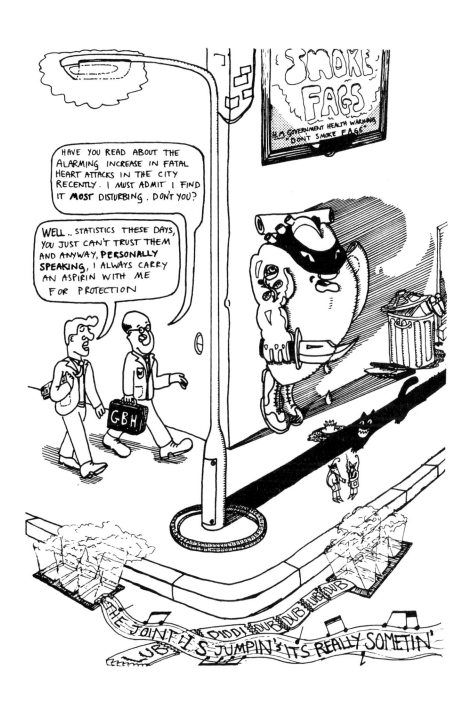

THE CARDIOVASCULAR SYSTEM

OVERVIEW

Heart Failure

Left ventricular failure/right ventricular failure

Ischaemic Heart Disease

Angina/myocardial infarction

Hypertension

Valvular Heart Disease

Infective Conditions

Rheumatic fever/infective endocarditis

Pericarditis:

Acute and chronic constrictive pericarditis

Cardiac Rhythm Disturbances

Extrasystole
Atrial fibrillation
Paroxysmal supraventricular tachycardia
Paroxysmal ventricular tachycardia
Ventricular fibrillation
Bradyarrhythmias

Congenital Heart Defects

Diseases of Heart Muscle (cardiomyopathies)

Peripheral Vascular Disease

Arterial obstruction
Deep vein thrombosis
Thrombophlebitis
Varicose veins/venous ulcers

It is important to realize that most diseases of the cardiovascular system described by orthodox medicine are closely related to one another ie –

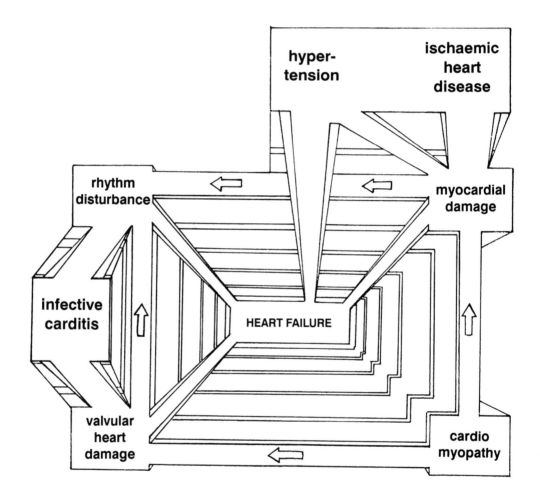

> Note that **heart failure** is the end result of most serious heart disease.

You should also remember that:

1) Cardiovascular disease is the main cause of death in Britain –

2) Atherosclerosis (+ thrombotic complications) and hypertension are the commonest "primary" CVS disease phenomena in the developed world. They are thus the commonest "causes" of ischaemic heart disease (angina, myocardial infarction and sudden death of cardiac origin) and of heart failure.

3) 95% of hypertension is "essential" (ie no known cause).

4) The following are regarded as risk factors for ischaemic heart disease:
   Smoking – 50% of smoking related deaths are from heart disease.
   Hypertension.
   High serum cholesterol ("hyperlipoproteinaemia").
   Being male (same risk in female after menopause).
   Getting older.
   Family history.
   High consumption of saturated fats
   Too much salt.
   Too little fibre.
   Emotional stress.
   Lack of exercise.
   Social deprivation.
   Obesity.
   Diabetes.
   Gout.
   Contraceptive pill.

There follows a brief review of common CVS diseases. Note that although congenital heart disease is relatively rare, it is important since about 50% is correctable by surgery.

HEART FAILURE

If the heart is unable to maintain sufficient circulation to provide adequate oxygenation of the tissues, it is said to have failed. Heart failure can be acute and immediately life threatening or may develop more slowly, producing a variety of symptoms and signs.

If heart failure is caused by diseased heart muscle, valvular damage or rhythm disturbance it is termed **low output failure**. Patients with low output failure tend to have cold, cyanosed peripheries.

If heart failure results from excessive workload it is called **high output failure**. In this case, the **output** of the heart is normal but insufficient to meet the oxygen demands of the body. It is thus seen in anaemia, hyperthyroidism, pregnancy etc and the affected patient will tend to have warm peripheries.

LEFT VENTRICULAR FAILURE

The clinical picture of **left ventricular failure** is dominated by **pulmonary oedema**:

left ventricle fails
↓
pressure in left atrium increases
↓
back pressure in pulmonary veins
↓
engorgement of pulmonary capillaries
↓
lung tissue becomes stiff
↓
fluid leaks out into alveoli = pulmonary oedema

Symptoms:

Breathlessness (including orthopnoea* and paroxysmal nocturnal dyspnoea**), wheeze, cough, fatigue and, sometimes, pink frothy haemoptysis.

---

*   Shortness of breath when lying flat.
**   Waking up in the middle of the night, desperately short of breath.

Signs:

Tachypnoea, dyspnoea, tachycardia, alternating strong and weak pulse beats and added heart sounds.

Important causes:

> › Hypertension
> › Myocardial infarction
> › Aortic valve disease
> › Mitral regurgitation
> › Fluid overload (eg kidney failure)

RIGHT VENTRICULAR FAILURE

Symptoms and signs:

Right ventricular failure produces back pressure in the vena cavae. This may result in:

> › Peripheral pitting oedema (ankles to sacrum)
> › Raised JVP
> › Engorged tender liver
> › Ascites
> › Pleural effusion (if severe)

NOTE:

The term "congestive cardiac failure" is used in different ways by different authorities. Some people would equate the term with right ventricular failure whilst others would only use it to describe severe combined LVF and RVF.

MANAGEMENT OF HEART FAILURE

a) Remove precipitating and exacerbating factors, eg treat anaemia, high blood pressure etc.
b) Reduce activity level.
c) Consider giving drugs (including diuretics, digoxin and vasodilators) to off-load the heart and improve myocardial function. Drugs may also be given to relieve fear and anxiety.
d) Consider whether surgery is necessary/feasible (eg valve replacements, heart transplants etc).

ISCHAEMIC HEART DISEASE

Heart disease caused by poor blood supply to the myocardium.

ANGINA

Central constricting chest pain precipitated by exercise and relieved by rest.

It is due to heart muscle ischaemia from coronary vessel atherosclerosis or spasms. Approximately 4% of patients with angina die each year from their IHD. The risk factors for arteriosclerosis have been described in chapter 6.

Symptoms:

Constricting retrosternal chest pain radiating in a characteristic manner,* precipitated by exercise, emotion, cold and other situations that make demands on the heart. Relieved by rest and nitrate drugs. There may also be dyspnoea, nausea and faintness.

Signs:

None in particular.

Management:

Encourage gentle exercise and maintenance of normal lifestyle. Reduce relevant risk factors if possible (eg STOP SMOKING). Sub-lingual and oral nitrates, β-blockers and Nifedipine all have a place in orthodox management.

Failure of drug therapy (ie serious disruption of lifestyle despite treatment) is an indication for coronary artery bypass surgery. (3.5% mortality; 70% improve or get complete relief; 50% have recurring angina within 7 years.)

---

*   Up to the throat and down the left arm (occasionally also the right).

NOTE:

1) "Unstable" angina is angina at rest or on minimal exertion. It indicates an increased likelihood of MI. It is treated in hospital with strict bed rest and vigorous drug therapy - possibly with coronary artery bypass surgery when pain has been controlled.

2) "Prinzmetal's" angina is recurrent angina at rest associated with a typical ECG pattern.

MYOCARDIAL INFARCTION

Necrosis of heart muscle due to lack of oxygen resulting from poor blood supply.

Each year, 5 people per 1000 of the UK population have myocardial infarcts. Most heart attacks are caused by coronary artery atherosclerosis/thrombosis (see chapter 6 for risk factors).

Symptoms:

Severe, crushing central chest pain radiating up into the throat and down the arms. Unlike angina, the pain of MI may well last for longer than 30 minutes. Breathlessness, fear and nausea ± vomiting are common. There may be a past history of angina.

Signs:

Heart attack victims look ill and frightened with cold, clammy hands and feet. The pulse rate will be raised and the blood pressure is often abnormal. The temperature may go up in the hours following the MI but rarely higher than 38.5°C.

Management:

Heart attacks are best managed in a calm, quiet atmosphere (not often found in coronary care units). Pain relief, oxygen, coronary artery vasodilators and anticoagulants are the mainstay of treatment (± life support as required). Patients are kept in bed until free of pain but should be gently mobilized as soon as possible and allowed home as soon as they are able to climb stairs without pain (hopefully about 2 weeks). The usual advice is to stay off work for 3 months.

Complications:

Early: Shock
                Heart failure
                Arrhythmia
                Cardiac arrest
                More infarcts

Later: Valvular dysfunction
                Ventricular aneurysm
                Heart rupture

Prognosis:

Roughly speaking, of 100 patients having a heart attack, 25 will die immediately and 75 will reach hospital alive. Of these, 1 will die in Accident and Emergency, 8 will die during the first week and 4 will die before discharge. 2 will need cardiopulmonary resuscitation at some point to keep them alive.

》 Of the 62 that leave hospital, 55 will still be alive after 1 year. The mortality rate is proportional to the number of coronary vessels blocked.

HYPERTENSION (high blood pressure)

There is no universally agreed definition of hypertension.* However, the higher the blood pressure, the greater the risk of stroke, heart attack, heart failure, kidney damage or eye problems. Over 20% of the UK population has been diagnosed hypertensive.

Approximately 90% of cases are given the label "essential hypertension" (ie of no obvious cause) and are treated symptomatically. The rest are associated with kidney disease, endocrine disorders, drugs (eg steroids and oral contraceptives), pregnancy or congenital abnormalities of the aortic arch.

Symptoms:

Usually none (but see notes 2 and 3 below).

Signs:

High blood pressure!
Other signs (heart failure, protein in the urine, papilloedema etc) only appear if organs are being damaged.

Management:

Measure the blood pressure on a number of different occasions with the patient fully relaxed.

If the diastolic pressure is consistently higher than 100mmHg (under 60s) or 105mmHg (over 60s), consider treating.

All patients with hypertension should stop smoking, lose weight, reduce dietary salt intake and learn a relaxation technique.

Many non-orthodox therapies offer effective treatment; orthodox management involves the lifetime use of beta-blockers, thiazide diuretics or other anti-hypertensive drugs.

---

*   The World Health Organisation defines it as a systolic pressure greater than 160 and a diastolic pressure greater than 95.

NOTES:

1) Systolic BP is governed by the elasticity and "stretchability" of arteries. Diastolic pressure relates to the peripheral resistance generated by arteriolar "tone". Degenerative changes in blood vessels as we get older mean that blood pressure always increases with increasing age. 170/90 would be an entirely acceptable BP for a healthy 75 year old.

2) High blood pressure associated with **symptoms** such as headache, visual disturbance, ringing in the ears, chest pain or breathlessness should be taken extremely seriously.

3) Severe hypertension (diastolic > 140 or systolic >220) needs emergency treatment since it may rapidly lead to heart failure, kidney failure, cerebral haemorrhage, retinal haemorrhage or fits.

4) Hypertension in a young person always merits full investigation since high blood pressure *secondary* to other (possibly treatable) disease is more common in this age group.

VALVULAR HEART DISEASE

If heart valves are damaged by disease they may become stenosed (orifice narrowed) **or incompetent** (allowing backflow).

Of the many diseases that may affect heart valves, rheumatic fever is still probably the most important (see below). Myocardial infarction, syphilis, endocarditis, hypertension and rheumatoid arthritis may all lead to valvular damage. Congenital valve defects are also quite common (but not all are serious).

Symptoms:

Range from nothing to fatigue, chest pain, dizziness and palpitations.

Signs:

Irregular pulse, displaced apex beat (from enlarged heart), thrills and **murmurs.** Signs of heart failure if severe.

Management:

The mainstays of management are:

1) Surgical valve replacement if appropriate.
2) Prevention of bacterial endocarditis.

INFECTIVE CONDITIONS

RHEUMATIC FEVER

Rheumatic fever is a disease of children and young adults that sometimes complicates streptococcal throat infection.

It is thought to result from an immunological cross sensitivity reaction in which antistreptococcal antibody acts against heart tissue. This may lead to permanent damage of **heart valves.** Note, however, that about 1/3rd of patients with chronic rheumatic valvular heart disease have no recollection of having had rheumatic fever in their childhood. Recognition and treatment of streptococcal sore throats (usually with penicillin) avoids the development of rheumatic fever.*

Clinical features:

10 days after a streptococcal throat infection, rheumatic fever presents with joint pain, stiffness, malaise and fever. After about 5 days, things improve only to get worse again in a cycle that repeats up to 3 times before the fever subsides. If heart tissue becomes inflamed, the fever is accompanied by chest pain. If cardiac damage is severe, heart failure may occur.

Red rashes and hard, painless nodules on the backs of elbows and wrists and the front of knees and ankles may also develop. These probably indicate severe carditis.

Treatment:

Is with oral penicillin for 10 days plus bed rest and aspirin for the joint pains. If there are signs of cardiac damage, it is usual to prescribe oral penicillin for between 5 and 20 years to prevent recurrence of a strep. throat since complications get worse with each attack. Antibiotic "cover" for surgical procedures is recommended for life.

---

*   Sydenham's chorea – also called St. Vitus' Dance –and acute glomerulonephritis are two other possible immunological sequelae of "strep. throats."

INFECTIVE ENDOCARDITIS

Is infection of a heart valve which has been previously damaged by rheumatic fever, cardiac surgery, cardiac investigations or syphilis etc. Congenitally abnormal and artificial (prosthetic) heart valves are also at risk.*

The infecting organisms usually come from the teeth, skin, gut or urinary tract and can be introduced into the blood stream by a variety of dental and surgical procedures (and by communal use of unsterilized needles in drug addicts). Rarely, acute endocarditis may be a complication of severe generalized infection (septicaemia). Bacterial endocarditis usually presents in a "subacute" form nowadays.

The symptoms and signs encompass 3 main areas:

> Signs of general infection (lethargy, malaise, low-grade fever, anaemia, clubbing, transient joint pain).
> Signs of underlying predisposing cardiac abnormality (eg murmurs).
> Embolic phenomena (strokes, occlusion of peripheral arteries, splinter haemorrhage under the nails).

Various other manifestations include enlarged liver and spleen and hard tender nodules on fingers. Untreated, 95% of cases will die from heart failure or cerebral embolus.

As a rule of thumb, fever in any patient with known heart disease (or who is known to be mainlining) should be regarded as bacterial endocarditis until proved otherwise.

Treatment:

Involves intravenous antibiotic therapy lasting for 4 weeks. In severe cases (those developing heart failure), surgery to remove and replace the damaged valve is often performed.

---

* Mainlining drug addicts also risk infective endocarditis since dirty needles can introduce bacteria directly into the blood stream near the heart.

Prognosis:

The mortality is about 30%, despite antibiotics. Less if diagnosed and treated early ....

» People with known heart valve damage would be given antibiotic prophylaxis before undergoing dental, surgical and invasive investigative procedures.

PERICARDITIS

Acute pericarditis means acute inflammation of the pericardium and is usually seen as a complication of myocardial infarction or as a benign idiopathic condition affecting young adults.

It sometimes accompanies other diseases such as severe chest infections, renal failure, lung cancer, SLE and RA.

Symptoms:

Gripping central chest discomfort, exacerbated by breathing, coughing and changes in posture (± symptoms of associated disease).

Signs:

A pericardial "friction rub" is sometimes heard (± signs of associated disease).

Treatment:

a) Benign idiopathic form: Bedrest + simple painkillers.

b) Secondary forms: Treatment of associated pathologies and complications.

Complications:

If a pericardial effusion develops, the normal action of the heart may be severely compromised producing shortness of breath, a raised JVP, tachycardia, low blood pressure and pulsus paradoxus. This state is known as "cardiac tamponade". Cardiac tamponade is a medical emergency and is treated by sucking out the fluid from the pericardial space via a needle passed through the chest wall.

CHRONIC CONSTRICTIVE PERICARDITIS

Is a rare condition in which scarring of the pericardial tissue produces chronic constriction of the heart and thus congestive heart failure.

It is seen as a complication of TB and may also follow episodes of acute pericarditis.

CARDIAC RHYTHM DISTURBANCES

Any disturbance of the regular activation of ventricular contraction is called an **arrhythmia.***

Background:

Orderly heart contraction depends on the myocardial properties of rhythmicity, conductivity and "refractoriness" – ie whichever tissue generates an activating impulse at the highest rate (normally the SA node) sets off the conduction of an electrical impulse to **all** myocardial cells which then depolarize, contract and repolarize (during which time they cannot contract again).

Exercise, catecholamines and sympathomimetics all increase impulse generation rate and conduction rate whilst decreasing refractoriness. Rest, vagal stimulation and drugs blocking sympathetic activity all diminish rhythmicity and conductivity and increase refractoriness.

Disturbances of heart **rate** and **regularity** both come under the heading "arrhythmia". "Normal" resting heart rates vary – in children a pulse rate of 100 bpm is usual whereas an Olympic athlete may have a pulse rate of 50!

Broadly speaking, rhythm disturbances may be caused in 3 ways:

a) **Severe myocardial disease** may depress the inherent rhythmicity of the heart. This state is usually terminal –

b) **Myocardial infarction, degeneration or cardiotoxic drugs** may block conductivity or increase refractoriness of myocardial tissues producing inefficient or inco-ordinate contractions. If, for example, myocardial disease blocks the transmission of SA generated impulses through the AV node, ventricular contraction has to be maintained by a slower *ventricular* "pacemaker" –

c) **An abnormal focus of impulse formation** (outside the SA node) – called an "ectopic focus" – may interfere with normal pacemaker activity by "capturing" the conducting system and activating a heart beat before the SA node discharges.

---

* Sinus arrhythmia is a misleading term used to describe the physiological observation that, in healthy people, heart rate increases slightly in inspiration and decreases during expiration.

Clinical examination:

May reveal normal heart rate with abnormal rhythm, abnormal heart rate with normal rhythm or combined disturbances of rate and rhythm.

Orthodox diagnosis and treatment of arrhythmias ultimately depends on the use of the electrocardiograph but you should be familiar with some of the commoner rate and rhythm disturbances and their implications.

EXTRASYSTOLES

Are premature, "ectopic" beats and may arise from anywhere in the myocardium. Patients may complain of sudden awareness of the heart beat or that the heart misses a beat and then starts with a sudden bump. The pulse will show occasional breaks in the normal "sinus" rhythm or may have a recurring pattern of irregularity.

Although such symptoms and signs merit a proper assessment of the cardiovascular system, occasional extrasystoles (usually generated by an ectopic *atrial* focus) are very common in normal people and are not "treated" unless they occur frequently enough to cause hypotension or heart failure. Frequent atrial ectopics may herald the onset of atrial fibrillation (see below). Ectopic beats after a myocardial infarction may arise from the ventricles and may precede life threatening ventricular fibrillation.

Note that digoxin therapy may cause ventricular ectopic beats.

ATRIAL FIBRILLATION

Is the commonest persistent arrhythmia seen in practice and occurs when disease of atrial myocardium produces an ectopic focus discharging at a rate of 500 beats per minute. This causes a haphazard spread of depolarization and stops concerted atrial contraction. The AV node only allows impulses to pass at a certain rate and thus the irregular high speed bombardment of the node by atrial impulses results in *total irregularity of ventricular rhythm.*

Clinical features:

Range from nothing to palpitations, breathlessness and heart failure but the important clinical sign is the **absolute irregularity of the pulse**. Common causes include mitral valve disease, **thyrotoxicosis**, hypertension, myocardial infarct and ischaemic heart disease affecting the SA node.

Management:

> Once again, the onset of atrial fibrillation demands a thorough CVS assessment (and exclusion of thyrotoxicosis). Persistent AF carries a risk of thrombus formation in the atria which may lead to systemic embolism. For chronic AF, the orthodox treatment is digoxin ± β-blocker (used here for its anti-arrhythmic properties). Recent onset of AF in a patient who is in heart failure or shock is usually managed by electric shock ("cardioversion").

PAROXYSMAL SUPRAVENTRICULAR TACHYCARDIA

> Is, as the name suggests, a sudden attack of rapid heart beat (100 up to 250 bpm) accompanied (sometimes) by dizziness, fainting, breathlessness and diuresis. Attacks switch off abruptly and may last minutes, hours or days. They result from rapid discharge of an abnormal atrial focus. They may have little significance in patients with normal hearts but, in the presence of heart disease, they may produce a serious (temporary) deterioration in cardiac function.
>
> Immersion of the face in cold water or performance of the Valsalva manoeuvre* may stop the attack. In more extreme or persistent cases, drugs or electric shock may be necessary.

PAROXYSMAL VENTRICULAR TACHYCARDIA

> Is a much more serious arrhythmia that may present in the same way as SVT. An ECG is necessary to distinguish between them. However VT usually only occurs in patients with known myocardial disease.

VENTRICULAR FIBRILLATION

> Is the complete disruption of orderly ventricular contraction. It causes an acute reduction in cardiac output and collapse of the patient. It is a common early complication of myocardial infarction.
>
> VF is a common cause of sudden death (though it sometimes stops spontaneously). Treatment is by electric shock (defibrillation).

---

*   Breathing out against a closed glottis.

BRADYARRHYTHMIAS (heart beating too slowly)

Bradyarrhythmias are only important when they cause symptoms. Severe bradycardia after an MI is life threatening and may require rapid, expert intervention (drugs, temporary pacemakers etc).

» β-blockers, verapamil and digoxin are common drugs that cause bradycardia.

CONGENITAL HEART DEFECTS

Is an enormous and complicated subject and will not be considered in any detail here. You could refer to a paediatric textbook for a more comprehensive account.

CHD is not rare –

Occurring in about 5 per 1000 live births.
1 out of 3 affected will not survive their first year.

May be an isolated cardiac abnormality or be part of a syndrome such as –

a) Maternal rubella affecting the foetus.
b) Down's syndrome.
c) Turner's syndrome.

Congenital heart defects may involve –

1) Stenosis of heart valves or the first part of the aorta.
2) Incompetence of valves with regurgitation of blood in the wrong direction.
3) Defects in the "walls" dividing the atria from each other or the ventricles from each other producing what are known as "shunts".

Names you may come across are –

> Atrial septal defect (ASD).
> Ventricular septal defect (VSD).
> Patent ductus arteriosus (PDA).
> Fallot's tetralogy.
> Pulmonary stenosis.
> Coarctation of the aorta.
> Eisenmenger's syndrome.

Symptoms:

Range from nothing through breathlessness and fatigue to angina, fainting, and retarded growth.

Signs:

Include heart murmurs, cyanosis, clubbing, heart enlargement, heart failure and pulmonary oedema.

Treatment:

Paediatric cardiac surgery to repair the plumbing defects is frequently extremely successful.

Prognosis:

Depends on the extent of the defect and the general health of the child.

DISEASES OF HEART MUSCLE (Cardiomyopathies)

A number of medical conditions (eg alcohol abuse, sarcoid, amyloid) and some orthodox drugs are associated with heart muscle damage but many cases of cardiomyopathy are of unknown cause.

Affected heart muscle may become weakened, stretched or hypertrophied This produces a variety of symptoms and signs including palpitations, breathlessness, angina and heart failure.

Management is symptomatic. If ventricular function deteriorates significantly, transplant surgery may be required to preserve life.

PERIPHERAL VASCULAR DISEASE

PERIPHERAL ARTERIAL OBSTRUCTION

There are 4 common clinical syndromes related to peripheral arterial obstruction:

> **Intermittent claudication**
> **Acute arterial obstruction**
> **Ischaemic foot**
> **Raynaud's phenomenon**

Raynaud's phenomenon is discussed in chapter 19 (in connection with connective tissue disorders).

INTERMITTENT CLAUDICATION:

Simply means intermittent limping. It is characterized by severe calf pain precipitated by exercise and relieved by rest and is the result of peripheral arterial obstruction, usually associated with widespread atheroma.

90% of sufferers are males over the age of 50.
Smokers and diabetics form the vast majority of cases.
80% of obstructions are in the femoral or popliteal arteries.

Clinical features:

Major peripheral arterial pulses will be reduced or absent depending on the site of obstruction. The involved limb will also be cold, pale or cyanosed and may be hairless and slightly wasted. There may also be ulceration and signs of gangrene (esp. toes and heel).
Intermittent claudication indicates widespread occlusive vascular disease and 80% of cases will go on to die from cardio- or cerebrovascular accidents.

Management:

Includes stopping smoking, reducing obesity, treating hypertension and diabetes if present, careful attention to foot hygiene and encouragement of gentle exercise. By-pass surgery is frequently necessary.

» Calf pain at rest (worse at night and relieved by hanging the legs over the side of the bed) indicates very severe obstruction.

ACUTE ARTERIAL OBSTRUCTION:

May be due to thrombosis or embolism (often associated with atrial fibrillation).

90% affects legs.

Clinical features:

Acute onset of pain, numbness, pallor and icy coldness of affected limb. Pallor is gradually replaced by cyanosis and then gangrene if untreated. Arterial pulses are absent distal to the site of obstruction.

Treatment:

Emergency surgery is the only treatment offering a real chance of survival.

ISCHAEMIC FOOT:

Is caused by chronic arterial obstruction below the knee and is usually seen in diabetics. Small vessels supplying toes are most often affected.

Clinical features:

Cold, painful, hairless, pulseless foot with areas of necrosis and ulceration. May be pale or cyanosed.

Treatment:

Is frequently ineffective. Includes "sympathectomy" to improve skin blood supply and drugs to relieve pain. Amputation is frequently necessary. Stopping smoking and scrupulous foot hygiene are essential.

DEEP VEIN THROMBOSIS

This is an important condition characterized by pain and swelling (usually in a leg) resulting from thrombosis of a deep vein.

The presence of DVT predisposes to **pulmonary embolism** and death, so recognition and prompt treatment is exceptionally important.

Risk factors include pregnancy, surgery, malignancy and immobility (hence the trend towards early post-operative mobilization in hospitals).

The following suggest a diagnosis of DVT:

> › Tenderness between the heads of the gastrocnemius.
> › Stiffness of the calf muscles.
> › Delayed cooling of the limb when exposed to the air.
> › Oedema, cyanosis and engorged superficial veins on affected limb.
> › Mild fever.

Treatment:

Follows hospital investigation by "venography" and involves enthusiastic anti-coagulant therapy.

THROMBOPHLEBITIS

Is the jargon name for superficial vein thrombosis associated with inflammation (usually due to infection) in or near a vein.

It is a common accompaniment to intravenous cannulation (drips) and also occurs in varicose veins. The affected vein feels like a hard cord under the skin and the surrounding area is inflamed and tender.

Treatment:

Involves the wearing of a gentle support stocking and a short course of antibiotics. Embolic complications are very rare but, untreated, infection can spread rapidly up a vein with more or less disastrous results.

SPONTANEOUS THROMBOPHLEBITIS:

(ie thrombophlebitis without an obvious cause) also occurs and may appear and disappear at different sites in a random manner (so called "thrombophlebitis migrans"). This may suggest the presence of a visceral carcinoma or be associated with polyarteritis, polycythaemia or Buerger's disease.

VARICOSE VEINS

Varicose veins are dilated, tortuous veins.

They frequently occur in the lower limbs (a penalty we pay for adopting an upright posture) but may also occur in spermatic, oesophageal and haemorrhoidal veins.

Efficient venous return from the lower limbs depends on the "muscle pump" and the competence of venous valves. If valves in the deep veins (or in the "communicating" veins between the deep and superficial vessels) become incompetent and allow high pressure leakage of blood from the deep system to the superficial, varicosity may result. Similarly, if there is any obstruction to venous return (eg tumours or pregnancy) varicosity may occur in superficial veins distal to the obstruction.

Symptoms:

Include a weary, aching sensation in the lower leg which gets worse as the day progresses. Sharp pains may occur over the varices. The ankles may swell and the skin may itch (due to leakage of red cells). Some people suffer calf cramps shortly after getting into bed at night.

Orthodox treatment:

Includes the use of support stockings, "injection-compression" treatments and various operative procedures including "vein stripping".

As well as thrombophlebitis, patients with varicose veins are prone to chronic dermatitis following minor trauma (eg scratching).

》 Note that varicose veins may rupture and cause profuse bleeding. Firm pressure and elevation are all that is required to stop the bleeding. A tourniquet should never be used.

VENOUS ULCERS

May complicate old "recanalized" deep vein thrombosis or varicose veins since in both conditions incompetent valves lead to venous stasis in the extremities with consequent oedema and local lack of oxygen. This produces superficial tissue necrosis and ulceration.

It is important to try and pinpoint the underlying pathology since venous ulceration following DVT is much harder to treat. It is also important to exclude *arterial* obstruction as a cause.

Treatment:

Elevation of the affected limb, exercise, massage and support bandaging will heal most venous ulcers (by improving venous return, reducing oedema, improving the muscle pump and softening hardened tissue). Once the ulcer has healed, treatment of the incompetent vessels should be considered.

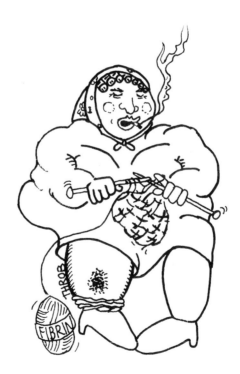

12. The Respiratory System

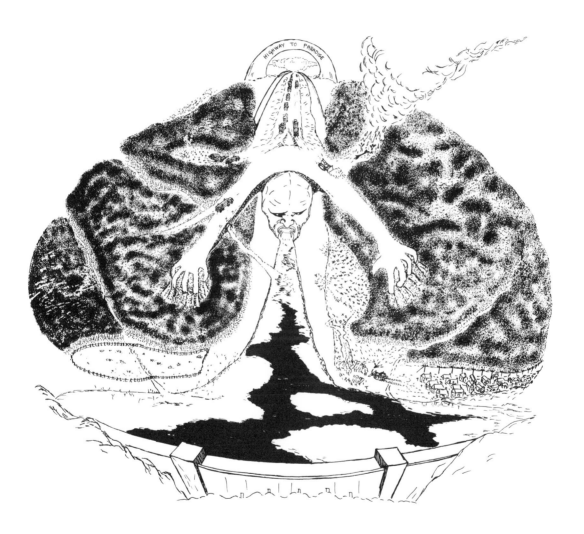

THE RESPIRATORY SYSTEM

OVERVIEW

Chronic Obstructive Airway Disease

| Chronic bronchitis and emphysema

Asthma

Carcinoma of the Bronchus

Tuberculosis

| Primary, post-primary and non-pulmonary TB

Pneumonia

| Lobar pneumonia
| Bronchopneumonia
| Viral pneumonias
| Aspiration pneumonia

Pleurisy

Acute Bronchitis

Influenza:

| A and B

Bronchiectasis

Pneumothorax

| Tension pneumothorax

Pulmonary Embolus

Childhood Diseases

| Bronchiolitis
| Croup/Epiglottitis
| Whooping cough
| Cystic fibrosis

CHRONIC OBSTRUCTIVE AIRWAY DISEASE – COAD

CHRONIC BRONCHITIS AND EMPHYSEMA

Chronic bronchitis is a chronic inflammatory condition of the bronchial tree. A person who has suffered daily cough with sputum for 3 months per year for at least 2 years is said, by definition, to have chronic bronchitis.

Emphysema is a histological (and thus often post-mortem) diagnosis. It is defined as enlargement of the air spaces distal to the smallest (terminal) bronchioles with accompanying destructive changes in the alveolar walls.

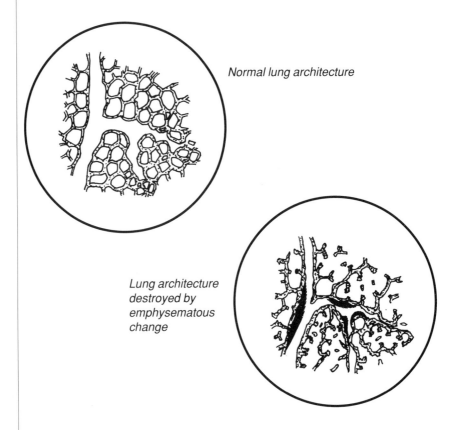

Normal lung architecture

Lung architecture destroyed by emphysematous change

The clinical complaint of chronic bronchitis is almost always accompanied by some degree of emphysematous change within the lung. The combination is generally referred to as **Chronic Obstructive Airway Disease (COAD)**.

Incidence:

30,000 (very unpleasant) deaths per annum in the UK.

Aetiological factors:

Smoking is the most important cause of COAD in the world today. The increased risk of dying from bronchitis = 1/2 x no. of cigarettes smoked per day.

Atmospheric pollution, "lower" social class, an industrial environment and being British also contribute. (A rare genetic enzyme disorder, α-1-anti-trypsin deficiency, causes emphysema in younger patients.)

Histology:

In chronic bronchitis, the bronchi become dilated and develop a rough, thickened mucosa containing increased numbers of mucous glands. A variable degree of chronic inflammatory change is seen under the microscope together with more or less widespread evidence of emphysema (see above). Note that the histological features do not always correlate clearly with the clinical pictures.

Clinical features:

The importance of the pathological changes outlined above is that they cause:

1) Obstruction of the airways (due to excess mucous secretion, bronchial spasm and destruction of alveoli by emphysema)

and

2) A decrease in the amount of lung tissue available for gas exchange and thus diminished oxygenation of the blood which, if severe enough, is termed **respiratory failure**.

In certain cases, these changes combine to cause compression of the capillaries in the alveolar walls leading to **pulmonary hypertension.** This can overload the right ventricle which enlarges and then fails. Right heart failure secondary to COAD is called **cor pulmonale**.

A common story might be as follows:

Initially, the patient has a "productive" morning cough and suffers frequent attacks of **acute** bronchitis (see later). As time goes on, there is increasing **dyspnoea** (shortness of breath) with wheezing and the acute infective episodes become more severe. Eventually, respiratory failure or chronic right heart failure (cor pulmonale) develop.

On examination, a chronic bronchitic will have a wheezing, hyperinflated chest and may be cyanosed. There may also be signs of right heart failure (peripheral pitting oedema, a raised jugular venous pressure, enlarged tender liver etc). The presence of clubbing would suggest more serious underlying pathology, eg lung cancer.*

Treatment:

Stop smoking and lose weight.
Consider treating acute exacerbations with antibiotics.
Use bronchodilators – inhalers ± tablets – as appropriate. Common ones include **salbutamol** (Ventolin), **terbutaline** (Bricanyl), **ipratropium** (Atrovent) and **theophylline**.
Right heart failure is treated with diuretics. Physiotherapy and home oxygen (low concentration, no smoking!) may also help.

Prognosis:

Is **poor** – only about 30% survive 5 years once respiratory failure/cor pulmonale develop.

---

*　A patient with clubbing always needs full investigation.

ASTHMA

A condition caused by bronchospasm and characterized by wheeze, cough and dyspnoea in any combination.

Clinically, asthmatic patients fall into two main groups:

1) **Extrinsic asthma** – begins in childhood, often with "allergic" family history or family history of asthma. Tends to be episodic. Often improves with age.

2) **Intrinsic (late-onset) asthma** – starts later in life, no allergic family history. Can be precipitated by infections (and also by taking aspirin). Tends to be chronic and hard to treat.

Aetiological factors:

› Heredity
› Reaction to common allergens (dust, pollen, some foods, drugs and bacteria) causing release of **histamine** etc from "sensitized" mast cells in the lung tissue
› Emotional difficulties
› Aspergillosis, filariasis, polyarteritis nodosa and pulmonary embolism may also present an asthmatic picture

Pathology:

Gross appearance: The lungs of an asthmatic usually look fairly normal but tenacious mucus and "plugs" of mucoid material are often found in the bronchi and bronchioles associated with small areas of lung collapse.

Microscopic appearance: The walls of the bronchioles are thickened and show some smooth muscle hypertrophy.

Clinical features:

Attacks are usually of sudden onset and may last hours or even days. They may be precipitated by specific allergens, exertion, excitement, cold air, respiratory infection or β-blocker drugs and are characterized by wheeze and tightness in the chest with inspiratory and expiratory difficulty (expiration is often more difficult). There may also be cough. The patient will be using the accessory muscles of respiration and may be extremely anxious. Sitting up eases things slightly. The pulse is rapid though the respiratory rate may not be increased.

Mild asthmatics usually have normal respiratory function between attacks but those with long-standing, severe asthma tend to suffer some degree of respiratory difficulty between acute episodes. Severe, prolonged asthma attacks* may lead to respiratory failure and sudden **death** within 24hrs if untreated.

Ominous signs are:

> › Inability to speak (and drink)
> › Wheeze getting quicker but patient getting iller
> › Low blood pressure
> › "Pulsus paradoxus"**
> › Any degree of drowsiness or confusion
> › Cyanosis (particularly worrying if the patient is known chronic bronchitic)

» | **SOMETHING SHOULD HAVE BEEN DONE BEFORE CYANOSIS AND DROWSINESS BECOME APPARENT.**

Treatment:

Orthodox treatment depends on a variety of drugs administered via inhalers:

Disodium cromoglycate *(Intal)* → Prophylactic mast-cell stabilizer
Salbutamol *(Ventolin)* → β2-agonist bronchodilator
Ipratropium *(Atrovent)* → Anticholinergic bronchodilator
Beclomethasone *(Becotide)* → Steroid

In severe cases, oral steroids and oral bronchodilators may be added. Avoidance of obvious allergens and desensitisation programmes may also play a part.

Intravenous bronchodilators, oxygen, antibiotics and artificial ventilation may all be used in the treatment of status asthmaticus.

---

* Known as status asthmaticus. See chapter 28.
** A decrease in blood pressure of more than 10mmHg during inspiration.

CARCINOMA OF THE BRONCHUS

Incidence:

35,000 deaths per year in UK, half of them under 65 years of age.

Population:

Age group: Average 55 years
             Range 18–80
Sex: M:F = 3.5:1
Occupation: Mining of radioactive ores, nickel refiners, arsenic expo-
             sure, haematite quarries, asbestos and chromate workers.

Aetiological factors:

Cigarette smoking – the increased risk of death is equal to the number
of cigarettes per day. Stopping decreases the risk by 1/2 in 5 years. In 15
years, the risk is only double that of a life-long non-smoker. Environmental
pollution is also an aetiological factor.

Types of cancer:

Squamous cell – 40%. Preceded by squamous metaplasia in bronchial
epithelium.*
Oat cell – 15%. Turnover may produce hormones including ACTH and
ADH.
Large cell undifferentiated – 25%.
Adenocarcinoma – 15%. More common in females. **Not** associated with
smoking.

Sites:

55% arise in large bronchi near the centre of the lung.
40% arise from smaller peripheral bronchi or bronchioles.
5% have a diffuse or "multifocal" origin.

---

*   See chapter 5.

Clinical features:

The patient is usually a **smoker** complaining of **worsening cough** and **haemoptysis**. Dyspnoea, central chest ache and **slowly resolving chest infections** are also common.

Patients may also present complaining of the effects of **metastases** involving brain, bone, liver, skin, kidney or adrenal glands. Some tumours are picked up on routine chest X-ray. Local extension of lung cancer causes various symptoms; anorexia, weight loss and fatigue imply advanced disease.

» Ca bronchus can produce a bewildering array of **"non-metastatic"** effects including **anaemia,** dementia, **cerebellar signs,** neuropathies, myopathies, **clubbing,** skin conditions, hormonal syndromes, thrombophlebitis, pericarditis and atrial fibrillation.

Treatment:

20% cases are "operable". Only 30% of these live for 5 years. Overall 5 year survival is under 10%. Average untreated survival after diagnosis is less than 6 months. Surgery is not contemplated if metastases are present.
Radiotherapy and chemotherapy may reduce distressing symptoms by reducing tumour size.

TUBERCULOSIS (TB)

Tuberculosis is the name given to infection with the micro-organism MYCOBACTERIUM TUBERCULOSIS.

> 50 years ago, TB caused 10% of *all* deaths in the UK and despite modern allopathic therapy (developed in the early 1950s), TB remains an important cause of death in many countries, especially those in which undernourishment is a major problem. Nowadays there are something over 10,000 new cases reported each year in Britain, many of whom come from immigrant and over 65 "populations".

PULMONARY TB

> Two main types of **pulmonary TB** are described – primary and post-primary.

PRIMARY TB:

> This is the syndrome produced by infection with TB bacilli in those who have not previously been infected (and thus is seen more often in children).

Pathology:

> There is a mild inflammatory response at the site of infection (usually the mid-zones of the lungs, the pharynx or the terminal ileum) followed by spread of infection to local lymph nodes. One to two weeks later, the reaction in the infected tissues changes to produce characteristic **caseating** (cheeselike) **granulomata.** This coincides with the development of a positive **Mantoux** test – a manifestation of a type 4 hypersensitivity reaction to TB bacterial protein.

Clinical features:

> Despite all this activity, primary TB is usually symptomless but may present as fever, lassitude and productive cough. Erythema nodosum is sometimes seen and lymph nodes in the neck may become enlarged. Even mild or symptomless infection can be spread via droplets from coughs and sneezes.

POST-PRIMARY TB:

This is the syndrome produced by reinfection with (or reactivation of) TB in a *previously infected* patient. Since the body is already "sensitized" to TB, this reactivation is followed by rapid granuloma formation in the infected area. This tends to localize the disease and thus regional lymph node involvement is uncommon.

The **upper** lobes of the lung are common sites of post-primary TB infection.

Clinical features:

Symptoms occur relatively late (after the disease has become well established) and are often non-specific: malaise, fatigue, weight loss, loss of appetite and night sweats. Cough, repeated small haemoptyses, slight fever and occasional chest pain may also occur.

Although the infecting organisms are present in the sputum of infected patients, it is often surprisingly difficult to diagnose a case of TB using laboratory tests. Thus a "high index of clinical suspicion" is necessary if the above symptoms are reported by someone in one of the "high risk" categories (down and outs, hostel dwellers, alcoholics, the malnourished, diabetics, people on steroids, health workers, Pakistani, Indian and Irish immigrants etc).

Treatment:

Consists of initial isolation (of doubtful value) and administration of various combinations of anti-tuberculous drugs for periods of up to 18 months. These drugs are undoubtedly effective but have an impressive list of side-effects. The favourites at the moment are isoniazid, rifampicin, ethambutol, streptomycin and pyrazinamide. Regular clinical assessments, chest X-rays and sputum cultures are used to monitor progress.

NOTES

1) Tuberculin tests:

Superficial (intradermal) injections of standardized preparations of protein derived from the capsule of the TB bacillus cause local inflammation and .a weal after 48-72 hrs in individuals **previously infected** with TB. The Heaf test and the Mantoux test are the most commonly used tuberculin tests. A strongly positive reaction in an unvaccinated person indicates the need for a period of treatment, even if no symptoms are present.

2) Prevention:

The **BCG** (Bacille Calmette-Guerin) is an attenuated bovine tubercle bacillus which confers a degree of immunity to TB infection when inoculated into human beings. It is currently administered to medical laboratory and heath care workers who are found to be Mantoux **negative** and also to the newborn infants of mothers with the disease. Although useful in many individual cases, it would not be cost effective to vaccinate the whole population since the incidence of TB in the UK is relatively low.

3) "Fate" of the tuberculous lesions in infected lung tissue:

› They may heal by **fibrosis**, often with calcification.
› They may spread and rupture into a bronchus causing tuberculous bronchopneumonia.
› They may "invade" blood vessels causing dissemination of organisms via the bloodstream causing **miliary** (seed-like) **tuberculosis** of the liver, spleen, lungs, bone, meninges etc – a very dangerous condition sometimes associated with immunosuppression.

NON-PULMONARY TB

Though uncommon, TB may occur as a **primary** phenomenon involving various organs other than the lung, eg TB meningitis, renal TB, TB of the spine, abdominal TB, TB pericarditis and TB of the adrenal gland (a cause of Addison's disease).

PNEUMONIA

Pneumonia means inflammation of the alveoli (inflammatory cells and exudate within the alveolar walls and air spaces).

Pathologists classify pneumonia as either bronchopneumonia or lobar pneumonia on the basis of the post mortem appearance of the infected lung tissue. However, it is more useful clinically to classify pneumonias on the basis of the causative organism or insult ie bacterial, viral, fungal, mycobacterial, protozoal, chemical, physical, allergic etc.

Before reviewing the features common to *all* pneumonias, it is worth sketching out the main features of the "classic pneumonias" as described by old-time physicians:

LOBAR PNEUMONIA

Was an acute disease of healthy adults caused by Streptococcus pneumoniae (pneumococcus) and preceded by exposure to cold and dampness. It lasted for 10 days and resolved by "crisis," after which the fever subsided and well being returned (thanks to the production of appropriate antibody). The mortality was between 20 and 50% and the tendency for doctors and nurses to wait up during the 10th night did much for the image of the medical profession, since they were at least on hand to share in the family's joy or sorrow (even if they had little to offer therapeutically except sympathy*).

BRONCHOPNEUMONIA

Was a killing disease of the young (eg a complication of measles or whooping cough), the very old (especially those with chronic bronchitis) and the debilitated and bed-ridden ("hypostatic" pneumonia) as well as being a serious complication of influenza. Most bacterial cases were caused by streptococci and staphylococci and those who recovered were left with some degree of permanent lung damage.

>> The advent of penicillin in 1943 greatly reduced the mortality in both these classical presentations but the descriptions and pathological observations still hold good today.

---

*   A quality undervalued by many modern medics.

Clinical features:

Clinically, all pneumonias are more or less similar. Presenting features include:

Fever, rigors, cough, sputum (purulent* in pyogenic bacterial cases), pleuritic chest pain,** dyspnoea at rest and confusion (particularly in the elderly). Various signs on percussion and auscultation reflect the underlying pathological processes and help confirm the diagnosis (along with appropriate x-rays).

Inflammation of the lung substance may also lead to inflammation of the adjacent pleura (pleurisy, pleural effusions etc).

Incomplete, ineffective, inappropriate or non-existent treatment may result in poor "resolution" leading to abscess formation or fibrosis of lung tissue.

Any acute pneumonia that fails to resolve after 6 weeks should be investigated for the presence of underlying carcinoma.

Management:

Drugs commonly used in combination in the treatment of pneumonias include benzylpenicillin, flucloxacillin, ampicillin, gentamicin and the newer cephalosporin class of compounds.

NOTES

Life threatening pneumonias causing rapid deterioration of the patient are likely to be due to staphylococci, pneumococci, Haemophilus influenzae or klebsiella.

Lobar pneumonia is usually caused by Streptococcus pneumoniae.

Pneumonia complicating debility or alcoholism is often due to Gram negative organisms.

---

*   Green and nasty.
**   Pain made worse by breathing and coughing.

---

which the symptoms, signs and results of clinical investigations (chest X-ray, sputum culture etc) do not form easily recognizable patterns.

VIRALPNEUMONIAS

Are more common in children and the virus most often involved is the RSV (respiratory syncytial virus). RSV pneumonia is hard to distinguish from other respiratory infections of infancy. Viral pneumonia in adults is rare but serious and can be a fatal complication of influenza.

ASPIRATION

Of food, vomit, chemicals or foreign bodies can cause serious bronchop-neumonia (so remember the recovery position* and never induce vomiting in someone who has swallowed a caustic liquid or petrol!).

* See chapter 29.

PLEURISY

Means painful inflammation of the pleural surfaces and is usually accompanied by the presence of fluid in the pleural space – a **pleural effusion**.

Irritation of the pleura and pleural effusions complicate a number of conditions (including acute and chronic lung infections, heart failure and malignancy).

Symptoms:

Dyspnoea and pleuritic pain.

Management:

Treat the underlying cause.

ACUTE BRONCHITIS

Minor acute respiratory tract infection (usually of viral origin) occurring in adults or children.

Symptoms:

Fever, cough, shortness of breath.

Signs:

Purulent sputum if secondary bacterial infection.
Diffuse wheezes and crackles.

Management:

Antibiotics may shorten illness if bacterial infection present.

INFLUENZA

A common epidemic infectious disease characterized by fever, malaise and respiratory symptoms.

The **Influenza A** virus causes widespread epidemics and has the habit of changing its antigenic nature from time to time. This makes it hard for the human population to develop resistance to 'flu since immunity to one antigenic variant (eg "Asian" 'flu) will not necessarily confer immunity to another (eg "Hong Kong" 'flu).

The **Influenza B** virus causes more localized outbreaks of a milder illness.

Epidemiology:

Influenza is a more serious disease than many people realize. It is highly infectious (via droplet infection) and, when complicated by secondary bacterial pneumonia, is an important cause of death amongst the elderly.*

Epidemics reach a peak between December and January with Influenza B outbreaks occurring every 2 years. A short incubation period aids the rapid spread of infection.

Clinical features:

Abrupt onset of fever, shivering and generalized aching of limbs and back followed by severe headache, sore throat, persistent dry cough, retrosternal discomfort and sore eyes. Sometimes vomiting and diarrhoea. Symptoms subside after 2 - 5 days, but cough may persist. Depression and tiredness are common during convalescence.

Unless an epidemic is known to be in progress, it is often hard to make a clinical diagnosis of influenza without microbiological or immunological evidence.

Complications:

The most common complication of influenza is secondary bacterial infection of the respiratory tract (anything from mild bronchitis to fatal pneu-

---

* The worldwide influenza "pandemic" of 1918-19 was responsible for over 20,000,000 deaths.

monia). Respiratory complications are much more likely in patients with pre-existing lung disease. Most serious of all is staphylococcal pneumonia, which presents as rapid onset of breathlessness, cyanosis, haemoptysis and shock.

Post infective encephalomyelitis is another (rare) complication of influenza.

Management:

There is no orthodox treatment for uncomplicated influenza. Respiratory complications are treated in hospital with antibiotics. The antigenic antics of the influenza virus make vaccination only partially successful and adverse reactions to the available vaccines are common.* There is, however, a case for immunizing the elderly and those with chronic heart, lung or kidney disease.

---

*   Allergy to egg is a contraindication to 'flu vaccination.

BRONCHIECTASIS

Bronchiectasis means dilation of the bronchi.

> It is a complication of respiratory tract disease and is often associated with a history of childhood chest infection (TB, pneumonia, whooping cough etc).

Clinical features:

> The dilated bronchi become stagnant backwaters of infected mucus and thus clinical features of bronchiectasis include recurrent chest infection, persistent cough, haemoptysis, clubbing and abnormal chest signs such as wheezes and crackles.

Management:

> Chest physiotherapy to drain sputum.
> Antibiotics and bronchodilators as required.

PNEUMOTHORAX

Pneumothorax means accumulation of air in the pleural space.

Tears in the pleura can be caused by trauma (eg stab wounds) or by lung disease (TB, lung cancer etc) but pneumothorax can occur spontaneously in fit young people.

Clinical features:

Air in the pleural space leads to lung collapse on the affected side. Small pneumothoraces may cause no symptoms at all but larger ones produce chest pain, shortness of breath and cyanosis.

In the condition known as **tension pneumothorax,** the pleural tear may act as a one way valve so that every inward breath draws more air into the pleural cavity. Since the air cannot escape, the chest contents are pushed progressively sideways and this may lead to cardiorespiratory arrest.

Management:

Small pneumothoraces resolve spontaneously.

Larger ones may require hospital treatment involving the insertion of a "chest drain", a tube which lets the air out and allows the underlying lung to reinflate.

Tension pneumothorax is an emergency requiring immediate insertion of a chest drain.

PULMONARY EMBOLUS

Embolus in the pulmonary circulation.

If a chunk of blood clot breaks off from a thrombus in a peripheral vein, it will travel via the inferior or superior vena cava to the right side of the heart and on into the pulmonary circulation. If it gets stuck, it will cut off the blood supply to a part of the lung and lung tissue will infarct. This may lead to respiratory failure and death.

Risk factors:

Deep vein thromboses (see chapter 10) are the main source of pulmonary emboli. Thus the risk factors for pulmonary embolus are immobility (eg post surgery), trauma, pregnancy, the oral contraceptive pill, heart attack and stroke.

Clinical features:

Pleuritic pain, shortness of breath, coughing up blood, cyanosis and shock.

Treatment:

Support vital functions.
Anticoagulants.

Prognosis:

Good if the patient survives the acute phase.

CHILDHOOD DISEASES

BRONCHIOLITIS

Is an epidemic disease of young children, common in the 3 months – 3 year age group (males more than females). Most cases are caused by the respiratory syncytial virus (RSV). Mortality is between 2 and 5%.

Symptoms result from widespread inflammation of the bronchial tree. Inflammatory oedema and thick bronchial secretions obstruct the airways.

Clinical features:

The illness starts with fever, catarrh and cough and, after about 24 hours, the child becomes extremely unwell with a respiratory rate of over 40/min. Expiration takes longer than inspiration and there may be intercostal recession* and an expiratory wheeze. Feeding becomes difficult and exacerbates the breathing difficulties. In severe cases, cyanosis may occur. Widespread fine crackles are found on auscultation. Secondary bacterial infection is common.

It is often hard to distinguish bronchiolitis from asthma (which tends to come and go) and bronchopneumonia (in which airway obstruction is less striking).

Management:

Since bronchiolitis is spread by droplet infection, more severe cases are isolated in hospital and nursed in an oxygen enriched, humid atmosphere. Tube feeding may be necessary. Antibiotics have no place in the management except in cases of bacterial superinfection. Steroids and artificial ventilation are used as a last resort.

» Since RSV is a relatively common cause of non-specific upper respiratory tract infection in all age groups, it makes sense to avoid exposing infants to adults with colds and 'flu.

---

* Sucking inwards of the intercostal muscles caused by the effort of inspiration.

CROUP & ACUTE EPIGLOTTITIS

Croup (acute obstructive laryngitis of viral origin) is an infrequent but dramatic complication of several childhood viral diseases (eg measles).It mainly affects children under 3.

Clinical features:

Hoarseness, barking cough and stridor.* Stridor is caused by inflammatory oedema of the vocal cords, epiglottis and pharynx which leads to narrowing of the upper airway. In severe cases, the respiratory effort needed to overcome this obstruction produces supraclavicular, thoracic and abdominal recession and there may even be cyanosis if airway obstruction is gross.

Differential diagnosis:

Although croup is usually self limiting and not life threatening, it is hard to differentiate it clinically from the much more sinister **acute epiglottitis,** a bacterial infection caused by Haemophilus influenzae. A child with bacterial epiglottitis will be extremely ill with a high fever and is in danger of *complete* airway obstruction.

The only sure way of differentiating between croup and epiglottitis is by laryngoscopic examination *in hospital* with artificial respiratory facilities readily available.

Management:

Epiglottitis is life threatening if untreated but can be cured by appropriate antibiotics.

Children with croup feel more comfortable when nursed in an atmosphere of high humidity.

» **NEVER ATTEMPT TO EXAMINE THE THROAT OF A CHILD WITH STRIDOR – YOU MAY PROVOKE COMPLETE RESPIRATORY OB-STRUCTION ....**

---

* A sound similar to that made by an unwell crow, caused by breathing in hard though a narrowed upper airway.

WHOOPING COUGH (Pertussis)

Whooping cough (pertussis) is discussed in greater detail in chapter 7. Only the main features are restated here.

Whooping cough is an infectious disease of children characterized first by catarrh and then by paroxysmal coughing fits (accompanied by the typical "whooops") and vomiting.

The causative organism is Bordetella pertussis (which is transmitted by droplet infection).

The disease is infectious from the onset of the catarrhal symptoms and remains so until the coughing fits have abated (4 to 6 weeks).

Complications:

Patchy lung collapse and pneumonia may lead to bronchiectasis. More rarely, pyrexia or cerebral anoxia may produce convulsions but lasting brain damage is very rare indeed.

Orthodox treatment:

Good nursing and prompt antibiotic treatment IF secondary bacterial pneumonia occurs.

CYSTIC FIBROSIS

A relatively common recessively inherited disorder affecting 1 in 3000 live births and characterized by the production of abnormally thick mucus. This causes damage to any tissue that depends on watery secretions for normal functioning, eg lung, pancreas and testis. It is also associated with a high salt content of the sweat.

Clinical features:

Presents in children as pancreatic insufficiency (foul fatty faeces), poor weight gain despite good appetite and repeated lower respiratory tract infections. Bronchial obstruction and bronchiectasis may occur. Clubbing is a prominent sign. Males are infertile.

Management:

Involves restricted fat diet, vitamin and pancreatic enzyme supplements, vigorous chest physiotherapy and continuous antibiotics. Vaccination against measles and avoidance of whooping cough are also important.

Prognosis:

Poor.

13. The Gastro-intestinal System

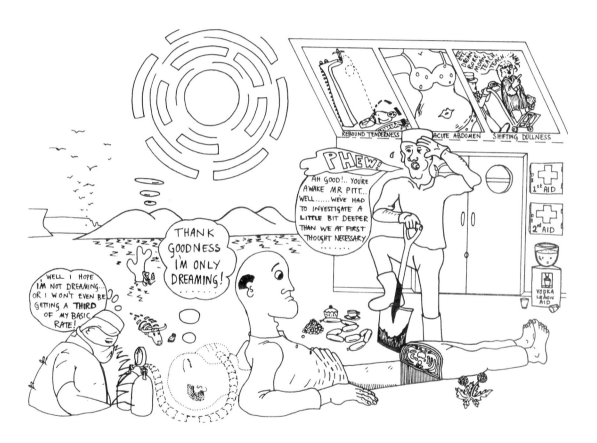

THE GASTRO-INTESTINAL SYSTEM

OVERVIEW

General

The acute abdomen
Peritonitis
Bowel obstruction

Gastrointestinal haemorrhage
Gastroenteritis

Mouth and Tongue

Stomatitis
Carcinoma of the cheek
Leucoplakia

Carcinoma of the tongue
Salivary gland disease

Oesophagus and Stomach

Hiatus hernia
Peptic ulcer

Small and Large Bowel

Inflammatory bowel disease
 (ulcerative colitis + Crohn's)
Diverticular disease
Irritable bowel syndrome
Malabsorption syndromes

Appendicitis
Hernias
Haemorrhoids

Liver and Pancreas

Jaundice (cholestasis)
Hepatitis
Cirrhosis

Gallstones
Pancreatitis

Gastrointestinal Neoplasm

Ca oesophagus
Ca stomach
Ca colon

Ca rectum
Ca pancreas
Ca liver

GENERAL

THE ACUTE ABDOMEN

A patient who becomes acutely ill with symptoms and signs relating to the abdomen is referred to* as "an acute abdomen".

Clinical features:

The spectrum of presenting symptoms and signs (plus results of basic investigations) *may* suggest a firm diagnosis but it is often surprisingly hard to choose from the following list of possible causes without performing laparotomy.**

› Rupture of an organ (spleen, aorta, ectopic pregnancy).
› Perforation of the bowel (peptic ulcer, appendicitis etc).
› Pancreatitis.
› Local peritonitis (diverticulitis, appendicitis, cholecystitis, salpingitis).
› Colic caused by muscular spasm (gall bladder, gut, ureter, uterus).
› Bowel obstruction.

The above are so-called **"surgical"** cases.

The following are possible "medical" causes of an acute abdomen:

› Myocardial infarction
› Gastroenteritis
› Urinary tract infection
› Diabetes
› Pneumonia
› TB
› Malaria
› Typhoid
› Cholera

---

*   by doctors.
**   Exploratory abdominal operation.

Management:

Whilst the Accident and Emergency doctors are deciding whether to operate or not, most "acute abdomens" will be put to bed "nil by mouth" with a drip to maintain fluid balance. Pain relief is only given when a course of diagnosis/action has been decided upon.

PERITONITIS

Peritonitis means inflammation of the tissue that lines the abdominal cavity and the outside of the viscera. It is potentially life threatening.

Peritonitis can be **localized** or **generalized** and is a potential complication of many abdominal conditions and surgical procedures. In other words, it is usually a **secondary** phenomenon.

Peritoneal inflammation leads to leakage of fluid into the abdominal cavity which causes a decrease in blood volume and possibly shock. The fluid acts as a culture medium for micro-organisms so the abdomen may end up filled with pus.

Furthermore, the gut tubing reacts to peritonitis by a short burst of hypermotility followed by paralytic obstruction (so called **paralytic ileus**). This further compromises the patient.

Common causes include –

> › Acute appendicitis
> › Acute cholecystitis
> › Acute salpingitis
> › Acute diverticulitis
> › Perforated peptic ulcer
> › Acute pancreatitis
> › Abdominal trauma (which includes surgery)
> › Ruptured ectopic pregnancy

Clinical features include –

> › Severe, sharp pain exacerbated by movement and coughing (pain may be referred to shoulder if diaphragmatic irritation)
> › Vomiting
> › Extreme tenderness of abdomen
> › Rigidity of abdomen (generalized peritonitis) or guarding (over areas of local peritonitis)

> › Diminished or absent bowel sounds

Management:

Resuscitation, fluid replacement, nasogastric suction and antibiotics followed by surgery (depending on underlying cause).

NOTE:

Consequences of localized peritonitis –

> › Area of inflammation may be "walled off" by surrounding tissue and eventually heal.
> › May be walled off with subsequent abscess formation.
> › May become generalized.

BOWEL OBSTRUCTION

Bowel obstruction may be either **mechanical** (in which the blocked bowel can still contract proximal to the obstruction) or **paralytic** (in which passage of bowel contents is obstructed by paralysis of the whole bowel). Paralytic obstruction is usually only seen as an early complication of abdominal surgery and thus will not be considered further here.

Mechanical obstruction of the bowel may be caused by:

> › Material getting jammed in the lumen of the gut (eg faeces, gallstones).
> › Disease of the bowel wall (eg inflammation, neoplasm).
> › Pressure on the bowel wall from outside (eg "adhesions", hernias).

Adhesions, hernias and carcinoma account for over 80% of cases of bowel obstruction.

Obstruction may occur in either the small or the large bowel –

90% of cases of small bowel obstruction are due to adhesions or "incarcerated" (jammed) hernias.

90% of cases of large bowel obstruction are the result of carcinoma, diverticular disease or volvulus (twisting of the bowel).

If the mechanical effect of the obstruction is to cut off the arterial blood supply, the affected portion of bowel will die and gangrene may follow. This state of affairs is referred to as **strangulation** of the gut.

The general clinical features of mechanical obstruction are:

› Anorexia
› Central cramp-like pain
› Nausea
› Vomiting
› Absolute constipation
› Abdominal distension and high pitched tinkling bowel sounds.

In small bowel obstruction, vomiting occurs earlier, the pain is felt more in the upper abdomen and distension is less marked.

Strangulation should be suspected if the patient is obviously very ill or shocked, if the pain becomes sharper or more constant or if signs of peritonitis develop.

Management:

Bowel obstruction is best managed in hospital where fluid replacement and nasogastric suction are the mainstays of management. Large bowel obstruction and strangulation always require surgery.

GASTROINTESTINAL HAEMORRHAGE

Vomiting of blood or the passing of blood or digested blood (melaena) rectally suggests gastrointestinal haemorrhage. Both presentations are serious; neither is much help in determining the site of the bleeding.

Diagnosis of the cause has been made much easier in recent years by the introduction of the fibre-optic endoscope and management consists of immediate resuscitation followed by medical or surgical treatment depending on the underlying pathology.

The commonest causes of upper GI tract bleeding are –

Peptic ulcers (80%).
Gastric erosions and the Mallory-Weiss syndrome* (15%).
Oesophageal varices in patients with chronic severe liver disease (5%).

---

*   Tearing the gastric mucosa by throwing up violently, eg after a drinking binge.

GASTROENTERITIS

Gastroenteritis means inflammation of the gastrointestinal tract causing diarrhoea $\pm$ vomiting and abdominal pain.

The term is commonly taken to mean "acute diarrhoea of infective origin" but, in practice, the differentiation between infective and non-infective causes of diarrhoea can only be made on the basis of a thorough history, examination plus relevant investigations.

The following points in the history are crucial:

› Is the attack an isolated event or part of a chronic history?
› If isolated and acute, is there a history of foreign travel, contact with other travellers returning from abroad, recent antibiotic therapy, or any possible relationship to food?
› If part of a recurrent pattern, has there been anorexia, weight loss, blood or mucous in the stool, laxative abuse etc?

The following causes should be considered:

Infectious:	Non-bacterial gastroenteritis (eg "travellers diarrhoea").
	Food poisoning (salmonella responsible for 75%).
	"Enteric" fevers (typhoid, paratyphoid).
	Dysentery (shigella or amoebic).
	Giardiasis.
	Campylobacter (often causes bloody diarrhoea).
Non-infectious:	Drugs (esp. antibiotics, laxatives, digoxin).
	Diverticular disease.
	Colonic carcinoma (diarrhoea may alternate with constipation).
	Irritable bowel syndrome.
	Inflammatory bowel disease.
	Malabsorption syndromes (eg coeliac disease).
	Diabetes.
	Thyrotoxicosis.

BLOODY DIARRHOEA SUGGESTS

> › Colonic carcinoma
> › Diverticular disease
> › Ulcerative colitis
> › Dysentery
> › Campylobacter enteritis
> › Ischaemic colitis

» Remember, however, that the commonest cause of **rectal** bleeding is **haemorrhoids.**

MOUTH AND TONGUE

STOMATITIS

Is the general term applied to inflammatory and ulcerative conditions affecting the mucous membranes of the mouth. (Gingivitis refers to inflammatory conditions of the gums.)

There are various types of stomatitis that you should know about:

› Aphthous stomatitis
› Herpes simplex infection
› Other viral infections
› Vincent's "angina"
› Oral thrush
› Angular stomatitis (cheilosis)
› Burns

You should also remember that the state of the oral mucosa tends to reflect general health and nutrition. Deficiencies of B vitamins, folic acid and iron may all be associated with mouth ulcers, angular stomatitis and a sore, smooth red tongue.

Immunosuppression and auto-immune disease are also often associated with stomatitis.

APHTHOUS STOMATITIS:

Refers to the periodic appearance of painful crops of small mouth ulcers which take about 2 weeks to heal. They are of varying size, round or oval in shape with a red margin and a yellowish base.

Aphthous ulceration in conjunction with conjunctival and genital lesions suggests a diagnosis of Behcet's syndrome (see chapter 24).

Aphthous ulcers plus arthritis, urethritis and conjunctivitis is called Reiter's syndrome (see chapter 18).

ORAL HERPES SIMPLEX INFECTIONS:

Include the common cold sore ("Herpes labialis") but may also present as a severe gingivostomatitis* (usually in children) in which the characteristic lesions are associated with malaise and fever.

OTHER VIRAL INFECTIONS:

Herpes zoster, chickenpox and hand, foot and mouth disease may all produce oral ulceration.

VINCENT'S ACUTE ULCERATIVE GINGIVITIS AND STOMATITIS:

This is a condition caused by Borrelia vincentii and Fusiformis fusiformis infection. If the tonsils are involved, the condition is known as **Vincent's Angina.**

In this country, Vincent's Angina is seen predominantly in young adults (sometimes associated with wisdom tooth problems) and presents with fever, malaise and pain in the mouth associated with oral ulceration. The ulcers bleed readily.

Management:

Must involve a dental surgeon. Untreated, the condition may cause severe damage to the attachment of the teeth and, in malnourished children, may even be fatal.

ORAL THRUSH:

Is seen in sick babies, the chronically ill, the immunosuppressed and the elderly. It produces thin, white, moist, cottage cheesy plaques that adhere to the oral mucous membranes (and possibly the tongue). The plaques rub off easily leaving red sore patches. Antibiotic therapy may produce atrophic candidiasis in which the main complaint is of a burning, red tongue. Poor denture hygiene may produce a similar (though less irritating) condition of the gums.

---

*   Gingivo = gums

ANGULAR STOMATITIS:

Produces moist, crusted, infected cracks at the corners of the mouth. It is often caused by toothlessness which deepens the creases at the mouth corners. The infecting organism is usually candida or Staphylococcus aureus. In fingersucking infants, the condition is referred to as *perleche.*

NOTE:

Single oral ulcers are most commonly caused by trauma (toothbrush, poor fitting denture, abrasive tooth edge etc) but remember that a persistent oral ulcer may be a malignant neoplasm.

CARCINOMA OF THE CHEEK

Is more common amongst those who smoke and drink spirits. It may also be caused by chewing tobacco or betel nut.

Management:

Radiotherapy. Surgery is performed to remove any residual or recurrent growth and to remove diseased regional lymph nodes. Skilled plastic surgery is required to achieve a reasonable cosmetic result.

LEUKOPLAKIA

Background:

Leukoplakia is the descriptive term used to describe roughened white patches on mucous membranes.

It is said that   SMOKING
SEPSIS
SYPHILIS
SPIRITS
SPICES
SHARP TEETH
LONGSTANDING THRUSH

all predispose to leucoplakia.

Management:

> **Leukoplakia is a pre-cancerous change** and an orthodox physician would advise the sufferer to give up irritant habits (ie stop smoking), and may also suggest referral to a surgeon for biopsy or excision of the lesions.

CARCINOMA OF THE TONGUE

> Has the same risk factors as leucoplakia.
>
> Occurs with equal frequency in women and men.
>
> Is often not diagnosed until late, because practitioners don't usually examine the tongue carefully.

Clinical features:

> Tongue cancer may present 1) as a raised oval plaque, an ulcer with everted edges and an indurated (hardened) base or 2) a deep infected split surrounded by an area of induration or 3) as a lobulated hardened mass. If the lingual nerve is involved, pain may be referred to the ear.
>
> Other presentations include pain in the tongue, inability to protrude the tongue, problems swallowing, problems with speech, offensive breath or a lump in the neck (caused by secondaries in regional lymph nodes).
>
> The tongue tip and edges are the most common sites.
>
> What is actually visible may be just "the tip of an iceberg."
>
> Up to 40% of cases have regional lymph nodes involvement at the time of presentation (particularly those with lesions on the posterior 1/3rd of the tongue). This carries a bad prognosis.

Orthodox management:

> Biopsy followed by a combination of radiotherapy and more or less radical surgery.

SALIVARY GLAND DISEASE

Salivary gland disease usually presents as salivary gland swelling. Salivary gland swelling may be caused by acute inflammation, chronic inflammation, tumour or retained salivary secretions.
Mumps is the commonest cause of acute salivary gland swelling.

Recurrent salivary gland swelling is usually due to salivary stones (calculi) ie **sialolithiasis.** Poor oral hygiene is a risk factor. The submandibular gland is most commonly affected since it secretes a thicker fluid than other salivary glands.

Chronic salivary gland swelling may be the result of chronic, non-suppurative infection but may also be due to tumour.

90% salivary tumours occur in the parotid gland and are more common in the over 30 age group.

The majority (up to 80%) of salivary tumours are benign and slow growing but pain, rapid growth, regional lymphadenopathy and facial nerve palsy (parotid tumours) would suggest carcinoma. Benign salivary gland tumours may undergo malignant change.

Malignant salivary gland tumours carry a poor prognosis.

Treatment of salivary neoplasm is by local excision (benign) or local excision plus radiotherapy (malignant).

You should also know about two specific salivary gland syndromes:

SJÖGREN'S* SYNDROME:

> A syndrome of unknown aetiology that often affects women close to the menopause. It is associated with connective tissue disease.
> Sufferers have red, dry eyes, arthritis, swollen parotid and lacrimal glands and a very dry mouth.

MIKULICZ** DISEASE:

> Enlargement of salivary glands associated with dry mouth.
>
> Usually affects young adults. Unknown aetiology.

---

*   A Swedish professor of opthalmology.
**   A nineteenth century Polish born surgeon.

OESOPHAGUS AND STOMACH

HIATUS HERNIA + REFLUX OESOPHAGITIS

If a part of the stomach herniates through the diaphragm into the thorax, the patient is said to have a hiatus hernia.

This causes incompetence of the oesophago-gastric sphincter mechanism which allows reflux of gastric acid into the oesophagus with consequent damage to the delicate oesophageal mucosa. Reflux may occur without hiatus hernia.

Hiatus hernia *without* reflux may not cause any symptoms.

Clinical features of reflux:

Acid regurgitation and heartburn (retrosternal burning pain) made worse by stooping.

It is often quite difficult to differentiate acid reflux from angina, peptic ulcer, diverticulitis and biliary disease.

Complications include:

Bleeding, stricture and aspiration* pneumonia (from aspiration of gastric acid).

Basic management includes:

› Losing weight
› Stopping smoking
› Raising the head of the bed
› Avoiding large meals, tight clothes and stooping

Antacids and "stomach coating" drugs like Gaviscon may help to protect the oesophageal mucosa. Surgery is sometimes attempted for intractable cases and complications.

---

* Sucking into the lungs.

PEPTIC ULCER

Ulcers may occur on the mucosal lining of the oesophagus, the stomach or the duodenum.

They may be single or multiple and vary from 1 mm to over 50 mm in diameter. They may bleed or perforate (especially the large ones) and may lead to pyloric obstruction. Gastric (stomach) ulcers may be malignant.

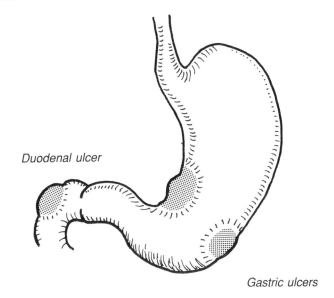

Duodenal ulcer

Gastric ulcers

Peptic ulcers are associated with –

> › Smoking
> › Blood group (duodenal → Gp O, gastric → Gp A)
> › High or low gastric acid secretion
> › NSAIAs*
> › Steroids
> › Stress
> › Hyperparathyroidism

*   Non Steroidal Anti Inflammatory Agents

Clinical features include –

> › Recurrent epigastric pain
> › A relationship of pain to food (mostly relieves)
> › Pain that wakes patient at night
> › Weight loss (usually suggests gastric ulcer)

Haematemesis, melaena and vomiting would suggest complications (haemorrhage or perforation). Definitive diagnosis depends on contrast radiography* and endoscopy with biopsy to exclude malignancy.

Management:

Depends on the site of the ulcer. Stopping smoking, losing weight, eating small amounts frequently, avoiding stress and taking simple antacids may all help. The orthodox drugs cimetidine or ranitidine will heal a large proportion of ulcers after about 8 weeks. Carbenoxolone (derived from liquorice) may help **gastric** ulcers to heal. Surgery may be life saving in complicated PU disease but is also used as an alternative to drug treatment in many cases (esp. intractable, recurrent disease).

Prognosis:

Ulcers tend to recur despite treatment. Over a 4 year period about 50% of duodenal ulcers will recur after drug therapy (but only 10% after surgical intervention).

---

*   Barium meal.

SMALL AND LARGE BOWEL

INFLAMMATORY BOWEL DISEASE

The term "inflammatory bowel disease" refers to two conditions, ulcerative colitis and Crohn's disease.

ULCERATIVE COLITIS:

Clinical features:

A recurrent inflammatory disease of the colon/rectum characterized by mucosal ulcers in the bowel wall. It presents as episodes of profuse diarrhoea (with blood, pus and mucus) plus fever, abdominal pain and dehydration. There may also be history of weight loss.

Complications:

Include bowel perforation and "toxic dilatation" of the colon (both of which may be fatal).

CROHN'S DISEASE:

A chronic inflammatory disorder affecting *any part* of the bowel* in a patchy manner. It is characterized by full thickness inflammation of the bowel wall plus submucosal ulcers and cracks.

Crohn's disease is becoming more common. The average age of onset is 27 years.

Clinical features:

Diarrhoea (usually no blood) plus fever.

Complications:

› Perianal abscesses and fistulae
› Bowel obstruction

---

*   but particularly the terminal ileum.

> › Bowel perforation with abscess formation; may produce fistulae into other parts of bowel, bladder or vagina
> › Symptoms and signs of malabsorption

It is sometimes hard to differentiate Crohn's from UC. It can also be confused with appendicitis.

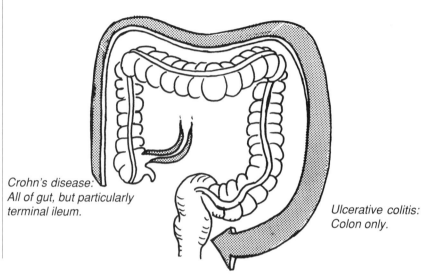

Crohn's disease:
All of gut, but particularly
terminal ileum.

Ulcerative colitis:
Colon only.

Aetiology:

The aetiology of inflammatory bowel disease is not understood. Infection, allergy, auto-immunity and psychogenic mechanisms have all been suggested.

Crohn's seems to be associated with the "western" lifestyle.

Both conditions can give rise to a strange spectrum of associated conditions including iritis, erythema nodosum, arthritis, skin rashes and hepatitis. Both conditions also carry a risk of colonic carcinoma depending on the duration of the illness (risk ↑++ after 10 years with UC).

Diagnosis:

Depends on contrast radiography* plus sigmoidoscopy with biopsy.

* ie barium meal or barium enema.

Management:

Consists of supportive treatment in hospital during acute exacerbations plus the use of **oral steroids** and **steroid enemas**. Salazopyrin (sulpha-salazine) can help prevent relapse.

Failure of medical treatment, complications and the risk or appearance of malignancy are indications for **surgery.** This may involve the removal of most of the large bowel. Faecal material is then eliminated via a **stoma** (ileostomy or colostomy).

About 70% of Crohn's patients eventually require surgery (20% in UC).

DIVERTICULAR DISEASE

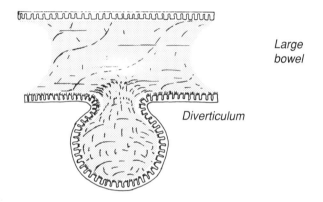

Large bowel

Diverticulum

A diverticulum is an outpouching of the gut wall.
Diverticular disease is the state of having diverticula in the bowel.
Inflammation of diverticula is called **diverticulitis.**

It is thought that the low fibre diet of many "civilized" countries causes high pressures within the gut which force the gastrointestinal mucosa to herniate through the muscle layers, producing diverticula. Most diverticula occur in the **sigmoid** colon.

Classic features of diverticulitis:

Lower abdominal pain + bloody diarrhoea. Diverticulitis may also cause profuse rectal bleeding. The syndrome may resemble appendicitis (but the pain is on the **left** side). Even without inflammation, the presence of diverticula may cause colicky abdominal pain.

Complications include:

> › stricture
> › obstruction
> › perforation
> › peritonitis
> › adhesions
> › fistulae into bladder or vagina

Perforation of a diverticulum is a relatively common cause of sudden death in the elderly.

Treatment of diverticular disease:

High fibre diet. Acute diverticulitis requires hospitalization, nil by mouth, antibiotics and pain relief. Complications will require surgical intervention.

IRRITABLE BOWEL SYNDROME

Is the label given to the syndrome of recurrent abdominal pain (± distension) with diarrhoea and/or constipation "in the absence of any demonstrable organic pathology."

Psychological factors are said to be important but symptoms can be triggered by antibiotic therapy, food poisoning and food intolerance. High fibre diet often helps but over 50% of sufferers find that orthodox therapy brings little or no relief.

MALABSORPTION SYNDROMES

There are many causes of gastrointestinal malabsorption. **Coeliac disease** is the major cause in the UK. Coeliac disease is caused by an intolerance to the wheat protein **gluten.** Gluten hypersensitivity causes the villi of the gut lining to atrophy with consequent malabsorption of food (including vitamins and minerals). It is usually diagnosed in childhood.

Clinical features include:

> › Loose, bulky foul smelling stools which are hard to flush away (fat malabsorption) –
> › Weight loss (fat/protein deficiency) –
> › Oedema (protein deficiency) –
> › Flatulence/abdominal distension (inefficient sugar breakdown) –
> › Anaemia (iron, folate and B12 deficiency) –

> › Peripheral "neuritis" (B-complex deficiency) –
> › Swollen red tongue, angular stomatitis (B-complex deficiency) –
> › Bone problems (calcium and vitamin D deficiency) –
> › Pins + needles or muscle spasm (calcium or magnesium deficiency) –
> › Bleeding (vitamin K deficiency) –
> › Weak muscles, heart arrhythmias (potassium deficiency) –
> › Low blood pressure (water and electrolyte deficiency) –
> › Clubbing (well, why not .....)

Coeliac disease is sometimes associated with an extremely itchy skin condition called **dermatitis herpetiformis**.

Management:

A gluten free diet .....

Other causes of malabsorption include:

Defective secretions:	Liver or biliary tract obstruction Pancreatic insufficiency
Inadequate digestion:	Gut "resection" Intestinal "hurry" following gastric surgery for PU disease
Damage to bowel lining:	Tropical "sprue" Crohn's disease
Infiltration of bowel wall:	TB Lymphoma Carcinoma Systemic sclerosis
Drugs:	Antacids Neomycin Cholestyramine Colchicine

Parasites in gut or change in intestinal flora from infection.

Enzyme deficiencies.

Intestinal ischaemia.

ACUTE APPENDICITIS

It is surprisingly difficult to diagnose this condition correctly.

As the name suggests, appendicitis results from inflammation of the appendix. It seems to be associated with low fibre diet, obstruction of the lumen of the appendix by faecal matter and eventual infection of the inflamed tissue by normal intestinal flora.

Clinical features:

As the inflammation begins, the patient experiences **central** colicky abdominal pain referred to the centre of the abdomen. Once the peritoneum becomes involved, the pain shifts to the **right iliac fossa.**

Abdominal pain may be accompanied by nausea and vomiting.

Signs:

Fever, fast pulse, furred tongue, flushed face, lying still, shallow breathing with acute tenderness in the RIF.

The differential diagnosis includes:

› Perforated peptic ulcer
› Food poisoning
› Cholecystitis
› Diverticulitis
› Cystitis
› Salpingitis
› Crohn's disease
› Inflammation of mesenteric lymph nodes

Complications include:

Perforation → peritonitis
Abscess formation

Treatment:

Surgical removal of the appendix (ASAP).

HERNIAS

A hernia is the protrusion of an organ (or part of that organ) through an abnormal opening.

5% of the population have external abdominal hernias –

> 73% in the inguinal region
> 17% through the femoral canal
> 8.5% umbilical
> 1.5% in other places

An external abdominal hernia usually consists of a peritoneal sac* covered by the layers of abdominal wall through which it passed and will contain a portion of bowel, bladder or whatever in a sac of peritoneum.

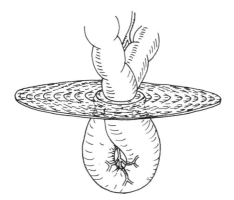

A loop of bowel herniating through an abnormal opening in a muscle. The peritoneal sac and other coverings are not shown.

Hernias may be **congenital** (primary) or **secondary.** Secondary hernias may be caused by raised intra-abdominal pressure (cough, constipation, pregnancy, carcinoma) or by old surgical incisions that produce abdominal wall weakness.

Hernias may be classified as:

Reducible → May only "come out" when patient stands up and can be "put back" relatively easily.

Irreducible → Can't be "put back".

---

* Often containing some bowel, bowel wall or bladder.

Complications:

Bowel obstruction
Strangulation
Perforation
Peritonitis

» A tender irreducible hernia in the absence of abdominal pain is simply a tender irreducible hernia. However, persistent abdominal pain, oedema and redness of skin over the hernia plus other symptoms and signs of intestinal obstruction may imply strangulation and hence constitute a surgical emergency.

Management:

Surgery is the recommended treatment for ANY external abdominal hernia (after appropriate attention to weight reduction, stopping smoking etc). Surgical supports are rarely of any use.

NOTE:

Femoral hernias often occur in females and are more prone to strangulation than inguinal hernias.

HAEMORRHOIDS (Piles)

Vascular swellings of the rectal mucosa caused by varicosities of the haemorrhoidal veins.*

Background:

The haemorrhoidal veins have no valves and are thus prone to become distended. In a person with chronic constipation, who has to strain to defecate, this tendency is much exaggerated and the veins may become varicose and inflamed. Thus **low fibre diet** could be said to be the main risk factor for piles. Pelvic tumours, pregnancy, heart failure and portal hypertension (see later) are also associated with haemorrhoids.

---

*   The haemorrhoidal veins drain into the inferior mesenteric veins which in turn connect with the portal vein.

Clinical features:

Bright red rectal bleeding, either coating the faeces or dripping/spurting out after defecation, is the principal complaint.

Frequent small bleeds can lead to anaemia. The increased mucus produced by the inflamed rectal mucosa over the piles may cause irritation and itchy bottom.

Piles may also prolapse out of the rectum on defecation and go back in afterwards ("second degree haemorrhoids") or may prolapse and stay prolapsed ("third degree haemorrhoids"). Prolapsed piles gripped by the anal sphincter can thrombose causing inflammation and intense pain. As with anal fissure,* this sets up a vicious circle where the constipated sufferer tries to avoid painful defecation and thus becomes more constipated, which further exacerbates the situation.

Management:

In the early stages, high fibre diet plus exercise usually resolves the problem. It is also important to treat any co-existing cough. Pain relieving suppositories and ointments may also help. However, many sufferers only find relief from one of the variety of surgical procedures available (ranging from injection of the piles with a sclerosant chemical – an outpatient procedure – to haemorrhoidectomy).

Remember, any patient complaining of rectal bleeding must have an abdominal examination and a rectal examination. Non-prolapsed piles are not palpable on rectal examination but many rectal cancers are and these must be excluded. Definitive diagnosis of internal haemorrhoids is made using a proctoscope (a small rigid tube that enables the examiner to see the rectal mucosa).

---

*   Small, acutely painful longitudinal split of the anal mucosa.

LIVER AND PANCREAS

JAUNDICE

Background:

When red blood cells die or are destroyed, bilirubin is formed from the breakdown of their haemoglobin. The body can't excrete bilirubin until it is made water soluble by a process called **conjugation,** which takes place in the liver.

After conjugation in the liver cells, bilirubin is released as a component of bile into the bile ducts and then passes either to the gallbladder for temporary storage or out via the common bile duct into the duodenum.

Bilirubin is converted in the gut to a substance called **urobilinogen**. Some of this passes out of the body with the faeces; the rest is reabsorbed into the bloodstream and is then excreted in the urine via the kidneys.

Jaundice means too much bilirubin in the blood which makes the skin and the sclerae go orangey-yellow. With a little thought, it becomes clear that there must be 2 basic situations in which jaundice will occur:

1) The liver may be unable to *conjugate* all the bilirubin presented to it (eg in **haemolytic** conditions such as malaria), in which case the excess bilirubin in the blood will be UNconjugated and thus INsoluble and will NOT appear in the urine – so called **acholuric jaundice**.

2) The liver may be unable to *excrete* the conjugated bilirubin produced by its cells. In this case the conjugated bilirubin formed within the cells regurgitates back into the bloodstream and (since it is water soluble) it eventually appears in the urine which is thus coloured dark brown – so called **cholestatic jaundice**. By the same token, since bilirubin isn't reaching the gut, the faeces will be the colour of putty!

Thus the first test which anybody can perform on a jaundiced patient is to see if there is any bilirubin in the urine (dip sticks available from chemists!).

A little bit more thought will show that cholestatic jaundice may be the result of either liver cell disruption as in hepatitis, primary biliary cirrhosis or drug damage (so called **intrahepatic cholestasis**) OR be the result of mechanical blockage of the biliary plumbing by gallstones, tumour, stricture, clot etc (so called **extrahepatic cholestasis**).

Some of the conditions causing jaundice will be described below but, as a rule of thumb, always ask jaundiced patients about:

› DRUGS
› FOREIGN TRAVEL (never forget malaria)
› ALCOHOL
› CONTACTS WITH OTHER JAUNDICED PEOPLE
› RECENT BLOOD TRANSFUSIONS
› SEXUAL BEHAVIOUR

In western medicine the treatment of acholuric and intrahepatic cholestatic jaundice is **medical** whilst the management of extrahepatic cholestatic jaundice is **surgical.**
A variety of sophisticated diagnostic techniques are available to try and make the necessary distinctions between the different types of jaundice.

HEPATITIS

Means inflammation of liver cells and has a variety of possible causes:

Viral: Hepatitis A, B and nonA-nonB
Other infections: Glandular fever
                        Leptospirosis
Alcohol:
Drugs: Paracetamol
                        Halothane
                        Methyldopa
                        Barbiturates

Only viral hepatitis is considered here.

HEPATITIS A:

"Infectious" hepatitis spread by faecal-oral route, common in institutions, often passes unnoticed in childhood.

› Incubation 2-6 weeks.
› Prodrome of anorexia, malaise, nausea, fever and joint pain.
› As fever settles, jaundice appears plus tender enlarged liver, enlarged spleen and lymphadenopathy.
› One attack probably gives life-long immunity.
› Passive immunization is available for 3-6 month protection.
› No specific treatment but avoid alcohol for 6 months.
› Mortality 0.5%.

HEPATITIS B:

"Serum" hepatitis. Spread by blood, secretions and sexual intercourse.

› Heroin addicts, haemophiliacs, homosexuals and haemodialysis patients and hospital staff are all at risk.
› Incubation period 1 to 6 months (some people are asymptomatic carriers).
› Prodrome as for hepatitis A followed by jaundice as patient starts to feel better. Jaundice lasts 4 weeks. Liver and spleen may be enlarged.
› Complex blood tests reveal disease type and indicate degree of infectivity of patient to others. One of the tests is referred to as the HBsAg or Australia antigen test.
› Active and passive vaccines available.
› Supportive treatment with barrier nursing and great care over handling blood and secretions is the basis of management.
› Prognosis generally good but may lead to chronic liver disease.

HEPATITIS nonA-nonB:

Is a "diagnosis of exclusion" and sometimes seen as a complication of blood transfusion. It is not as serious as hepatitis B.

CIRRHOSIS

The term **cirrhosis** implies that the architecture of the liver has been irreversibly damaged by fibrosis (scarring).

In 50% of cases, a cause is not found.
25% of cases are the result of **alcohol abuse**.
Hepatitis B infection may also lead to cirrhosis and there are a number of other possible causes, all rare, which will not be discussed here.

Background:

To understand the effects of cirrhosis it is necessary to review some basic liver anatomy, histology and physiology:

1) The liver is supplied with oxygenated blood via the **hepatic artery**.

2) *All* the blood from the gut (from the lower oesophagus to the anus) flows into the **portal vein** and is carried to the liver for "processing".

3) The many terminal branches of the portal vein and the hepatic artery run next to each other within the liver substance and eventually drain

into **sinusoids** which are minute channels passing between the sheets of liver cells.

4) After passing amongst the liver cells in this way, blood passes into small **central veins** which eventually unite to form the large **hepatic vein** which then drains "processed" blood into the **inferior vena cava**.

5) The **portal** venous system is **connected** (through the diaphragm) with oesophageal tributaries of the **azygos** vein thus forming a **porto-systemic** connection. Other porto-systemic connections exist eg between the portal system and the veins of the abdominal wall in the para-umbilical region.

6) The main functions of the liver are **synthesis, detoxification and secretion.**

Clinical features:

The destruction of liver cell architecture that develops in cirrhosis has two serious consequences:

1) portal venous obstruction

2) liver cell failure

» *Portal venous obstruction* produces high pressures in the portal venous system (ie portal hypertension) and may result in:

› Ascites (fluid in the abdominal cavity).
› Enlarged spleen.
› Oesophageal varices (may cause acute massive haemorrhage and haematemesis if they burst).

Oesophageal varices

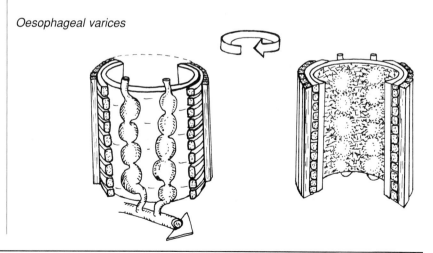

» *Partial failure of liver cell function* may produce:

› Jaundice (often associated with itching).
› Red palms.
› White nails.
› Gynaecomastia.
› Palmar contracture affecting the little and ring fingers (Dupuytren's contracture).
› Clubbing.
› Testicular atrophy.
› More than 5 spider naevi.

In **early cirrhosis,** further damage can be avoided by abstinence from alcohol and avoidance of damaging drugs and chemicals.

Severe cirrhosis may ultimately result in *complete liver failure* manifested as **"hepatic encephalopathy"** ie –

› Flapping tremor.
› Lethargy and amnesia progressing through delirium to stupor.
› Coma and death.

Hepatic encephalopathy is irreversible and its hospital management is directed towards relieving symptoms.

Note that certain drugs (eg paracetamol, methyldopa, halothane anaesthetic), poisons (eg carbon tetrachloride) and infections (eg viral hepatitis) can cause *acute* massive liver cell death and thus acute liver failure. Although the symptoms and signs of liver failure are the same in either case, the patient with cirrhosis has a **chronic** condition with symptoms and signs of liver failure that develop in an insidious manner.

Note also that patients with cirrhosis have an increased risk of developing liver cell carcinoma (10% cases).

PRIMARY BILIARY CIRRHOSIS

Is a progressive disease of unknown aetiology characterized by the gradual destruction of the intrahepatic bile ducts and liver cells. It may be of auto-immune origin.

Clinical features:

The "classic" presentation is of **a middle aged woman complaining of itching**. Other clinical features include enlargement of liver and spleen, skin hyperpigmentation and obstructive jaundice. Clubbing, hairyness, xanthelasma, bone problems and signs of other auto-immune syndromes may also occur.

Orthodox management:

Drug treatment with penicillamine and cholestyramine plus vitamin K, D and A supplements may help to relieve symptoms. However, death from liver failure or general infection is usual within 10 years of diagnosis.

GALLSTONES (cholelithiasis)

Up to 15% of the population in western developed countries have gall-stones. The majority of these are asymptomatic.

Bile contains cholesterol, bile pigments from broken down haemoglobin and phospholipids. If the relative concentrations of these components are altered for any reason, various types of gallstones may form.

In conditions causing **haemolysis** small "pigment" stones (invisible on X-ray) are common.

In the **elderly,** the **obese** and people on **oral contraceptives** or **steroids,** there is a tendency towards the formation of large "cholesterol" stones (also invisible on X-ray).

Many gallstones are a mixture of components, and are called "mixed" stones; about 10% of these will show up on X-ray.

Various other factors predispose to gallstone formation, particularly the western high protein, high fat diet. Infection and stasis of bile flow due to anatomical anomalies of the biliary tree are also aetiological factors. Diabetics and patients with Crohn's disease have a particular tendency to develop gallstones.

Gallstones may produce a variety of clinical pictures:

The most common are:

> › Acute cholecystitis*
> › Chronic cholecystitis
> › Biliary colic
> › Obstructive type jaundice from obstruction of common bile duct

Other presentations include:

> › Cholangitis (infection of the bile ducts which presents as jaundice accompanied by septicaemia)
> › Empyema (a very ill patient and a gallbladder filled with pus)
> › Gallstone ileus (where a gallstone perforates out of the gallbladder and into the gut, possibly causing obstruction)
> › Chance finding on routine X-ray.

ACUTE CHOLECYSTITIS:

Presents with right sided upper abdominal pain, fever, vomiting and signs of localized peritonitis (extreme tenderness, rebound tenderness and localized "guarding").

Lay two fingers on the middle of the right hypochondrium and ask patient to breathe in. If this causes considerable discomfort, it suggests an inflamed gallbladder (Murphy's sign). It is often hard to differentiate acute cholecystitis from peptic ulcer, pancreatitis, appendicitis and hepatitis. Even myocardial infarction, pneumonia and pleurisy may be confused with it.
A variety of diagnostic imaging techniques are employed in hospital to help visualize gallbladder/biliary tree pathology. Ultrasound is one of the most popular and least dangerous investigations used.

Management:

Nil by mouth, pain relief and intravenous antibiotics in the acute phase followed by early or delayed removal of the gallbladder (cholecystectomy) to avoid recurrence. Operative mortality up to 1%. Early operation avoids risk of perforation.

---

*   Cholecystitis means inflammation of the gallbladder.

CHRONIC CHOLECYSTITIS:

Presents as intermittent colicky abdominal pain due to chronic inflammation of the gallbladder.

Management:

Investigation.
Cholecystectomy.

BILIARY COLIC:

Severe, colicky, right upper abdominal pain radiating to the back (sometimes), often accompanied by jaundice.

Management:

Pain relief followed by investigation, operative exploration of biliary plumbing and, usually, removal of gallbladder.

PANCREATITIS

May be ACUTE or CHRONIC.

ACUTE PANCREATITIS:

An acute inflammatory reaction affecting the pancreas and surrounding tissues. This may result in large amounts of enzyme rich fluid leaking into the abdominal cavity.

Common causes include **gallstones** and **alcohol excess** but many cases are **idiopathic**.

Rare causes include **mumps**, surgical trauma, steroid therapy, diuretic therapy, polyarteritis nodosa, hyperlipidaemia and any blockage of the pancreatic duct (stones, tumours, worms).

Considering the nature of the chemicals produced by the pancreas in health, it is not surprising that inflammation of the organ can result in haemorrhage and necrosis of pancreatic tissue.

Death (around 17% cases) may be caused by shock or renal failure, overwhelming infection of the damaged tissues or respiratory failure (from "shock lung").

Clinical features:

Central abdominal pain radiating to the back associated with vomiting and varying degrees of abdominal tenderness.
May go into shock.
Signs may be relatively few even in serious disease.

The appearance of "bruised" looking discoloration around the umbilicus or on the flanks (a reflection of the internal haemorrhagic process) would imply very serious illness.*

Once again, it can be hard to differentiate acute pancreatitis from any other cause of acute abdomen (or from MI for that matter) but a blood test showing a high level of the enzyme **serum amylase** would be highly suggestive of the diagnosis.

Management:

› Admission to hospital.
› Urgent correction of shock with intravenous fluids.
› Nil by mouth.
› Pain relief.
› Frequent assessment.

"In extremis", surgery to wash out the abdomen ("peritoneal lavage") may be performed.

---

* and is extremely rare.

CHRONIC PANCREATITIS:

Associated with	$\rightarrow$	**Alcoholism**
		Malabsorption syndromes
		Hyperparathyroidism
Characterized by	$\rightarrow$	Prolonged ill health
		Recurrent central abdominal pain
		(radiating to back)
		Steatorrhoea (fatty stools)
		Diabetes

Management:

› Pancreatic enzyme supplements
› A low fat diet
› Avoidance of alcohol
› Vitamin supplements

Intractable pain may be relieved by surgery to remove part or all of the offending organ.

GASTROINTESTINAL NEOPLASM

CARCINOMA OF THE OESOPHAGUS

An unpleasant disease with a very poor prognosis.

Mostly affects males over 65.
Alcoholism, tobacco, previous corrosive damage to oesophagus and long standing anaemia (in women) are all risk factors.
It is more common in South Africa, the Caspian and some parts of mainland China.
It mostly occurs at the lower end of the oesophagus.
It is usually a squamous cell carcinoma which may spread up and down the oesophagus and locally to involve the trachea.
Metastasis is via the lymphatics.

Clinical features:

Progressive dysphagia and weight loss.
Occasionally aspiration pneumonia.

Management:

Aim is to restore the power of swallowing using a combination of surgery and radiotherapy. Only 70% are fit enough for an operation.

Prognosis:

The average post-operative survival is about 15 months.
Oesophagectomy has a 15% mortality.

CARCINOMA OF THE STOMACH

Accounts for 10 deaths per 100,000 population per year in the UK.

Associated with → gastric polyps
chronic (atrophic) gastritis
blood group A
pernicious anaemia
(and possibly eating smoked fish,
the use of food preservatives
and a number of other environmental factors).

Stomach cancers may take a variety of forms but are all **adenocarcinomas**. 50% involve the pyloric region.

Clinical features:

> ›
> ›
> › appetite   weight   (341)
> ›
> › *Extradural space   (382)*
> ›
> ›
> › Enlarged left supraclavicular lymph node

Management:

Contrast radiography and endoscopy + biopsy provide the diagnosis but treatment is often directed towards relieving symptoms since surgery will be of no use in at least 60% of patients (in whom the cancer will have spread to other organs by the time a diagnosis is made).

Prognosis:

15% of cases are alive 5 years after diagnosis .....

CARCINOMA OF THE COLON/RECTUM

Predisposing factors:

> › Ulcerative colitis
> › Crohn's
> › Polyps
> › Low fibre diet

May cause:

> › Rectal bleeding
> › Change in bowel habit
> › Pain
> › Anaemia
> › Weight loss
> › Obstruction
> › Perforation
> › Fistulae
> › Ascites
> › Jaundice

Diagnosis:

> Rectal examination.*
> Barium enema and sigmoidoscopy.

Management:

> Surgical but depends on the extent of disease at diagnosis.

Prognosis:

> Caught early, 90% will be alive 5 years after surgery.
> If there are widespread metastases at presentation, 5 year survival is only 5%.

---

* 70% occur at the junction between the sigmoid colon and rectum.

CARCINOMA OF THE PANCREAS

Background:

The incidence of Ca pancreas is increasing in developed countries. It is seen in smokers and diabetics, often between 50 and 60 years of age.

Pathology:

80% are adenocarcinomas, 2/3rds of which are found in the **head** of the gland. They tend to be poorly differentiated and to spread quickly. Local spread may involve all nearby structures (including common bile duct, producing jaundice). Liver and lymph node metastases are early features.

Clinical features:

› Weight loss
› Epigastric pain (relieved by sitting forward)
› Jaundice
› Fatty stools
› Sudden onset diabetes
› Migratory spontaneous peripheral vein thrombosis
› Acute pancreatitis

Since the pancreas sits behind the peritoneum, symptoms are often rather vague, which delays diagnosis and hence worsens the prognosis.

Management:

Symptom relief.

Prognosis:

The overall 5 year survival is 2%.

NEOPLASTIC DISEASE OF THE LIVER

May be primary or secondary:

Secondary growth (from lung, breast, stomach, colon etc) is more common than primary cancer.

Primary liver cancers (the commonest are known as a **hepatomas**) have a dreadful prognosis and are more common in Africa, Malaya, China and Japan than in Europe.

Risk factors for hepatoma include cirrhosis and persistent hepatitis B infection.

Clinical features of liver secondaries:

> Enlarged, hard, irregular liver
> Jaundice
> Liver failure
> Ascites
> Inferior vena cava obstruction (eg leg oedema)

Treatment:

There is no completely effective orthodox treatment for liver malignancy. Liver transplant is a singularly heroic undertaking for all concerned.

14. The Endocrine System

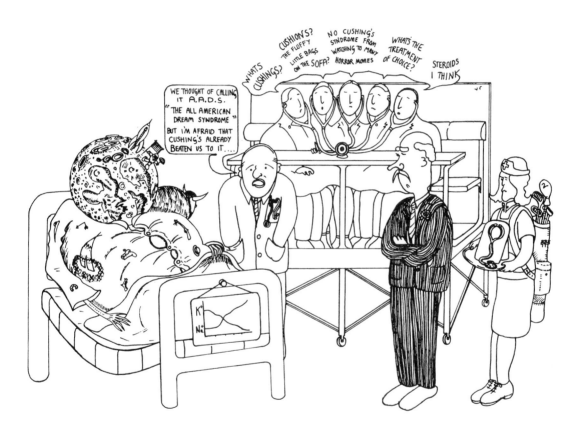

THE ENDOCRINE SYSTEM

OVERVIEW

Thyroid Disease

Hyperthyroidism
Hypothyroidism
Thyroid malignancy

Pituitary Problems

Pituitary tumours
Hyperprolactinaemia
Acromegaly
Hypopituitarism
Diabetes insipidus

Adrenal Problems

Cushing's disease
Adrenal insufficiency (Addison's disease)
Conn's syndrome
Phaeochromocytoma

Parathyroid Problems

Hyperparathyroidism
Hypoparathyroidism

NOTE:

Growth problems, gynaecomastia, hirsutism and impotence are complaints frequently referred to endocrinologists. Their differential diagnosis is considered in chapter 30.

A number of endocrine conditions are also classed as organ specific auto-immune disorders – ie Addison's disease, Hashimoto's disease, idiopathic hypoparathyroidism and premature ovarian failure.

THE PITUITARY AND ITS TARGET ORGANS

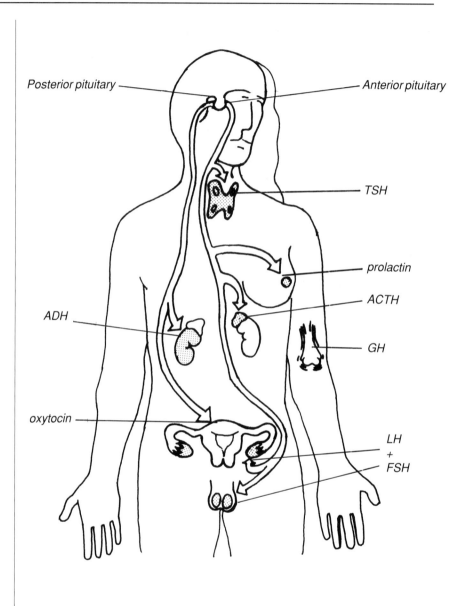

THYROID DISEASE

Thyroid problems are relatively common.

Background:

Thyroid enlargement* may be associated with hyperthyroidism or hypo-thyroidism or may simply be caused by a "non-toxic" goitre which neither under- nor over-produces thyroid hormones.

Thyroid problems usually present either with the symptoms and signs of hyper- or hypothyroidism or as a complaint of a lump in the neck (± symptoms and signs of hormone disturbance).

If the thyroid is enlarged, the problem is to exclude **malignancy** (which may be amenable to orthodox management). Unfortunately, it is very difficult to rule out thyroid cancer by clinical examination.

HYPERTHYROIDISM

Hyperthyroidism (**thyrotoxicosis**) is the clinical syndrome produced by excess blood levels of T4** (± T3).

Aetiology:

By far the commonest cause of thyrotoxicosis is **Graves' disease*** – an auto-immune condition that runs in families and is 5 times more common in females than males.

Rarely, "toxic" single (or multiple) thyroid nodules may produce thyrotox-icosis. Overmedication with T4 in hypothyroid patients (and illicit self medication by doctors and nurses) also occurs. There are about 9 other possible causes, all of which are rare.

---

* Also known as "goitre".
** T4 = Thyroxine.
*** After a 19th century Irish physician.

Pathology:

In Graves' disease, hyperthyroidism results from the presence in the blood of IgG antibodies which bind to the TSH receptors of the thyroid follicular cells. This antibody/receptor binding stimulates thyroid hormone production. Separate immunoglobulins seem to be responsible for the thyroid enlargement and eye changes characteristic of Graves' disease (see below).

Clinical features:

The clinical features of hyperthyroidism can be worked out from a knowledge of the physiology of T4 (thyroxine).

General: Weight loss with normal appetite.
                 Fatigue.
                 Intolerance of heat.
                 Excessive sweating with warm, moist skin (esp. palms).
                 Nervousness and irritability (even apparent psychosis).

Goitre: **Diffuse thyroid swelling.**
                 Nodular thyroid swelling.

Eye: Lid retraction (sclera visible below upper lid).
                 Lid lag (eyelids lag behind sclera when patient looks down).
                 Exophthalmos (sclera visible above lower lid).
                 Periorbital puffiness.
                 Gritty feeling eyes with red, oedematous conjunctiva (chemosis) – **perhaps corneal ulceration** .
                 Impaired movement of extra-ocular muscles – may cause double vision (ophthalmoplegia); **particular problems looking upwards.**

Cardiovascular: Palpitations, shortness of breath, tachycardia, peripheral vasodilation, atrial fibrillation, heart failure.*

GI: Diarrhoea.

---

*   If ↑ BP, consider associated phaeochromocytoma and check visual acuity – may be papilloedema.

NS/MS:	Generalized muscle weakness.
	Fine tremor.
	Brisk tendon jerks.
	Association with myasthenia gravis.

Skin:	Itching, palmar erythema, spider naevi.
	Pretibial myxoedema. *

Reproductive:	Disturbed menstruation.
	Infertility.
	Loss of libido.
	Gynaecomastia.

In the above list, features characteristic of (but not always present in) Graves' disease are written in bold type. Thus –

Graves' disease produces hyperthyroidism associated with diffuse thyroid enlargement, eye abnormalities (exophthalmos etc) and swelling of the lower legs called pretibial myxoedema.

A typical case of thyrotoxicosis would present as:

> › Nervousness
> › Tiredness
> › Palpitations
> › ↑ appetite
> › ↓ weight
> › Excessive sweating
> › Heat intolerance

Always consider thyrotoxicosis in a middle aged patient with tachycardia or atrial fibrillation.

Differential diagnosis:

Thyrotoxicosis is hard to differentiate from so called "anxiety states". Orthodox diagnosis depends on blood tests of T4, T3 and TSH levels plus appropriate investigation of thyroid swellings by scans etc.

---

*   Non pitting swelling of lower legs.

Orthodox management:

1) Antithyroid drugs such as carbimazole taken for up to 18 months. 2/3rd relapse within 2 years after therapy ceases in which case surgery or radio-iodine is tried. Propranolol (a β-blocker) is sometimes used to control cardiac symptoms.

2) Radioactive iodine – simple and effective but often produces hypothyroidism! Also risk of carcinogenesis.

3) Surgery (subtotal thyroidectomy) is used after failure of drug therapy or if goitre is large or causing pressure symptoms. 80% have good result, 15% end up hypothyroid and 5% relapse. Complications of procedure include recurrent laryngeal nerve palsy and hypoparathyroidism (ie parathyroid tissue may be removed accidentally).

NOTE 1:

Although lid retraction usually responds to above treatments, exophthalmos and ophthalmoplegia may not. Correction of these may need the help of an ophthalmic surgeon.

NOTE 2:

Thyrotoxic crisis is a rare complication of uncontrolled severe hyperthyroidism with a mortality rate of 10%.
Features include hyperpyrexia, extreme muscle weakness and heart failure. Orthodox management involves emergency IV fluids, oxygen, steroids, β-blockers, carbimazole and iodine.

In patients taking carbimazole, thyrotoxic crisis may be precipitated by infection.

HYPOTHYROIDISM

Hypothyroidism is the clinical syndrome produced by decreased blood levels of T4 and T3.

It is sometimes referred to as **myxoedema** since there is a characteristic deposition of mucopolysaccharide beneath the skin which produces swelling (non-pitting) of subcutaneous tissues.

Aetiology:

Without goitre:

1) Spontaneous primary auto-immune atrophic hypothyroidism (!).
   (More common in women, may be associated with diabetes or other organ specific auto-immune disorders.)

2) Complication of thyroid surgery or radio-iodine treatment.

With goitre:

1) Hashimoto's disease (auto-immune thyroiditis + goitre).
   Usually afflicts women over 60 years old; doesn't necessarily produce hypothyroidism).

2) Drugs, especially "anti-thyroid" drugs. Also lithium, phenylbutazone.

3) Dietary iodine insufficiency.

4) Inherited problems of iodine metabolism.

Hypothyroidism may also be secondary to pituitary failure.

This is rare.

Thyroid agenesis may produce "cretinism" in infants.

(see growth problems).

Clinical features:

Symptoms develop insidiously and include:

> › Tiredness
> › Depression
> › Weight gain
> › Constipation
> › Cold intolerance
> › Hoarse voice
> › Heavy periods

Signs:

> › Typical facial appearance (periorbital puffiness and pallor)
> › Coarse cold skin, coarse dry hair
> › Slow pulse
> › Non-pitting swelling of hands, feet etc
> › Goitre (sometimes)
> › Reflex jerks have slow recovery phase (best seen with ankle jerks)

» Ischaemic heart disease often accompanies hypothyroidism.

» Hypothyroidism in an elderly person is sometimes misdiagnosed as dementia .....

» Severe hypothyroidism can produce "myxoedema madness" or even coma.

Diagnosis:

Depends on blood tests of T4, T3 and TSH levels.

Orthodox management:

Involves oral thyroxine replacement therapy – often for life. If goitre, must exclude thyroid malignancy.

THYROID MALIGNANCY

If a patient presents with a lump in the neck remember:

› Examine lump (or lumps) for tenderness, surface contour, consistency and fixity to underlying tissues.
Check if there is any regional lymphadenopathy.

› If you think there is thyroid enlargement, assess the patient's thyroid status.

› Thyroid lumps move up and down on swallowing.

› Smooth, non-painful, non-"toxic" thyroid enlargement is most unlikely to be malignancy (it is probably either Graves', Hashimoto or iodine deficiency).

› Painful thyroid swelling may be due to inflammation from a viral thyroiditis but may also relate to malignancy.

› In orthodox practice, virtually all patients with thyroid enlargement are sent for thyroid "scans".
"Hot" nodules found in scans are **not** malignant.
Cold nodules may be (but usually are not).

ALL thyroid malignancies are rare and each carries a different prognosis:

PAPILLARY CARCINOMA:

The most common. May affect young adults.

Management:

Thyroidectomy and thyroxine replacement.

Prognosis:

Quite good.

FOLLICULAR CARCINOMA:

Relatively common. Secondaries appear early and may secrete thyroxine (producing thyrotoxicosis).

Management:

Thyroidectomy plus radio-iodine to destroy metastatic lesions.

Prognosis:

Again, quite good (50% ten year survival).

ANAPLASTIC CARCINOMA:

Highly malignant, usually afflicts elderly.

Management:

Palliative radiotherapy.

Prognosis:

Dreadful.

MEDULLARY CARCINOMA:

Rare tumour that secretes calcitonin (and also ACTH, 5HT and prosta-glandins). It may coexist with phaeochromocytoma. Typical presentation would be firm thyroid swelling associated with regional lymphadenopathy and diarrhoea.

Management:

Surgery.

Prognosis:

Variable.
Close relatives should be checked for same condition.

PITUITARY PROBLEMS

Pituitary disease is rare.

PITUITARY TUMOURS

Histology:

There are three histological types of pituitary tumour, all "adenomas".

Clinical features:

The clinical features of pituitary disease depend on the nature of the pathology and the part of the gland affected.

The pituitary lies directly below the optic chiasma and pituitary tumours tend to grow upwards.

Pituitary tumours may produce illness by:

> › Local pressure
> › Secretion of hormones in unusual amounts
> › Producing hypopituitarism

Clinical features of local pressure effects:

> › Headache
> › Visual field defects (particularly bitemporal hemianopia)
> › III, IV and VIth cranial nerve palsies
> › Papilloedema (if growth obstructs CSF flow into the 3rd ventricle producing $\uparrow$ ICP*).
> › Pressure on hypothalamus may produce sleepiness, weight gain, problems in temperature control and even diabetes insipidus (see page 352).

Clinical features of abnormal hormone secretion:

> › Pituitary tumours secreting abnormal amounts of ACTH are responsible for about 10% of cases of **Cushing's syndrome.**

---

*   ICP = intracranial pressure.

› Abnormal secretion of growth hormone produces **acromegaly** (or "gigantism" in children).
› Abnormal secretion of prolactin produces the clinical syndrome of **hyperprolactinaemia**.
› **"Prolactinomas"** are the commonest hormone secreting pituitary tumours.

Clinical features of hypopituitarism:

See page 351.

Treatment:

Excess hormone secretion and pressure symptoms can be relieved by surgical removal or irradiation of the gland supplemented by drug treatment. Hypopituitarism is managed by hormone replacement.

Notes:

Deterioration of vision not correctable with spectacles and not due to eye pathology should always raise the suspicion of pituitary tumour.

Although pituitary adenomas are "benign", it is obvious from the above that they may cause severe problems; some adenomas do, in fact, take on the features of malignancy in that they start to invade the surrounding tissues.

Other tumours may affect the pituitary; craniopharyngiomas are congenital tumours that arise between the pituitary and the floor of the third ventricle and present in childhood with the effects of local pressure. Secondary tumours and meningiomas also occur in this region.

HYPERPROLACTINAEMIA

Hyperprolactinaemia is the commonest condition caused by pituitary dysfunction. It usually presents to the gynaecologists in the guise of menstrual disturbance, hirsutism and infertility. Increased blood prolactin levels also produce acne, galactorrhoea,* ↓ libido and (in males) impotence and mild gynaecomastia.

If caused by a pituitary prolactin secreting adenoma ("prolactinoma"), there may be associated local pressure effects.

Other causes of ↑ prolactin are:

› Pregnancy, breast feeding, stress and sleep (so called "physiological" causes).
› Drugs, including the phenothiazines and haloperidol (both used in the control of psychosis), methyldopa and oestrogens.
› Chronic renal failure.
› Hypothyroidism.
› Sarcoid.

Management:

Depends on underlying cause.

In practice, it may be impossible to make a firm diagnosis of the underlying cause in which case the drug bromocriptine may be used to decrease pituitary prolactin secretion. Prolactinomas are removed surgically.

---

* Milk discharge from the nipples.

ACROMEGALY

A rare condition caused by the hypersecretion of **growth hormone**, usually from a pituitary adenoma. It affects adults between 20 and 40 years of age.

Clinical features (which develop slowly):

› Increase in size of skull, supraorbital ridges and mandible (producing separation of the teeth and jutting jaw).
› Thick, spade shaped fingers, increasing shoe size and vertebral enlargement (producing kyphosis).
› Enlarged tongue, heart, liver and thyroid.
› Headache (the dura is stretched as skull enlarges).
› Skin becomes coarse and oily.
› Voice deepens.

Hypertension,heart failure, diabetes, joint pain, proximal muscle weakness and pins and needles may also develop.

If caused by pituitary tumour, pressure effects may occur.

Management:

Destruction of the tissue producing the excess hormone is the goal of orthodox management. The choice between surgery, external irradiation and radioactive implant depends on the age and health of the patient. Untreated, the life expectancy of a person with acromegaly is halved by the cardiovascular complications.

Bromocriptine also reduces GH levels and is thus a useful additional treatment.

HYPOPITUITARISM

Underactivity of the pituitary gland.

Aetiology:

> Surgery
> Radiation
> Adenoma
> Post partum* haemorrhage
> Secondary malignancy

Clinical features:

Children → "Peter Pan" dwarfism (look young when old).

Adults → A variety of hormonal problems including menstrual disturbance, adrenal insufficiency, hypothyroidism and decreased body hair.

As a general rule, the effects of GH, FSH and LH deficiency appear early.
TSH and ACTH deficiency manifests later.
Deficiencies of posterior pituitary hormones are rare.

Treatment:

Hormone replacement (eg "the pill", cortisone, thyroxine).

---

* After giving birth.

DIABETES INSIPIDUS

A rare condition caused by decreased antidiuretic hormone (ADH) secretion from the posterior pituitary.

Aetiology:

› Idiopathic
› Familial (ie inherited)
› Secondary malignancy
› Surgery
› Head injury

Clinical features:

Thirst producing polydipsia (drinking a lot) + polyuria (weeing a lot) – up to 20 litres of urine a day. The urine produced is very dilute (ie its specific gravity is very low).

Treatment:

Vasopressin (an artificial ADH) administered by intra nasal spray. Carbamazepine* may be used to improve the response of the kidney to ADH.

Note:

Diabetes insipidus is sometimes of psychogenic origin.

There is also a rare inherited condition called nephrogenic diabetes insipidus.

---

*   An anti-epileptic drug.

ADRENAL PROBLEMS

Background:

The adrenal medulla secretes adrenaline and noradrenaline (catecholamines).

The adrenal cortex produces steroid hormones (corticosteroids) in 3 main groups:

1) Glucocorticoids (eg cortisol) which raise blood sugar, antagonize insulin, facilitate the action of catecholamines on the heart and blood vessels, suppress the inflammatory response, break down protein, reduce the white cell count and cause sodium retention and potassium loss.

2) Mineralocorticoids (eg aldosterone) which cause sodium retention and potassium loss.

3) Sex hormones, including androgens and oestrogens.

CUSHING'S DISEASE

The clinical syndrome produced by corticosteroid excess.

Aetiology:

Usually the result of **steroid therapy**.

Rare causes:

› Alcohol excess.
› Pituitary adenoma.*
› Primary adrenal adenoma or carcinoma.
› Non-metastatic systemic effects of carcinomas such as oat cell carcinoma of the lung.

---

* Excess corticosteroid produced from a pituitary adenoma is called **Cushing's disease** after the eminent American surgeon and professor Harvey Cushing – the man who described the pituitary as "conductor of the endocrine orchestra".

Clinical features include:

> › Moon face
> › Acne
> › Fat body ± "buffalo" hump on back
> › Muscle weakness
> › Purple stretch marks (striae) on abdomen, thighs and buttocks ("normal" stretch marks are pink)
> › Easy bruising
> › Osteoporosis (leading to back ache and, sometimes, vertebral collapse)
> › Diabetes
> › Sodium retention
> › Potassium loss
> › Kidney stones
> › Hypertension
> › Mental disturbance
> › Masculinization of females

Management:

Depends on diagnosis of the underlying cause (which involves a whole battery of blood tests). Possibilities thus include withdrawal of steroid therapy, pituitary surgery and bilateral adrenalectomy with hormone replacement.

Prognosis:

Cushing's syndrome can kill within 5 years if untreated.

ADRENAL INSUFFICIENCY

May present as an acute "adrenal crisis" or as a chronic condition*.

ADRENAL CRISIS:

May be associated with trauma, severe hypotension, sepsis or surgical adrenalectomy. Patients on (or recently taken off) steroid therapy are at risk of adrenal crisis if subjected to stress such as surgery, trauma or infection. Adrenal crisis may also be precipitated by rapid withdrawal of steroid therapy.

Clinical features:

Apathy and epigastric pain. Low blood sugar. Coma.

Management:

IV hydrocortisone, fluids and glucose (+ treatment of infection if present).

CHRONIC ADRENAL INSUFFICIENCY (ADDISON'S DISEASE):

Is well known by students of medicine but is rare in practice.
80% of cases are "idiopathic" – presumed auto-immune and often associated with other organ specific auto-immune conditions.
Also caused by TB and metastatic tumours in adrenals.

Clinical features:

> Insidious onset
> Weakness
> Apathy
> Anorexia
> Weight loss
> Abdominal pain
> Menstrual disturbance

There may be hyperpigmentation of the inside of the cheeks and palmar skin creases as well as vitiligo and postural hypotension.

---

*   Called **Addison's disease** after Thomas Addison, the 19th century "founder of endocrinology".

Management:

Depends on cause but basically requires steroid replacement therapy and careful follow up.

Prognosis:

A well managed patient with Addison's disease has a normal life span.

CONN'S SYNDROME

Conn's syndrome is the eponym for **primary hyperaldosteronism**. It is *very* rare.

Aetiology:

Usually caused by a benign adrenal adenoma producing excess aldosterone.

Clinical features:

Excess aldosterone secretion causes a decrease in blood potassium levels. This causes weakness, polyuria and polydipsia.
Sodium retention produces **hypertension**, but usually no oedema because of the polyuria.

Conn's syndrome is thus one of the differential diagnoses of high blood pressure.

Management:

Adrenal adenomas are removed surgically. Aldosterone antagonists (eg spironolactone) may also help.

PHAEOCHROMOCYTOMA

A benign tumour of the adrenal medulla, which produces excess amounts of catecholamines. It is *extremely* rare.

Aetiology:

Idiopathic, but associated with thyroid carcinoma and parathyroid adenomas.

Clinical features:

Result from stimulation of α- and β-adrenoreceptors.
α-receptor stimulation produces $\uparrow$ blood pressure (systolic and diastolic) + $\downarrow$ heart rate. β-receptor stimulation causes $\uparrow$ blood pressure (systolic), $\uparrow$ heart rate and an $\uparrow$ in cardiac output.

The main feature of phaeochromocytoma is **hypertension**, but some people present with attacks of
› pallor
› palpitations
› anxiety
› headache

Diagnosis:

Excessive amounts of the breakdown products of catecholamine metabolism appearing in the urine suggest the diagnosis.

Management:

Removal of the tumour $\pm$ α- and β-blocking drugs.

PARATHYROID PROBLEMS

HYPERPARATHYROIDISM

Means increased levels of circulating PTH.

PRIMARY HYPERPARATHYROIDISM:

Results from inappropriate overproduction of PTH from one or more parathyroid glands and is usually due to the presence of a single **benign parathyroid "adenoma"**. Multiple adenomas, parathyroid hyperplasia and carcinoma also occasionally produce the condition.

Clinical features:

50% of sufferers (about 1 person in every 800, women more than men) are asymptomatic. In the other 50%, increased bone resorption leads to **hypercalcaemia** and may thus produce the classic clinical picture of **"bones, stones, abdominal groans and psychic moans"** – in other words, bone erosions and cysts plus hypercalcaemia leading to kidney stones, peptic ulcer, depression and confusion. Nowadays, the common-est presentation is tiredness, muscle weakness and vague ill health.

» **Hypercalcaemia** may, in addition, produce anorexia, nausea, vomiting, thirst, polyuria, constipation and muscle fatigue.

Management:

Parathyroidectomy.

SECONDARY HYPERPARATHYROIDISM:

Is really nothing to do with primary hyperparathyroidism. It is simply an appropriate physiological response to **hypocalcaemia** in conditions such as osteomalacia (vitamin D deficiency) and chronic renal failure. Unfortu-nately, the extra PTH may cause bone resorption and thus bone disease.

TERTIARY HYPERPARATHYROIDISM:

May occur after a long period of *secondary* hyperparathyroidism. The chronically overstimulated parathyroid tissue develops autonomous adenomas which oversecrete PTH.

HYPOPARATHYROIDISM

Means decreased levels of circulating PTH.

Aetiology:

Primary idiopathic → Associated with Addison's disease and other auto-immune conditions.

Secondary   →   Inadvertent (or overenthusiastic) surgical removal of parathyroid tissue.

Clinical features:

Result from decreased blood calcium levels and include

› Pins and needles around the mouth
› Muscle cramps and spasms
› Fits
› Poor condition of skin, teeth, hair and nails.

Hypoparathyroidism is also associated with cataract.

Diagnosis:

› Blood calcium ↓
› Blood phosphate ↑
› Blood alkaline phosphatase level normal.

Treatment:

Vitamin D and calcium supplements

Note:

Vitamin D deficiencies may cause decreased blood calcium (see chapter 20).

15. Metabolic Disorders

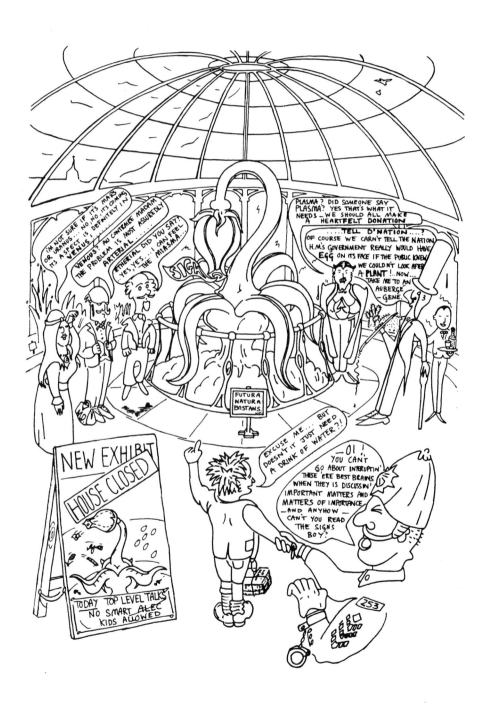

METABOLIC DISORDERS

OVERVIEW

Diabetes Mellitus

Type 1 (IDD)
Type 2 (NIDD)
Diabetic coma

Disorders of Lipid Metabolism

Type IIa
Type IIb
Type IV

Porphyrias

» Gout, pseudo gout and metabolic bone diseases (osteoporosis, osteomalacia, Paget's disease of bone and renal osteodystrophy) are dealt with in chapters 18 & 20.

DIABETES MELLITUS

A state of persistent hyperglycaemia* due to lack or diminished effectiveness of endogenous insulin.

Diabetes may be primary (idiopathic) or secondary to pancreatic disorders, drug therapy (eg thiazide diuretics and steroids) or other disease (eg acromegaly). Secondary diabetes is relatively rare, but there are over 500,000 cases of primary diabetes diagnosed in the UK at the present time.

Clinically, diabetes may be classified as insulin dependent (IDD) and non-insulin dependent (NIDD).

TYPE 1 OR INSULIN DEPENDENT DIABETES (IDD):

Usually develops in childhood and may be associated with a genetic predisposition plus viral infection (? mumps, ? Coxsackie) and subsequent auto-immunity. About 0.2% of the population under the age of 30 have IDD, with up to 30 per 100,000 new cases diagnosed each year.

TYPE 2 OR NON-INSULIN DEPENDENT DIABETES (NIDD):

Has a strong genetic component, is associated with obesity and usually appears in middle to late middle age, more commonly in women than men. Approximately 1% of the population has NIDD.

Pathophysiology:

Insulin increases the rate of glucose transport out of the blood, across cell membranes into liver, fat and muscle cells.

IDD is associated with:

A marked decrease in the number of pancreatic β–cells.
It is thought that, in genetically susceptible individuals, a seemingly inconsequential viral infection may cause the immune system to attack and destroy pancreatic cells. Under the microscope, inflammatory cells can be seen infiltrating and surrounding the Islets of Langerhans.

---

* Increased blood sugar.

NIDD is associated with:

↓ cell sensitivity to the effects of insulin.
↓ sensitivity of pancreatic cells to increased blood glucose.

Note that in NIDD, the pancreatic cells appear normal and secrete a biologically normal insulin. However, obesity produces insulin insensitivity since the fat cells of obese people appear to have fewer insulin "receptors" than those of thin people.

Biochemical changes and clinical effects of insulin lack:

1) Inability to control **carbohydrate metabolism**
2) Increased **fat breakdown**
3) Increased **amino acid breakdown**

1) Leads to hyperglycaemia and glycosuria.* The increased plasma osmolarity associated with hyperglycaemia stimulates thirst. Glycosuria causes an "osmotic diuresis"** thus reducing body fluid volume which exaggerates thirst.

2) Leads to excess "ketone bodies" (such as acetone) in the blood – hence the breath will smell of acetone and (since ketone bodies are acidic) the patient will become "acidotic".

3) Prevents proper protein synthesis and may lead to weight loss.

Clinical features:

› Weight loss
› Polyuria
› Polydipsia
› Lethargy
› Pruritus vulvae (itchy vulva)
› Infections and boils

The complications of diabetes may affect **any** organ and can be minimized by good management (ie meticulous control of blood glucose levels).

---

*   Sugar in the urine.
**   The sugar in the glomerular filtrate "sucks" water out of the blood and into the urine as it passes through the renal tubular system.

Management:

A patient with diabetes requires careful blood sugar level monitoring and dietary manipulation and may need either oral hypoglycaemics* (Type 2 DM) or subcutaneous insulin injections (Type 1 DM).

Management by a team that includes experienced nurses, eye specialists, dieticians, chiropodists** and experienced practitioners is the most effective. Regular (annual) check ups are an absolute necessity and should include the following:

› Check visual acuity
› Examine the fundi for retinopathy
› Check BP
› Assess renal function by checking for proteinuria (and, if possible, by testing blood urea and creatinine).
› Examine the feet for arterial problems (pulses, temperature of feet), neuropathy (↓ sensation, ↓ ankle jerks), and nail infection etc.

Orthodox management of NIDD involves diet (1200/1500cal per day) until weight loss relieves the symptoms. If this is not effective, oral hypoglycaemic agents are used.

The management of IDD involves subcutaneous self injection of insulin combined with dietary advice (low fat, high fibre, calorie controlled) and home assessment of blood (or urine) glucose.

Complications:

› Vascular
› Eye
› Kidney
› Neuromuscular
› Skin infection
› Diabetic coma
› Complications of diabetic pregnancy

---

* Blood sugar lowering drugs.
** The importance of care of the feet and nails cannot be overstressed and can avert major complications (infected ulcers etc).

Vascular:

Vascular complications account for up to **75% of diabetic deaths**. Large vessels are affected by widespread atheroma thus greatly increasing the incidence of IHD and occlusive vascular disease. Small vessels undergo pathological changes which damage the "microcirculation" of vital organs.

Eye:

Diabetes is assoicated with retinal degeneration, retinal detachment, vitrous haemorrhage and cataract. 20% of diabetics suffer eye complications but good diabetic "control" seems to slow the development and progress of eye pathology.

Diabetic "retinopathy" is a reflection of capillary damage and consists of retinal haemorrhages, exudates, aneurysms, infarcts and new capillary proliferation.

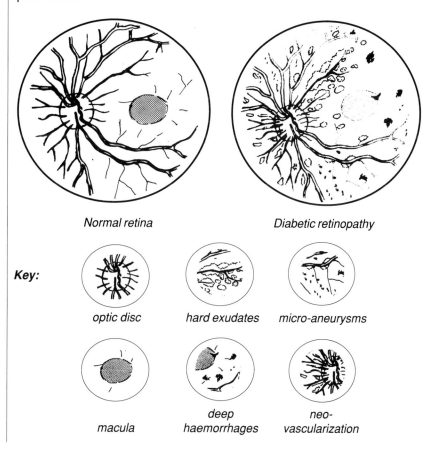

Normal retina   *Diabetic retinopathy*

Key:

optic disc   *hard exudates*   *micro-aneurysms*

macula   *deep
haemorrhages*   *neo-
vascularization*

Kidney:

> Diabetes causes characteristic glomerular damage and also predisposes to pyelonephritis (sugary urine makes good culture medium ....). Thus **diabetic renal disease** may cause hypertension, the nephrotic syndrome or renal failure and **accounts for up to a third of diabetic deaths occurring under 40 years of age.**

Neuromuscular:

> Neuromuscular complications afflict about a third of diabetics. The commonest is **a sensory peripheral neuropathy in which vibration sense is lost in the lower limbs** accompanied by ↓ ankle jerks and eventually ↓ pain perception. Patients complain of pins and needles or numbness/cramps in the feet that is worse at night. Once pain perception is lost, chronic ulcers may form over pressure points which are singularly difficult to heal.
>
> Autonomic neuropathy is also quite common, producing erectile impotence (males), postural hypotension, nocturnal diarrhoea and urinary retention etc. Single nerve palsies and painful asymmetrical quadriceps wasting (called mononeuritis multiplex and diabetic amyotrophy respectively) may also occur.

Skin:

> Some patients starting insulin therapy suffer from tender skin lumps after each injection for a few weeks; the problem usually resolves spontaneously. Many patients also experience painless fat atrophy at injection sites (less likely if human insulin used).
>
> **Necrobiosis lipoidica diabeticorum** is a rare condition in which there is atrophy of subcutaneous collagen over the shins. This causes unpleasant looking violet/yellowish discoloration of the skin of the lower leg.

Infection:

> **Urinary tract infection**, skin infection, TB and **thrush** are all more common in diabetics.

Diabetic coma:

There are two types:

› Hypoglycaemic coma
› Hyperglycaemic ketoacidotic coma

Hypoglycaemic coma:

Usually the result of excess antidiabetic medication combined with exercise, ↓ food intake or ↑ alcohol intake. Symptoms come on rapidly and may be relieved by eating a couple of sugar lumps.

Before having a fit or going into a coma, the patient becomes agitated, sweaty, confused and aggressive. The pulse will be fast. If not treated rapidly (intravenous glucose) hypoglycaemic coma may cause irreversible brain damage.

Hyperglycaemic coma:

Caused by insulin lack and progressively increasing blood glucose. Slow onset, often precipitated by infection or the cessation of insulin therapy.

Patient bone dry, overbreathing, breath smelling of acetone, vomiting, confused, ↓ BP and eventually coma.

Management requires much experience and involves IV insulin, fluid replacement, correction of electrolyte and acid/base imbalances and treatment of infection (if present).

Complications of diabetic pregnancy:

See chapter 27.

DISORDERS OF LIPID METABOLISM (hyperlipidaemias)

Hyperlipidaemia means too much fat in the blood (cholesterol, triglycerides etc).

Background:

The classification of hyperlipidaemias appears confusing (the WHO classifies them into 6 categories: Type I, IIa, IIb, III, IV and V) but only 3 of these are important in day to day practice (IIa, IIb and IV) because they are both common and treatable.

» In a patient suspected of having ischaemic heart disease, always consider the possibility that hyperlipidaemia is part of their problem.

Aetiology:

Hyperlipidaemias may be primary (hereditary) or secondary to other diseases, eg:

Type II hyperlipidaemias:	Type IV hyperlipidaemias:
hypothyroidism	diabetes
hypertension	alcoholism
the nephrotic syndrome	oestrogen therapy
diabetes	renal failure
cholestatic jaundice	gout
	pancreatitis

» Hyperlipidaemias seem to be associated with western diet and lifestyle.

Clinical features:

Type IIa: Women are affected more than men.
Blood cholesterol and LDL ↑.
Corneal "arcus senilis" (a pale ring around the cornea)
Xanthomas (fatty yellowish lumps) in tendons (eg Achilles tendon, extensor tendons on hands) and on extensor surfaces over joints.
Associated with severe occlusive (atheromatous) coronary artery disease.

Type IIb: Blood cholesterol, triglycerides and LDL ↑.
Xanthelasma (yellow fatty deposits under skin, especially around eyes).

Arcus senilis.
Also leads to ischaemic heart disease.

Type IV: Commoner in women.
Usually no symptoms or signs (but occasionally xanthomas).
Again, associated with premature atherosclerosis.

Management:

› ↓ weight
› ↓ saturated fats, sugar and alcohol in diet
› Stop smoking
› Control hypertension

Drugs can be used to lower blood triglyceride and cholesterol levels.

PORPHYRIAS

The porphyrias are a group of six peculiar syndromes related to disturbance in porphyrin production.

Porphyrins are intermediate products in the multi-enzyme process from which haem is made. (Haem production occurs mostly in the liver and the bone marrow.)

If any particular porphyrin is overproduced (eg because of a deficiency of a particular enzyme) various bizarre clinical effects are seen due either to direct toxicity or to the fact that porphyrins react to exposure to light. Four types of porphyrias are related to excess porphyrin production in the liver; two (much rarer) types relate to increased production in red cells.

Aetiology:

Porphyrias may be inherited or secondary to liver disease. They may also be precipitated by drugs (eg antibiotics, oral contraceptives, alcohol) or severe fasting.

Clinical features:

The clinical features vary between the different syndromes but nerves, heart, gut, blood, skin and mental state may all be affected, eg –

› Abdominal pain, vomiting and constipation
› Peripheral neuropathies, weakness and paralysis
› Confusion, psychosis and epilepsy
› Tachycardia and hypertension
› Photosensitive skin rashes with blistering of exposed areas
› Haemolytic anaemia
› Fluorescent pink discoloration of teeth

Management:

› Remove obvious precipitants
› Fluid replacement
› High carbohydrate diet
› Symptomatic control of pain, nausea etc

Note:

Congenital erythropoietic porphyria, the one characterized by haemolytic anaemia, photosensitive blistering skin rashes and fluorescent pink teeth, could be taken as quite a good description of a vampire and may account for the legends that have grown up in various parts of the world ....

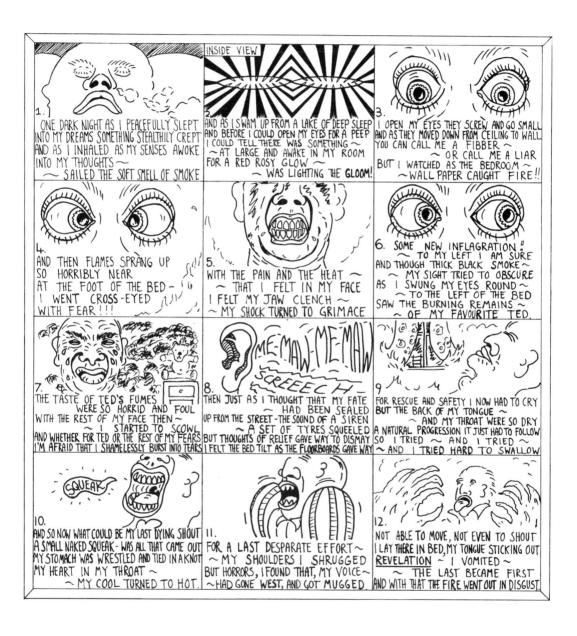

INSIDE VIEW

1.
ONE DARK NIGHT AS I PEACEFULLY SLEPT
INTO MY DREAMS SOMETHING STEALTHILY CREPT
AND AS I INHALED AS MY SENSES AWOKE
INTO MY THOUGHTS ~
~ SAILED THE SOFT SMELL OF SMOKE

2.
AND AS I SWAM UP FROM A LAKE OF DEEP SLEEP
AND BEFORE I COULD OPEN MY EYES FOR A PEEP
I COULD TELL THERE WAS SOMETHING ~
~ AT LARGE AND AWAKE IN MY ROOM
FOR A RED ROSY GLOW ~
~ WAS LIGHTING THE **GLOOM!**

3.
I OPEN MY EYES THEY SCREW AND GO SMALL
AND AS THEY MOVED DOWN FROM CEILING TO WALL
YOU CAN CALL ME A FIBBER ~
~ OR CALL ME A LIAR
BUT I WATCHED AS THE BEDROOM ~
~ WALLPAPER CAUGHT FIRE!!

4.
AND THEN FLAMES SPRANG UP
SO HORRIBLY NEAR
AT THE FOOT OF THE BED —
I WENT CROSS-EYED
WITH FEAR!!!

5.
WITH THE PAIN AND THE HEAT ~
~ THAT I FELT IN MY FACE
I FELT MY JAW CLENCH ~
~ MY SHOCK TURNED TO GRIMACE

6. SOME NEW INFLAGRATION "
~ TO MY LEFT I AM SURE
AND THOUGH THICK BLACK SMOKE ~
~ MY SIGHT TRIED TO OBSCURE
AS I SWUNG MY EYES ROUND ~
~ TO THE LEFT OF THE BED
SAW THE BURNING REMAINS ~
~ OF MY FAVOURITE TED.

7.
THE TASTE OF TED'S FUMES
WERE SO HORRID AND FOUL
WITH THE REST OF MY FACE THEN ~
~ I STARTED TO SCOWL
AND WHETHER FOR TED OR THE REST OF MY FEARS
I'M AFRAID THAT I SHAMELESSLY BURST INTO TEARS

8.
THEN JUST AS I THOUGHT THAT MY FATE
~ HAD BEEN SEALED
UP FROM THE STREET - THE SOUND OF A SIREN
~ A SET OF TYRES SQUEELED
BUT THOUGHTS OF RELIEF GAVE WAY TO DISMAY
I FELT THE BED TILT AS THE FLOORBOARDS GAVE WAY

9.
FOR RESCUE AND SAFETY I NOW HAD TO CRY
BUT THE BACK OF MY TONGUE ~
~ AND MY THROAT WERE SO DRY
A NATURAL PROGRESSION IT JUST HAD TO FOLLOW
SO I TRIED ~ AND I TRIED ~
~ AND I TRIED HARD TO SWALLOW

10.
AND SO NOW WHAT COULD BE MY LAST DYING SHOUT
A SMALL NAKED SQUEAK - WAS ALL THAT CAME OUT
MY STOMACH WAS WRESTLED AND TIED IN A KNOT
MY HEART IN MY THROAT ~
~ MY COOL TURNED TO HOT.

11.
FOR A LAST DESPARATE EFFORT ~
~ MY SHOULDERS I SHRUGGED
BUT HORRORS, I FOUND THAT, MY VOICE ~
~ HAD GONE WEST, AND GOT MUGGED.

12.
NOT ABLE TO MOVE, NOT EVEN TO SHOUT
I LAY THERE IN BED, MY TONGUE STICKING OUT
REVELATION ~ I VOMITED ~
~ THE LAST BECAME FIRST
AND WITH THAT THE FIRE WENT OUT IN DISGUST.

DISEASES OF THE NERVOUS SYSTEM

OVERVIEW

Infectious Diseases

Meningitis, encephalitis and
myalgic encephalomyelitis (post-viral syndrome)

Circulatory Disorders

Extracerebral haemorrhage and stroke syndromes

Headache Syndromes

Migraine and trigeminal neuralgia

Balance Disorders

Meniere's disease

Movement Disorders

Parkinson's disease

Neuromuscular Disorders

Myasthenia gravis and muscular dystrophy

Facial Palsy

Bell's palsy

Demyelinating Diseases

Multiple sclerosis and motor neurone disease

Degenerative Conditions

Dementia

Neoplastic Conditions

Cerebral tumour

Electroconvulsive Disorders

Epilepsy

INFECTIOUS DISEASES

MENINGITIS

Infection of the arachnoid and pia mater. It can be caused by a variety of micro-organisms.

Incidence:

Difficult to assess but causes about 300 deaths per year in England and Wales.

Causative organisms:

The commonest **bacteria** causing meningitis are:

Meningococcus (aka Neisseria meningitidis)
Pneumococcus (aka Streptococcus pneumoniae)
Haemophilus influenza (more common in small children)
E. coli (more common in neonates)

The **TB bacillus** and some **viruses** also cause meningitis.

Aetiological factors:

> Skull fracture
> Severe middle ear or sinus infections
> Pneumonia and other severe infections
> Overcrowding (for meningococcal meningitis)

Tuberculous meningitis is commoner in Asian communities.

Pathogenesis:

Having reached the meninges via the bloodstream or by direct spread from a nearby focus of infection, micro-organisms spread through the sub-arachnoid space and provoke a gross **inflammatory reaction**.

The pus in the CSF creates a good culture medium for the further multiplication of bacteria or viruses.

Untreated, this can lead to thrombosis of cerebral veins, infarction of brain tissue, hydrocephalus, circulatory collapse and death. Patients that survive may be left with permanent brain damage.

Transmission:

Meningococcal meningitis sometimes causes epidemics in closed communities since the organism lives in the **nasopharynx** and can be spread by **droplet infection**.

Pathology:

Exudate accumulates within the **sulci** of the brain and around the **optic chiasma**. The CSF looks cloudy.

Under the microscope, infected tissue shows intense inflammatory reaction (particularly around blood vessels) with numerous organisms present.

In severe **meningococcal** meningitis, the heart, joints, adrenal glands and skin may also become involved.

Clinical features:

> Increasingly severe bursting **headache** with **photophobia**.
> Patient lies curled up and has **fever**.
> Signs of **meningeal irritation**, ie neck rigidity and pain on passive extension of knee with hips flexed.

As the condition gets worse, drowsiness, confusion, fits and cranial nerve palsies may develop.

In **meningococcal** meningitis, a characteristic **haemorrhagic rash** is seen particularly on the lower limbs.

Management:

If meningitis is suspected, a diagnostic **lumbar puncture** is always performed and a sample of CSF is sent for "culture". Treatment then depends on the type of organism found, but a combination of **benzyl penicillin** and **chloramphenicol** will deal with most bacterial causes.

There is no treatment for **viral** meningitis (which is usually less severe).

Tuberculous meningitis (which often has an *insidious* onset with signs developing *late*) requires prolonged, specialist treatment.

Prognosis:

Overall mortality (despite treatment) for bacterial meningitis is 10% (80% in newborn infants). The complications of epilepsy, deafness and mental retardation are much more likely to occur in children. Most patients with viral ("aseptic") meningitis make a complete and uncomplicated recovery but tuberculous meningitis has a 15-20% mortality and high risk of post-infective complications.

ENCEPHALITIS

Many viruses including mumps, rubella, varicella (chickenpox), influenza and herpes simplex can cause acute inflammation of the brain, which is called **encephalitis.**

This can be very difficult to distinguish from meningitis. However, since the main pathological effect of encephalitis is to cause **swelling** of the brain, signs of **raised intracranial pressure** (falling pulse rate, rising blood pressure, coma, strange breathing patterns and cranial nerve palsies such as pupillary abnormalities) predominate over signs of **meningeal** irritation (although both may occur).

Note:

If infection spreads to the brain directly from the middle ear or nasal sinuses or indirectly via the bloodstream from some distant focus, a brain abscess may form.

Differentiation of brain abscess from encephalitis, meningitis and cerebral tumour can be very difficult.

Nowadays, **brain scans** (CT or CAT scans) are of primary importance in the diagnosis of intracerebral pathology.

MYALGIC ENCEPHALOMYELITIS (post-viral syndrome)

A poorly understood syndrome characterized by a multitude of symptoms and signs.

Aetiology:

Not known, but perhaps relates to the immune system's difficulty in handling viral infections when already overburdened by "environmental" stress. ME does not seem to be related to any **specific** viral infection (although the clinical picture is similar, in some respects, to that caused by the Epstein-Barr virus*).

Clinical features:

The most common symptoms are generally agreed to be:

› Severe fatigue precipitated by minimal exertion and not relieved by rest
› Generalized aches and pains (sore muscles in particular)
› Depressed mood
› Problems adjusting to changes in temperature
› GI disturbance

There may be a variety of "neurological" signs (eg tremor in one hand) not explainable in terms of a more straightforward neurological diagnosis.

Diagnosis:

Is usually by exclusion of other possibilities. A variety of non-specific blood tests (to determine IgM levels, helper/suppressor cell ratios and levels of viral proteins) may be used to support the clinical suspicion of ME.

Management:

The objective should be to tailor the approach to the individual's whole problem. Diet, vitamin and mineral supplementation and complementary medicine all have a place in management. Orthodox approaches include the use of antihistamine drugs, immune system modulators and immuno-globulin injections.

* Infectious mononucleosis.

CIRCULATORY DISORDERS

EXTRACEREBRAL HAEMORRHAGE

Extracerebral haemorrhage can occur from blood vessels located in the "space":
1) between the skull and the dura (**extradural haemorrhage**),
2) between the dura and the arachnoid (**subdural haemorrhage**),
3) between the arachnoid and the pia/brain substance (**subarachnoid haemorrhage**).

Subarachnoid haemorrhage is sometimes considered to be one of the "**stroke**" syndromes, in as much as it presents as a **neurological deficit of relatively sudden onset,** but it is probably better to reserve the term "stroke" for conditions in which there is **ischaemic damage to a part of the brain itself**.

EXTRADURAL HAEMORRHAGE:

Is caused by **trauma** (especially to the side of head) damaging the **middle meningeal artery** as it passes upwards on the inside of the temporal bone.

Clinical features:

A classic history would be of trauma causing a momentary loss of consciousness followed by apparent recovery. Signs of raised intracranial pressure then develop with death occurring after about 7 days. You must know the **danger signs of raised ICP** viz: –

> **headache**
> **drowsiness**
> **vomiting**
> **falling pulse rate**
> **rising blood pressure**
> **pupillary abnormalities**
> **strange respiration patterns**
> **various cranial nerve palsies**

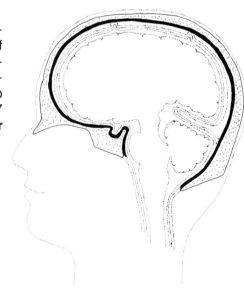

Extradural space

Management:

> The standard treatment is neurosurgical removal of the clot and tying off of the bleeding artery through "burr holes" drilled in the skull.
>
> Steroids are sometimes given to reduce brain swelling.

Prognosis:

> Early recognition of extracerebral haemorrhage should lead to a good recovery. Untreated, the condition is nearly always fatal. **Thus any moderately severe head injury probably warrants a skull X-ray.**

SUBDURAL HAEMORRHAGE:

> Is caused by bleeding from "bridging" veins which pass from the cerebral cortex to the dural venous sinuses. Though presumably caused by trauma, the injury responsible may not have been noticed by the patient.*
>
> The elderly, alcoholics, epileptics and children are all at risk of subdural haemorrhage after even **trivial** head injury.

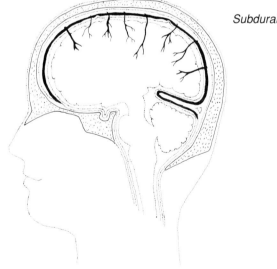

Subdural space

---

*   Only about 50% of cases will report previous trauma.

Clinical features:

Problems may develop over a period of **weeks or months** after the precipitating event and consist of headache, confusion and **fluctuating or decreasing levels of consciousness**. Other neurological signs, including those of ↑ ICP, may also develop.

Prognosis:

Neurosurgery and removal of the clot usually results in **complete recovery**.

SUBARACHNOID HAEMORRHAGE:

Bleeding into the subarachnoid space.

80% result from **rupture** of congenital **"berry"** aneurysms (so-called because they look like berries!) somewhere in the Circle of Willis*. They may also be caused by rupture of other congenital arterial malformations and are more likely to occur in patients who have a bleeding tendency (such as those on **anticoagulants**). **High blood pressure** greatly increases the chance of having a subarachnoid haemorrhage.

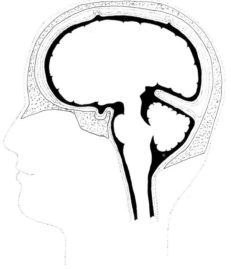

Subarachnoid space

---

* Thomas Willis (1621-1675), son of a Wiltshire farmer and founder member of the Royal Society. Well known for his charitable works, he was the first to describe a number of conditions (eg whooping cough). He also was the first to use the terms "reflex" and "neurology" in their modern senses.

Clinical features:

The symptom is **severe headache of sudden onset, as if hit on the back of the head**.

There may also be (in increasingly sinister order) **neck stiffness, cranial nerve palsies, drowsiness, hemiplegia and coma**.

› One third of patients die in the first attack
› Another 1/3rd have a second bleed within days
› If you survive the first month, you have a 90% chance of surviving a year or more
› Of those that survive a year, a 1/3rd live out their life well and symptom free

Management:

After various investigations (including, possibly, **arteriography** – which can be both dangerous and unpleasant), just a few cases are considered suitable for surgery. Various drugs have also been tried but the results have proved unpredictable.

STROKE SYNDROMES

Stroke is the relatively sudden onset of neurological deficit resulting from ischaemic infarction of a part of the brain.

It is the major neurological problem of our age and produces enormous suffering through immobility, loss of sphincter control, loss of independence and loss of dignity.

Epidemiology:

› Approx. 1 patient on a GP list per 500 patients per year suffers a stroke
› 50% of victims are dead after 6 months
› One third of the survivors will need continuous nursing

Risk factors:

› Hypertension
› Angina
› Diabetes (and other causes of peripheral vascular disease such as **smoking**).
› Oral contraceptives

+ Possibly

› Obesity
› Physical inactivity
› High blood lipid levels

Pathology:

80% of cases result from **thrombosis** or **embolus*** (see chapter 6).

20% of cases are due to **intracerebral haemorrhage** resulting from "spontaneous" rupture of an intracerebral vessel or vessels. Occasionally, intracerebral haemorrhage is due to vasculitis, brain abscess, anticoagulant therapy or blood disease.

---

*   Emboli are small clots – sometimes mixed up with other material – which form in one part of the circulation and then travel in the bloodstream to another part where they may get jammed in a vessel of small diameter, thereby cutting off the blood supply.

The mortality from haemorrhagic strokes is very high with 80% of patients dying within one month.

Clinical features:

In the clinical situation, it is extremely difficult to distinguish between the different underlying pathologies. The commonest stroke presentation is **hemiplegia**, but there is enormous variation with some strokes evolving slowly, some coming on quickly, some remaining "static" after the initial event and some progressing inexorably towards death.

Nevertheless, involvement of certain arteries does produce particular clinical patterns, ie:

Middle cerebral artery:
> contralateral hemiplegia*
> variable sensory loss
> possibly dysphasia**

Anterior cerebral artery:
> contralateral weak leg

Posterior cerebral artery:
> contralateral homonymous hemianopia***

Mid-brain infarction:
> coma
> pupil + gaze abnormalities
> paralysis

Pontine infarction:
> quadriplegia****
> pinpoint pupils
> coma or "locked in" syndrome+

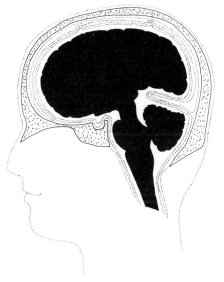

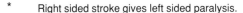

*	Right sided stroke gives left sided paralysis.
**	Can't speak properly.
***	Loss of vision in half the visual field.
****	All four limbs paralysed.
+	Patient conscious and aware but complete loss of motor and sensory function.

Management:

If, during the unconscious phase of a stroke, there are signs of ↑ICP (and CT scan evidence of haemorrhage), surgical "decompression" may be considered.

The presence of atrial fibrillation (in the absence of CT scan evidence of haemorrhage) suggests thrombo-embolic stroke and may be an indication for anticoagulant therapy.

Otherwise, immediate management is directed towards maintaining respiration, hydration and nutrition and to preventing bed sores.

Thereafter, management involves relieving distress, vigorous rehabilitation and prevention of future strokes as far as is possible (by better management of diabetes if present, consultation with a cardiologist if heart disease is suspected, control of hypertension if present, treatment of blood disorders and stopping smoking etc).

» The management of stroke patients should be a team effort utilizing the skills of many practitioners (including natural therapists), in close co-operation with relatives if possible. There has been little success with drug treatment of the complications of strokes. It has been shown, however, that rehabilitation such as passive physiotherapy should be started as **soon** as possible (preferably as soon as the patient is in bed) if it is to achieve maximum effect.

TRANSIENT ISCHAEMIC ATTACKS (TIAs):

TIAs are defined as transient focal neurological deficits caused by vascular pathology and lasting less than 24 hours with no **residual neurological deficit**. "Mini strokes", in other words.

People who have TIAs are at slightly increased risk of suffering a future major vascular accident such as stroke or heart attack.

Remember that similar transient focal neurological deficits may occur in migraine, severe hypertension, epilepsy, hypoglycaemia and several other conditions, so a thorough general assessment is indicated in every case.

One particular type of TIA, characterized by hemiparesis, speech problems and a misty blindness in one eye, is sometimes caused by micro-emboli (coming from an internal carotid artery thrombosis) lodging briefly in a cerebral artery. The chances of a future more serious stroke may be averted in these patients by surgery to remove the clot from the carotids; but up to 40% will have had a major stroke within 3 years.

When the source of a TIA lies in the vertebro-basilar arteries, patients may complain of deafness, dizziness, fainting attacks, vomiting etc. These patients have a better prognosis.

Management:

It is obviously important to control hypertension and other risk factors (if present) but otherwise, the most effective orthodox "preventive" medicine appears to be the taking of one low dose aspirin tablet daily after the first attack.

Driving is not permitted for 6 months after a TIA.

HEADACHE SYNDROMES

MIGRAINE

Recurrent headache with visual and/or gastrointestinal disturbance affecting about 10% of the population.

Epidemiology:

More common in females.
Often family history.
Various foods, emotional states and times of the day or week may precipitate migraines.

Pathology:

The initial "aura" is thought to be caused by cerebral vasoconstriction producing localized brain hypoxia.
Subsequent vasodilation produces the characteristic throbbing headache.

Clinical features:

› Classical attacks start with a visual **aura** in field opposite to that of succeeding headache
› This is followed by ɔ throbbing **unilateral** headache associated with nausea, vomiting and photophobia
› There may be **transient** hemiparesis or sensory disturbance

Migraine is **rarely** associated with serious underlying pathology.

Treatment:

The "first line" treatment involves simple analgesics (often with metoclopramide (Maxolon) to reduce nausea). Clonidine (Dixarit), methysergide (Deseril) and pizotifen (Sanomigran) are sometimes prescribed prophylactically. Ergotamine preparations* (eg Cafergot, Lingraine and Migril) may abort attacks.

---

*   Powerful vasoconstrictors.

MIGRAINOUS NEURALGIA (cluster headaches):

This is a clinical syndrome of **unknown** cause characterized by attacks of severe paroxysmal pain in the face and eye that may wake the patient up at night and last for up to 2 hours.

The attacks are associated with reddening of the eye and blocking of the nose on the affected side.

Since the attacks occur in clusters (eg nightly for several weeks then about a year symptom free), the syndrome is also referred to as "cluster headaches".

Treatment:

The drug **ergotamine** (Cafergot, Lingraine, Migril etc) given at night during a bad patch may diminish the severity of the attacks and **methysergide** (Deseril) is also used prophylactically.

Both these drugs have unpleasant side effects and are potentially toxic.*

OTHER HEADACHE SYNDROMES

Headache is one of the commonest presenting complaints in medicine and, whilst the acute headaches associated with subarachnoid haemorrhage or acute meningitis rarely produce diagnostic confusion, a history of **chronic** headache may relate to any one of a large number of disorders.

The vast majority of chronic headaches are of "benign" origin but you should nevertheless study the relevant parts of chapters 10 and 30 which give a framework for separating the serious from the less serious (in terms of orthodox prognosis).

In particular, you should have a thorough working knowledge of the presentation and implications of the condition known as **temporal arteritis**, a connective tissue disorder discussed in chapter 19.

Hypertension, sinusitis and "eye strain" are probably the most common **diagnoses** made in cases of chronic headache and all are discussed elsewhere. The following are relatively common **causes.**

---

*   Prolonged use of **Deseril** is no longer considered justified because of the potential for serious complications.

TENSION HEADACHE:

Probably the commonest form of chronic headache. It relates to chronic tension in the muscles of the scalp and neck.

Tension headaches are usually generalized, may last for several hours at a time and can be complicated by sharp stabbing pains.
The scalp may be tender.

COUGH HEADACHE:

Severe generalized headache precipitated by a bout of coughing.
It has no sinister significance.*

DEPRESSION:

Headache is a common presentation of depression.

COSTEN'S SYNDROME (temporomandibular joint syndrome):

Costen's syndrome causes more or less severe shooting pains felt in front of the ear and radiating to other parts of the face or scalp.
It may relate to a history of night time teeth grinding and can be precipitated by chewing.
The underlying mechanism is unclear but dental correction of the "bite" and the wearing of a "brace" on the teeth at night may bring dramatic relief.

TRIGEMINAL NEURALGIA (Tic Douloureux)

Very severe stabbing pain in the face affecting one or more of the divisions of the trigeminal nerve **but not extending outside this area**.

Population:

Tends to affect older people.

Aetiology:

Underlying pathology usually unknown.
Occasionally a symptom of multiple sclerosis or brain tumour.

* In most cases ....

The appearance of trigeminal neuralgia in a person under 60 years of age should raise the suspicion of MS.

Clinical features

Very severe, sharp, stabbing pains in the face, often precipitated by touch, movement or cold winds. There are sometimes **trigger** areas which, if touched, will produce the pain. There may also be prolonged, dull, "background" ache. Symptoms are often (not unreasonably) accompanied by depression.

The pain may be bad enough to cause suicide.

There are usually no obvious physical "signs".

Management:

Reassurance that the condition is not "serious"* plus assurance that it tends to come and go with long periods of remission between attacks is often helpful.

Beyond this, there are a whole range of orthodox approaches ranging from the prescription of **carbamazepine**** ("Tegretol") to various surgical procedures designed to block or divide affected nerves. Few are effective.

Addictive pain killing drugs (opiate derivatives) are avoided if possible, but simple analgesics have little or no effect on the acute pain of this condition.

It is usually recommended that any coexisting "depression" should also be treated.

NOTE:

There are many causes of facial pain (often *described* by patients as "headache") relating to the nasal sinuses, the ears and the teeth (see chapter 30) but it is often impossible to correlate the complaint of facial pain to an orthodox diagnosis.

---

*   In the sense that it is not life threatening.
**   See epilepsy.

You should, however, be aware of the condition known as **post herpetic neuralgia.**

This presents as severe facial pain following herpes zoster (shingles) infection of the trigeminal nerve.

It can be a distressing and intractable problem causing increased sensitivity of the involved skin accompanied by a continuous, deep, pain that can lead to depression and despair.

Conventional medical treatment only brings limited relief for most sufferers.

BALANCE DISORDERS

MENIERE'S DISEASE

In 1861, the French physician Prosper Meniere* described the syndrome of **progressive deafness associated with episodic vertigo, tinnitus and vomiting** that we now refer to as Meniere's disease.

It is probably the best known (if not the most common) disorder of balance described by the orthodox tradition.

Background:

The onset is usually between the ages of 40 and 50.

The cause is unknown.

Pathology:

Increased pressure in the endolymph of the inner ear causes dilation of the endolymphatic system and degeneration of the hair cells of the organ of Corti.**

Clinical features:

› The condition is characterized by sudden attacks of vertigo (an hallucination of movement) with unsteadiness and vomiting.
› Nystagmus (flickering movements of the eyes) may be observed during an attack.
› Each episode may last for several hours.
› Attacks recur at intervals of days, weeks, months or years until (in some cases) complete deafness ensues (at which point the attacks of vertigo usually stop).

---

*   Meniere was the casualty officer on duty on a day in 1830 when 2000 rioters were admitted to Paris hospitals in just 24 hours. He was an expert on orchids and died of influenzal pneumonia at the age of 63.

** Alfonso Corti (1822-1888), Sardinian anatomist and histologist.

Management:

Orthodox treatment of Meniere's disease is frequently unsatisfactory. It relies in the first instance on tranquillizers and anti-emetics and progresses to ultrasound destruction of the labyrinth or surgical section of the vestibular nerve (in severe, intractable cases).

» **Before undertaking any form of treatment of a disorder of balance, the practitioner should assess the patient's hearing since underlying hearing loss has important implications for the site and nature of the pathology.**

Differential diagnosis:

There are many causes of vertigo and deafness and a knowledge of the anatomy and physiology of the ear and auditory and vestibular pathways often helps to pinpoint a diagnosis.

Deafness will be dealt with as a separate topic in chapter 25, but the common causes of vertigo (other than Meniere's disease) are important, and should be learnt:

› **PROBLEMS AFFECTING THE LABYRINTH:** a) Streptomycin (an antibiotic) is "ototoxic".* b) "Benign postural vertigo" – benign attacks of vertigo occurring when the head is held in a certain position. Probably due to minor abnormalities of utricle and saccule.
› **BRAIN STEM ISCHAEMIA:** Vertigo is a common symptom of vertebro-basilar artery insufficiency.
› **MULTIPLE SCLEROSIS** and any other condition affecting the cerebellum. May cause balance problems.
› **TEMPORAL LOBE EPILEPSY**
› **MANY DRUGS** – including alcohol
› **MIGRAINE**
› **ACUTE VESTIBULAR NEURONITIS:** A self limiting disorder, presumably of viral origin. It sometimes occurs in epidemics characterized by vomiting and vertigo.

---

*   Damages ears.

MOVEMENT DISORDERS

PARKINSON'S DISEASE*

A common condition of middle aged/elderly people in which abnormalities in the **basal ganglia** produce the characteristic trio of **tremor, rigidity** and **akinesia** with progressive disability leading to dementia and death ...

Epidemiology:

Responsible for around 2000 deaths per annum in the UK.

Aetiology:

In most cases, the aetiology is entirely unknown but the following can produce Parkinsonism to a greater or lesser degree:

> **Drugs** (phenothiazines especially)
> The aftermath of **encephalitis**
> **Arteriosclerosis** affecting brain blood vessels
> **Carbon monoxide poisoning**

Pathogenesis:

It is thought that a relative deficiency of "dopaminergic"** neurones in the **basal ganglia** causes the problem.

Pathology:

The brain looks more or less normal, in the absence of other pathology.

Under the microscope, loss of neurones can be seen in the basal ganglia.

---

*   James Parkinson – 1755-1824. Born in East End of London, practised in Shoreditch. Keen on politics and palaeontology. He named the condition **paralysis agitans**.
** Dopamine producing.

Clinical features:

> › Pin rolling tremor
> › Rigidity of all muscles (described as "lead pipe" or "cogwheel" if tremor is bad)
> › Expressionless face
> › Monotonous speech
> › Slowness in initiating and executing movements *unless* uncommonly urgent motivation*
> › Shuffling, bent walk

Treatment:

> If the cause is a drug, reducing the dosage will help.
>
> Otherwise, **L-dopa** (plus a dopa-decarboxylase inhibitor) can help relieve rigidity and akinesia for a time.
> Anticholinergic drugs help tremor.
>
> The common anti-Parkinson drugs are
> › **Levodopa**
> › **Levodopa** with **carbidopa** (Sinemet)
> › **Bromocriptine** (Parlodel)
> › **Benzhexol** (Artane). Benzhexol is an anticholinergic drug.

Prognosis:

> The benefit of drugs diminishes after about 4/5 years.
> Eventually the disease progresses to immobility, contractures, incontinence and dementia with death occurring in 10/12 years (but with a wide variation). However, early experiments with foetal brain tissue transplants have produced dramatic relief in some cases.

*   eg being suddenly and unexpectedly thrown in a swimming pool.

NEUROMUSCULAR DISORDERS

MYASTHENIA GRAVIS

A strange disease, probably of **auto-immune** origin and characterized by **weakness and easy fatiguability of skeletal muscles.**

The **proximal** limb muscles and the muscles concerned with chewing, swallowing, speech, eye movement, keeping the eyelids open are most affected. The weakness improves after **rest** and after administration of drugs called **anticholinesterases.**

Population:

Female/male = 2/1.

Aetiology:

About 10% of patients have a **thymic** tumour. Otherwise, the aetiology of the condition is unknown.

Pathogenesis:

As we have already mentioned, immunological factors are important. In 85% of patients with MG, blood tests show the presence of **auto-anti-bodies** against acetylcholine receptors which effectively reduce the number of functioning ACh receptors in skeletal muscles. The **thymus** appears to be **hyperplastic** in 75% of cases. Under the microscope, voluntary muscles appear abnormal with atrophy of muscle fibres and abnormalities of nerve endings and motor end plates.

Clinical features:

Symptoms may develop towards the end of the day or after physical exertion and include:

> Double vision (diplopia)
> Drooping eyelids
> Problems chewing
> Problems swallowing
> Regurgitation of fluids through the nose
> Slurred speech
> Problems combing hair and climbing stairs

The muscular weakness that these symptoms represent can be confirmed by physical examination but tendon reflexes are **normal** and there is **no** sensory deficit. Muscle wasting may be noticeable later.

» Note that **severe MG** is a medical emergency characterized by inability to breathe, cough or swallow.

Management:

Surgical removal of the **thymus** (in severe cases) and regular treatment with an anticholinesterase drug such as **pyridostigmine** taken daily. Too much of this drug paradoxically **increases** weakness. Its GI side effects can be eased by administration of **atropine**.

Steroids and **immunosuppressant** drugs are used if the response to pyridostigmine is inadequate.

Prognosis:

Many patients present with just the ocular manifestations of the disease. About 10% of these go on to develop generalized myasthenia.
The severe form of the disease can be managed reasonably effectively by the measures outlined above.

MUSCULAR DYSTROPHIES

A group of inherited disorders characterized by weakness and degeneration of skeletal muscles.

There are 4 common types:

›   Duchenne muscular dystrophy
›   Limb girdle muscular dystrophy
›   Facio-scapulo-humoral muscular dystrophy
›   Dystrophia myotonica

The age of onset and prognosis is different for the different types.

Only Duchenne muscular dystrophy will be described here.

DUCHENNE MUSCULAR DYSTROPHY*:

Inheritance:

X-linked recessive (~70%) or the result of "spontaneous" mutation (~30%)

Population:

Boys. The disease is usually apparent before 4 years of age.
Female carriers occasionally show mild symptoms.

Clinical features:

Weakness/degeneration of pelvic girdle muscles → problems running/walking → problems getting up from sitting (have to "climb up legs" to get upright) → weakness spreads to arms → totally disabled within a few years with contractures of arms and legs → death from chest infection or heart failure (heart muscle eventually becomes involved in degenerative process).

Management:

› General support
› Everything possible to maintain mobility
› Genetic counselling to family

Prognosis:

Most sufferers die by age 20.

---

*   Guillaume Duchenne 1806-1875, French neurologist working in Boulogne and Paris.

FACIAL PALSY

BELL'S PALSY*

Used to be considered as **idiopathic paralysis of the facial nerve** but it is now thought of as a **virally induced "polyneuropathy"** with inflammatory demyelination extending from brainstem to periphery.

The 5th, 7th, 9th and 10th nerves may all be involved.

Clinical features:

Presents with abrupt (often painful) onset of sagging mouth, dribbling, impaired taste and sometimes dry eye, **all** on one side of the face.

Examination reveals unilateral inability to wrinkle forehead, whistle or blow out the cheek on the affected side.

Management:

There is no treatment except to protect the eye (if necessary) with dark glasses and artificial tears. Those who are going to recover completely usually regain facial movement within 4 weeks.

Occasionally, for the first few weeks after recovery, patients complain of unilateral tears when they eat. This is thought to be due to aberrant regeneration of branches of the superficial petrosal nerves.

You should refer to chapter 30 for a list of other causes of facial palsy.

---

*   Sir Charles Bell, 1774-1842, a kindly Scottish surgeon and anatomist. Founder of the
     Middlesex Hospital Medical School.

DEMYELINATING DISEASES

MULTIPLE SCLEROSIS

A chronic relapsing disorder of unknown aetiology characterized by patches (plaques) of myelin loss in the CNS. It causes about 100 deaths per year in England and Wales.

Population:

Age group: Between 20 and 40 at onset.
Sex: Slightly more common in women.

Geography:

More common in temperate zones.
More common in Orkney and Shetland than in England.
Children "acquire" the risk of the population they are raised in.

Pathogenesis:

Perhaps an immunological response to myelin previously altered (? in childhood) by virus infection (? measles).

Pathology:

Patchy loss of myelin is seen in the CNS, particularly in the **optic nerves, brainstem** and **cervical spinal cord**. The myelin sheath around peripheral nerves is **unaffected,** hence muscle bulk is usually normal (though tendon jerks are sometimes increased).

Clinical features:

Usually presents as a **single focal neurological deficit** eg:

› rapid deterioration of central vision (optic neuritis)
› isolated numbness of legs
› progressive weakness of legs

Also

› vertigo
› cerebellar signs

> increased reflexes
> upgoing plantar response
> impotence
> incontinence
> pain
> pins and needles in arms or legs on flexing neck
> nystagmus

Diagnosis is suggested by abnormalities of CSF composition and by alterations in the speed of conduction along optic pathways (assessed using a non invasive test, a bit like an EEG, to measure "visual evoked potentials").

Late features:

> disturbance of mood
> intellectual deterioration
> speech disorder
> tremor
> paralysis of legs ± spasticity

Management:

Many interventions have been tried but there is no conventional cure. Symptomatic management of movement, bowel and bladder problems is important and involves co-operation between medical, nursing and community services.

Prognosis:

Relapses last a few months, remissions after many years.
A first presentation of optic neuritis is usually associated with a very long period of subsequent remission.
After 20 years, 20% are dead and only 35% are still working.
5 years after diagnosis 70% are still working or getting on normally.

MOTOR NEURONE DISEASE

A progressive, degenerative disease involving the pyramidal tracts, the anterior horn cells of the spinal cord and the lower cranial nerve nuclei.

Epidemiology:

Rare – 1.5 cases per 100,000 population per year.
Affects older people.

Clinical features:

Muscular weakness and fasciculation* but **no sensory deficit**.

There are 3 classical presentations:

a) Weakness, wasting and fasciculation of the small muscles of the hand followed by upper limbs.

b) Weakness, wasting and fasciculation of the tongue and muscles of the pharynx.

c) Spastic weakness of the legs, later spreading to the arms.

Thus the neurological deficits can be **lower motor neurone or upper motor neurone** in type and combinations of all the above may occur in any one patient.

Treatment and prognosis:

There is no conventional treatment and death occurs (usually from aspiration pneumonia) within about 2 years of presentation. Mental alertness is preserved throughout ....

---

*   Trembling.

DEGENERATIVE CONDITIONS

DEMENTIA

**Progressive brain atrophy due to nerve cell loss leading to a charac-
teristic worsening of memory and global intellectual deterioration
without impairment of consciousness.** If it occurs before age 65, it is
called "presenile" dementia. Idiopathic presenile dementia is named after
Alois Alzheimer*.

Epidemiology:

More common in the elderly, but also seen in middle age.

Aetiology:

Many theories have been advanced to explain dementia, including a
genetic model, an accumulation of abnormal proteins model, an infectious
disease model and an aluminium poisoning model None has gained
universal acceptance to date.

Pathology:

The brain undergoes diffuse atrophy with relative enlargement of the
ventricles. Under the microscope, brain tissue is seen to be disrupted by
plaques of fibrillary protein and neurofibrillary tangles.

Clinical features:

› Insidious onset
› Personality changes, including unprovoked anger, hoarding of money
  and possessions etc
› Gross impairment of recent memory
› Declining intellectual function
› Persecutory delusions
› Episodes of nocturnal wandering
› Eventual reversion to a childlike state – bed ridden and doubly incon-
  tinent – until death from a variety of causes

---

*   A Bavarian neurologist and pathologist who correlated the clinical picture of progressive
      dementia with certain microscopical changes in brain tissue. His original description was
      published in 1906.

Treatment:

1) Exclude any **"treatable"** organic cause (including **hypothyroidism, vitamin B12 + folate deficiency, syphilis, thiamine deficiency, cerebral tumour, subdural haematoma and certain types of hydrocephalus**).
Remember that **depression** may mimic or complicate dementia.

2) Treat any coexisting physical condition (especially diabetes, urinary tract infections and pneumonia).

Prognosis:

Ultimately gloomy, but mobilization of community support services plus holiday hospital admissions etc may help the patient and the family to retain reasonable quality of life.

NEOPLASTIC CONDITIONS

CEREBRAL TUMOURS

Background:

Rare – 1 in 20,000 of the population.

80% are primary,
20% are secondary (from bronchus, breast, kidney, colon, ovary, prostate or thyroid).

Most primary tumours arise from **covering** or **supporting** brain tissues rather than from neuroglia.

Clinical features:

People with brain tumours usually present with signs of increasing intra-cranial pressure* and, in 30%, epilepsy.

The appearance of progressive "focal" neurological signs depends on the site of the growth.

Management:

A brain scan may reveal an operable tumour.
Angiography may be necessary to determine the safest way to perform the operation.

Prognosis:

Secondary worse than primary.
Inoperable much worse than operable.

---

*   Beware throbbing bilateral frontal headache worse in the morning and exacerbated by bending, coughing and straining.

ELECTROCONVULSIVE DISORDERS

EPILEPSY

Epilepsy is the diagnostic label given to a variety of self-limiting **seizures** ranging from momentary staring into space to generalized **convulsions**.

Epileptic seizures are associated with abnormal electrical activity in the brain. This can often be demonstrated on an **electro-encephalogram** (EEG).

Epidemiology:

At least 6% of the population will suffer a single (non-febrile) convulsion at some point during their lives.

In any given population of 100,000, there will be about 900 people with established epilepsy, about half of whom will have had a seizure in the past 2 years.

Approximately 30 new cases per 100,000 people are diagnosed each year.

Classification:

1) IDIOPATHIC –

a) Primary generalized major seizures ("Grand Mal")
b) Absence attacks ("Petit Mal")

2) SYMPTOMATIC –

a) **Focal brain disease**
   Brain abscess
   Tumours (about 10% of middle aged people presenting with seizures will have a tumour)
   Trauma (including birth trauma)
   Cerebrovascular disease

b) **Infection**
   Meningitis
   Encephalitis

Febrile convulsions (about 10% of children who have a febrile convulsion will go on to have seizures later in life).

c) **Anoxia**
"Stokes-Adams" attacks
Fainting
Strokes etc

d) **Metabolic and toxic**
Hypoglycaemia
Hypocalcaemia
Kidney failure ("uraemia")
Drug overdose
Drug withdrawal (eg alcohol, anticonvulsants, barbiturates)

Clinical features:

GRAND MAL:

› Sometimes momentary premonition or "aura".
› Then sudden loss of consciousness (± cry) → generalized rigidity of body (**tonic phase**) → generalized jerking (**clonic phase**).
› Frequently accompanied by sweating, incontinence and tongue biting.
› Period of flaccid unconsciousness after attack.

PETIT MAL:

› Usually begins in childhood.
› Often just a few seconds of unexpected "absence" (staring into space) but may be some jerking or even falling to the ground without warning.*

FOCAL SEIZURES:

Patient usually remains conscious.

Three patterns recognized:

a) Regular jerking of a limb which may spread to another limb or to the face on the same side of body –

---

* So called akinetic seizure.

b) Tingling or spreading sensory disturbance on one side of body –
c) **Temporal lobe epilepsy,** which causes abnormal emotional experiences, taste and smell hallucinations, deja vu, and feelings of unreality.

» **Focal fits should always be fully investigated.**

Diagnosis:

> › Be aware that **stress** can precipitate epilepsy (as can flashing lights, flickering TVs etc).
> › Check if there is a family history.
> › Make sure that you have excluded the easily treatable or the very serious.

Treatment:

The commonest drugs used to control fits (in various combinations) are:

Carbamazepine (Tegretol)
Phenytoin (Epanutin)
Sodium valproate (Epilim)
Ethosuximide (Zarontin)

Treatment is usually continued for many years.

» ALL these drugs have many side effects. **None of them should be "stopped" suddenly** (because of the danger of precipitating **status epilepticus** – see chapter 28).

It is important to discuss employment and driving with anyone suffering from epilepsy. (In UK, epileptics need to be free of attacks whilst awake for **two years** in order to obtain a licence.)

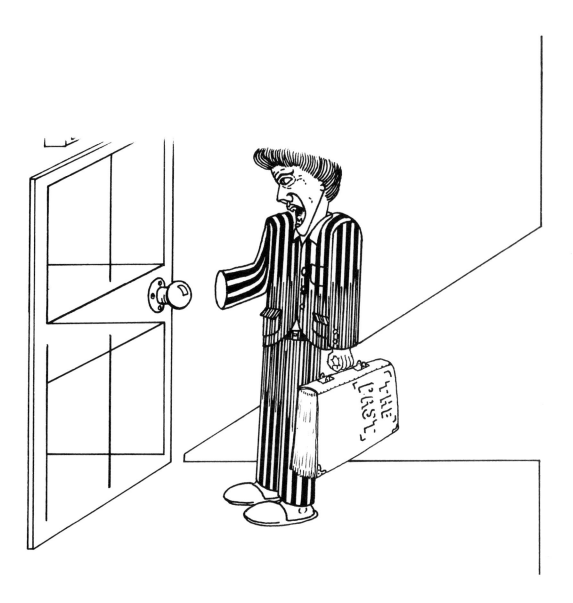

MENTAL HEALTH

OVERVIEW

Introduction

The Language of Psychiatry

Psychosis

Definition   Hypomania
Schizophrenia   Bipolar disorder
Psychotic depression

Neurosis

Definition   Obsessive/compulsive neurosis
Neurotic depression   Hysterical neurosis
Anxiety states

Personality Disorders

Schizoid   Obsessional
Cyclothymic   Psychopathic
Histrionic

Organic Brain Syndromes

Korsakoff's psychosis
Acute organic syndromes

Eating Disorders

Anorexia nervosa
Bulimia

Treatment in Psychiatry

Psychiatry and the Law

Case Taking in Psychiatry

The Assessment of the Mental State

» | Alcohol/drug dependence, psycho-sexual disorders and mental impairment (subnormality) are specialist topics outside the scope of this book. They are nevertheless interesting and important and you are encouraged to investigate them in your own reading.

INTRODUCTION

The current orthodox "medical model" (see chapter 1) has proved surprisingly durable as a way of approaching the classification and management of organic disease in developed western countries.

However, the powerful reductionist tools of conventional allopathy have only partial relevance to the complexities of thought and emotion encountered in psychiatric practice and there is a wealth of psychiatric literature explaining how best to describe roses with rulers.

It is important to realize at the outset that there is much argument about what really constitutes mental illness. When it comes down to it, a person is likely to be labelled mentally ill if their thought patterns, speech or behaviour lie outside commonly accepted limits of normality. Psychiatrists, therefore, have the unenviable task of arbitrating on what is "normal" and they work very hard to try and maintain a consensus on what constitutes psychiatric illness. This is, in fact, extremely important since they have considerable statutory power to detain people for treatment should their mental derangement constitute a danger to themselves or others.

It is likely that you will find much of what follows in the next few pages unsatisfactory and that is probably because it *is* unsatisfactory! Nevertheless, as anyone who has experience of severe mental disturbance knows, psychiatric illness can be profoundly painful and the sufferer is likely to find her/himself shunned by most of those s/he comes into contact with.

Psychiatrists and their co-workers in mental health take on the sort of problems most people instinctively run away from – the following is a brief introductory outline to their approach.

THE LANGUAGE OF PSYCHIATRY

The following are common terms used in psychiatry. They represent only a small part of a complex language.*

DELIRIUM:

An extreme state of organic brain dysfunction (characterized by disorientation, illusions, hallucinations, overactivity and changes of consciousness level).

DELUSION:

A delusion is a fixed, firm, false belief, inappropriate to a person's ethnic, social or religious background and held in the face of logical argument.

Delusions are important markers of **psychotic** illness and come in many forms, eg delusions of –

› Thoughts being interfered with.
› Thoughts being put into your head.
› Thoughts being "broadcast" to outsiders.
› Thoughts being spoken aloud.
› Thoughts being echoed.
› Thoughts being taken out of your head.
› Being controlled.
› Everything referring to you** (newspaper headlines, TV broadcasts etc).
› Paranoia
› Guilt
› Grandiosity
› Nihilism
› Misinterpretation
› Hypochondriasis
› Religious significance

etc, etc.

---

*   "A Glossary of Mental Disorders and Mental Health Legislation" – published by Wyeth
     Laboratories – is a useful dictionary of current psychiatric terms.
**   So called "ideas of reference"

DEPERSONALIZATION:

The feeling of not being oneself/feeling unreal.

DEREALIZATION:

The feeling that everything around you seems strange or somehow dreamlike.

FLIGHT OF IDEAS:

A way of talking* in which the topics change at an alarming rate.
The change from one topic to another may be sparked off by a rhyme, a pun or any other loose association of ideas.
With a little concentration, it is usually possible to travel with someone on their flight of ideas (ie to more or less understand what they're talking about).

HALLUCINATION:

An hallucination is a sensory perception that occurs without an obvious external stimulus (eg hearing voices coming from **outside** your head).
Auditory and visual hallucinations are more common than taste and smell hallucinations. Auditory hallucinations are a common accompaniment to "schizophrenia".

ILLUSION:

An illusion is a **misinterpretation** of a sensory perception; eg thinking that the doctor coming towards you is a werewolf (unless, of course ....).

Illusions are features of **organic mental states**.

PARANOIA:

Para-nous means "beyond reason" and thus, strictly speaking, paranoia is a psychiatric term used to describe the classic features of psychosis. Since persecutory delusions are common features of psychosis, the term is often taken to mean oversuspicion but the formal definition is "syn-

---

* Speech is taken in psychiatry – by and large – to represent thought.

dromes characterized by persecution, grandeur, litigation, jealousy, love, envy, hate or the supernatural".

PSYCHOSOMATIC:

Simply means the influence of mental function on body function.

It is sometimes used (in a derogatory sense) to imply that an apparently organic condition (eg asthma or peptic ulcer) is "all in the mind" (as if that somehow makes the complaint less deserving of attention!).

STEREOTYPIES:

Stereotyped, repetitive, voluntary movements not due to neurological disorder, eg head banging, rocking and eye poking.
They often occur in cases of mental retardation.

TICS:

Quick, involuntary, repeated, purposeless movements not caused by an obvious neurological disorder.

PSYCHOSIS

DEFINITION:

Psychosis means disturbance of thought, emotion and volition severe enough to distort a person's awareness of the world.
A catch phrase definition is that psychosis represents a "break down in reality testing".
A lay definition would be "completely mad".

Psychotic people frequently suffer hallucinations and delusions.

CLASSIFICATION:

Schizophrenia – a psychotic disorder of **thought**
Psychotic depression ⎫
Hypomania   ⎬   psychotic disorders of **emotion**
Bipolar disorder   ⎭
(manic depression)

SCHIZOPHRENIA

> › A psychotic disorder of thought.
> › Tends to affect younger people.
> › Usually chronic with periods of remission and relapse.
> › Thought disordered and confused by delusions.
> › Emotional responses blunted or inappropriate.
> › Behaviour apathetic, indecisive and withdrawn and sometimes bizarre.
> › Thus becomes virtually impossible to function in "normal" society.
> › Auditory hallucinations (discussing the sufferer or commenting on what they're doing) are common, as are delusions of thought interference and persecution.
> › The disturbance of logical thinking is often manifested in speech which, though grammatical and apparently fairly normal, often makes no sense when studied more closely.
> › "Schizophrenics" also complain that their thoughts sometimes "stop dead" leaving their mind a complete blank. This is referred to as **"thought block"**.

PSYCHOTIC (endogenous) DEPRESSION

> › Severe depressive disturbance of emotion more common from middle age onwards.

> The depressed mood often appears "spontaneously" and is so profound that there may be delusions of guilt or hypochondriasis ("I am being punished for being evil" or "my insides are rotting away with cancer").
> **Suicide is a real risk.**
> The sufferer may be agitated or may be so withdrawn and lacking in energy that they just sit immobile in a chair not bothering to eat or go to the toilet .....
> Bowel habit, appetite and sleep may all be disturbed.
> Feelings of depression are often worse first thing in the morning.

HYPOMANIA*

> A state of extreme overactivity, elation and excitement (sometimes accompanied by hallucinations and delusions).
> Tends to be self limiting but recurs at intervals.
> Delusions tend to be of a grandiose nature.
> Thoughts race at such a speed that speech shows "flight of ideas".
> Overactivity leads to progressive decrease in sleep.
> Tendency to start many projects, completing none.
> Dress becomes more extravagant, social/sexual inhibitions diminish, tendency to spend money unwisely.
> Behaviour eventually disruptive and possibly a danger to sufferer and others.

BIPOLAR DISORDER (manic depression)

> Alternating phases of mania and depression with normal periods in between.
> Affects males and females equally and seems to run in families.
> Tends to get worse as age increases.
> A surprising number of extremely successful people suffer from degrees of manic depression.

---

* The term hypomania is used to imply something slightly less than mania, although in practice it is hard to tell the difference.

NEUROSIS

DEFINITION

There is no universally accepted definition of neurosis but the term is usually taken to include psychiatric conditions in which **contact with "reality" is maintained** (ie no delusions and hallucinations).

Neurotic psychiatric illness (non-psychotic depression, anxiety states, obsessional disorders etc) is no less painful, however, since the sufferer usually has an acute awareness of the nature of his/her condition.

NEUROTIC ("reactive") DEPRESSION

Neurotic depression is classically defined as depressed mood in reaction to some external problem (eg bereavement). It is supposedly less severe than psychotic depression and is not necessarily accompanied by bowel, sleep and appetite disturbance. However, neurotic depression is frequently accompanied by symptoms of anxiety.

Many psychiatrists feel that the trivial distinction between endogenous and reactive depression is artificial and unhelpful.

ANXIETY STATES

A state of anxiety becomes a psychiatric problem i) when the symptoms and signs of anxiety are out of proportion to its causes or ii) if anxiety starts to appear independently of obvious precipitants.

Individuals prone to anxiety often have a past history of difficulty coping with stress, and typically recognize their fears as "irrational". Anxiety states may be dominated by "autonomic" symptoms (fast pulse, sweating, butterflies in stomach, light headedness etc) or by unbearable mental feelings of apprehension and fear.

They may represent a generalized reaction to stress or be concentrated into a "phobic" condition, eg
Claustrophobia – fear of being shut in.
Agoraphobia* – fear of being in a crowd, away from the safety of home.

---

*　Literally fear of the market place.

OBSESSIVE/COMPULSIVE NEUROSIS

Although not common, this is a relatively clear cut syndrome, common in people with a long history of obsessional traits.

It is characterized by feelings of being compelled to "carry out some action, to dwell on an idea, to recall an experience or to ruminate on an abstract topic".

Unwanted thoughts or ideas seem to intrude on normal thought but are recognized as being inappropriate or nonsensical.

The attempt to get rid of these urges and thoughts may produce severe anxiety, which may be relieved somewhat by performing little rituals (washing hands a certain number of times, checking several times that the windows or doors have been closed, touching every lamp post you pass etc).

Ultimately, the need to perform these rituals may become quite disabling in the context of a normal working life.

HYSTERICAL NEUROSIS (conversion hysteria)

Despite its common usage, hysteria has a fairly precise meaning in psychiatry.

In hysterical neurosis, the patient may develop a physical or psychological symptom which (in the patient's mind) mimics a "real" disease. Although the symptoms and signs may bear only a slight resemblance to typical "organic" illness, the patient's suffering will be real to them and the mechanism producing the state seems to be unconscious (ie hysterical conversion is NOT just a posh name for malingering!).

You should bear in mind, however, that many people labelled "hysterics" subsequently *do* turn out to have organic disease.

PERSONALITY DISORDERS

Personality is defined (by psychiatrists) as "the sum total of characteristics that determine the unique adjustment of an individual to life circumstances".

"Abnormal" personalities only become medically relevant if i) they cause an individual suffering; ii) they cause society to suffer or iii) they predispose to the development of a more serious psychiatric disorder.

The following personality types are often referred to:

SCHIZOID:

Withdrawn, sensitive, reclusive, stubborn.
Tend to fantasize.
Possible predisposition to schizophrenic disorders.

CYCLOTHYMIC:

Marked fluctuations between elation and depression.
Work output tends to increase dramatically in "up" phases.
Commonly seen in doctors, artists, comedians etc.
Possible predisposition to manic depression.

HISTRIONIC:

Attention seeking, manipulative, self indulgent, egocentric.
Problems establishing lasting relationships.

OBSESSIONAL (anankastic):

Perfectionist, tendency to check things, constant feeling of "could do better".
May develop opposing characteristics to compensate (eg unpunctuality.....).

PSYCHOPATHIC:

a) Aggressive –

Seriously irresponsible, antisocial, impulsive.
Inability to tolerate frustration which may lead to explosive/aggressive behaviour.

Tends to exploit personal relationships in unscrupulous way.
Often ends up in conflict with law.
Thought to be result of failure of "social maturation".

b) Inadequate –

Again irresponsible and immature.
Tends to neglect responsibilities and duties rather than become aggressive.
Again, tendency to conflict with law.

NOTE:

There is some evidence that dietary changes and vitamin supplementation may help the maturation/integration of "inadequate" personality types.

ORGANIC BRAIN SYNDROMES

Organic damage to brain tissue produces changes in cognitive ability (memory, orientation and concentration) and consciousness level. **Severe** brain degeneration can produce breakdown of emotional and physical control mechanisms and disorganization of personality.

Any patient showing a disturbance of memory, orientation (who am I, where am I) or consciousness must be investigated to exclude treatable causes of organic brain damage.[*]

> The major chronic organic brain syndrome is dementia, and this has been described in chapter 16. Only Korsakoff's psychosis and acute brain syndromes will be considered here.

KORSAKOFF'S PSYCHOSIS[**]

> A syndrome characterized by specific **loss of short term memory** capacity in the absence of generalized dementia.
> Often linked with chronic alcoholism.
> Thought to be irreversible.

ACUTE (organic) BRAIN SYNDROMES

> States where systemic disturbance (fever, poisoning, cerebral anoxia etc) cause clouding of consciousness and visual hallucinations.
> The extreme form is referred to as delirium.
>
> **Delirium tremens** (DTs) is the organic brain syndrome provoked by acute withdrawal from alcohol (and some drugs).

---

[*]   Note that organic brain damage does NOT, per se, produce hallucinations, delusions or other psychotic features.

[**] Which is not, in fact, a psychosis according to our formal definition

EATING DISORDERS

ANOREXIA NERVOSA

A syndrome characterized by persistent, active refusal to eat. This leads to profound weight loss.

› Most common in young women.
› Weight loss produces physiological changes including amenorrhoea, slow pulse, decreased body temperature.
› Strange eating habits, alterations in body image (thinking you look fat even if everyone else thinks you're thin) and an unusual attitude to food are common.
› May be accompanied by depression.
› The problem often seems to have its roots entangled in a rigid family situation and is notoriously difficult to manage.
However, **without treatment, anorexia nervosa frequently proves fatal.**

BULIMIA

A syndrome related to anorexia, with similar problems of self image and attitude to food, in which the sufferer repeatedly "binges" and then induces vomiting.

TREATMENT IN PSYCHIATRY

There is really no such thing in psychiatry as specific treatment for specific illness.

The objectives are i) to ease the disruption caused by an altered mental state and ii) to help the patient regain or maintain a more or less normal life within the community.

The options available are:

Psychological:

> › Simple counselling
> › Psychotherapeutic techniques
> › Behavioural therapies

Physical:

> › Electroconvulsive therapy
> › Major tranquillizers (eg chlorpromazine, trifluoperazine and haloperi-dol)
> › Minor tranquillizers (various benzodiazepines)
> › Antidepressants (tricyclics such as amitriptyline and imipramine; mono-amine oxidase inhibitors such as phenelzine and tranylcy-promine)

All psychotropic drugs have impressive side effects, particularly:

1) "Phenothiazine" type major tranquillizers such as chlorpromazine (Largactil):

   Restless legs
   Involuntary mouth movements
   Parkinsonism
   Odd movements of head and neck

2) Tricyclic antidepressants:

   Hypotension
   Palpitations
   Dry mouth
   Constipation
   Blurred vision
   Urinary retention

Confusion
Insomnia
Rashes

3) Benzodiazepine tranquillizers (eg Valium):

Withdrawal of the drug exaggerates the symptoms for which it was
originally prescribed

Occupational:

›   Occupational and industrial therapy, in which the patient is given a
    chance to re-learn life and work skills in a sheltered environment.

PSYCHIATRY AND THE LAW

The history of the care of the mentally ill is littered with stories of neglect, illtreatment and indifference and it was only with the **1959 Mental Health Act** that the emphasis finally changed to care and rehabilitation rather than incarceration and restraint.

The Act* contains sections governing the role of the various caring agencies, voluntary and compulsory admission to hospital, the management of criminal patients and special hospitals, the management of patient's property.

The sections covering compulsory admission ("sectioning") of the severely mentally ill (against their will if necessary) for observation or compulsory treatment are particularly interesting. "Sections" are usually applied for by the patient's own doctor or by a near relative or social worker and most require approval by 2 doctors, one of whom has a specialist training in psychiatry. They range from emergency admissions (up to 72 hours) via compulsory detention for observation (28 days) to 6 month admissions for compulsory treatment.

Copies of the 1959 Act and its 1983 amendments are available from HMSO, London.

---

*   Modified in 1983 by the Mental Health Amendment Act.

CASE TAKING IN PSYCHIATRY

OUTLINE

Presenting problem

Factual personal history:
(no waffle!)

> Birth – date/place/details
> Developmental landmarks (walking, talking etc)
> School record
> Higher education
> Occupation
> Sexual relationships
> Marriage
> Children

Present circumstances:

> Job
> Housing
> Finances
> Hobbies
> Friends

Family history

Past medical and psychiatric history:

> Including "forensic history" ie brushes with law etc

Drugs, allergies, smoking, drinking

Patient's view of his/her own personality type

Rest of general medical history

THE ASSESSMENT OF THE MENTAL STATE

The "mental state examination" in psychiatry takes the place of the physical examination in general medicine.

It is an attempt to make some *objective* assessment of the patient's mental processes and does not rely on the patient's co-operation (for the most part).

OUTLINE

Non-verbal behaviour:

Dress (cleanliness, colour, unusual accessories etc)
Walk (fast, slow, odd etc)
Motor activity (tics, mannerisms etc)

Social manner:

Aggressive
Withdrawn
Open
etc

Non-verbal expressions of mood:

Miserable
Anxious
Cheerful
etc

Speech (taken to reflect thought processes):

Form: Rate
            Quantity
            Volume
            Tone
            Flight of ideas
            Neologisms
            Schizophrenic speech disorder etc

(continued next page)

Content: Any suggestion of: Delusions
                                   Hallucinations
                                   Mood disturbance (depression, elation)
                                   Anxiety
                                   Obsessive/compulsive phenomena

Cognitive ability:

Conscious level

Orientation: Space (where am I)
              Time (what day is it)
              Person (who am I)

Recent memory

Past memory

Concentration

Failure to answer several of the following questions probably indicates a
defect in cognitive ability:

          How old are you?
          What day is it?
          What's your address?
          What year is it?
          Where is this place we're in now?
          Who am I?
          What year did the second world war start?
          Who's the prime minister/monarch at the moment?
          Can you subtract 7 from 100 in your head and keep doing it?

18. Joint Disease

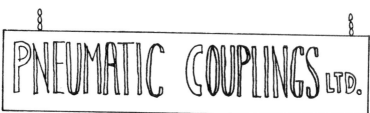

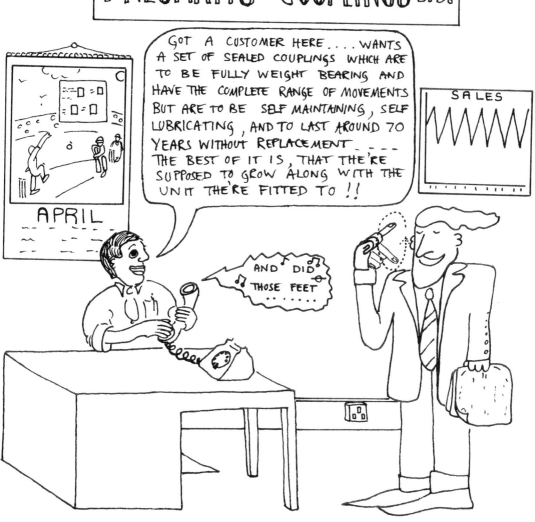

JOINT DISEASE

OVERVIEW

Classification of Arthritis

Introduction to Arthritis

Rheumatoid Arthritis

Osteoarthritis

Comparison of the Main Features of RA and OA

Seronegative Arthritides

Ankylosing spondylitis
Reiter's disease
Psoriatic arthritis
Arthritis associated with inflammatory bowel disease

Crystal Deposition Diseases

Gout

A Classification of Low Back Pain

Conditions Associated with Arthritis and Connective Tissue Disorders

Carpal tunnel syndrome
Raynaud's phenomenon

CLASSIFICATION OF ARTHRITIS

MULTISYSTEM:

Rheumatoid arthritis

Seronegative arthritides: Ankylosing spondylitis
                              Reiter's syndrome
                              Psoriatic arthritis
                              Arthritis associated with
                              chronic inflammatory bowel disease

Connective tissue diseases

OTHER:

Osteoarthritis

Crystal deposition disease: Gout
                                Pseudo-gout

Infective arthritis

Back pain

Soft tissue damage

NOTE:

Sarcoidosis and amyloidosis are two other "multisystem" diseases which may occasionally present as "arthritis".

INTRODUCTION TO ARTHRITIS

Background:

Arthritis means joint disease associated with inflammation. It produces a clinical picture of **pain, stiffness and loss of function** with **signs of inflammation** at one or more joints.

The term **"arthrosis"** refers to NON-inflammatory joint disease.

"Rheumatic" complaints are the cause of at least 35,000,000 working days lost a year in Brittain. They account for about 20% of a GP's workload and 30% of the disabled population. Many rheumatic diseases involve **several body systems** and the **pattern** of disease distribution often provides major diagnostic clues.

General investigation of arthritis:

1) It is important to examine all joints for:
   heat
   tenderness
   swelling
   deformity
   loss of function

2) Joint "imaging" of various kinds (X-rays etc).

3) Non-specific blood tests for inflammation including:
   > ESR* – a measure of blood viscosity, frequently raised in inflammation.
   > Haemoglobin – anaemia is a frequent accompaniment to chronic inflammatory disease (see chapter 23).

4) Analysis of synovial fluid taken from joints.

5) Immunological tests to detect **antibodies** such as **rheumatoid factor** and **anti-nuclear factor** (both evidence of an underlying **auto-immune** process).
   The terms **seropositive** and **seronegative** refer to the presence or absence of **rheumatoid factor** in the blood of a patient with arthritis.

---

*   erythrocyte sedimentation rate.

RHEUMATOID ARTHRITIS

An idiopathic, chronic, generalized inflammatory disease affecting many parts of the body and particularly the synovial membranes of joints and tendons. Persistent "synovitis" eventually destroys joints and damages the surrounding tissues.

Prevalence:

Affects 1% of males and 3% of females in UK.

Population:

Most frequent onset at about 40 yrs, rare in children.

Aetiologicalfactors:

› Positive family history in about 10%.
› Strong association with particular "tissue type" (known as HLA-D4).
› Seems to be a recent disease (post 1800).
› Auto-immune mechanisms appear to be responsible for maintaining the disease process, but the initial "trigger" may be **infective**.

Geography:

Worldwide, but rare in isolated African communities.

Pathogenesis:

The principal pathologies are **synovitis, nodules, vasculitis** and hyperplasia of lymphoid tissue.

Pathology:

RA causes extensive hypertrophy of synovial tissue associated with a layer of inflammatory tissue (called **pannus**) growing across the joint surface and eating into bone and cartilage at joint edges.

Nodules (30% of patients) develop at subcutaneous pressure points, on tendons and in some internal organs (lungs, eyes etc).

Under the microscope, chronic inflammatory cell infiltration is seen in synovial tissue. Nodules also have characteristic appearance.

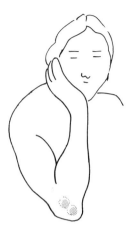

Rheumatoid nodules

Clinical features:

RA starts with weeks or months of general malaise ± weight loss and mild fevers.

Joint symptoms often begin in the hands or feet in **symmetrical** way, but almost any pattern is possible.

Joints become painful, swollen and stiff, worse in the morning.

Advanced disease produces joint deformity (often accompanied by muscle wasting and nerve entrapment).

"Tenosynovitis" may cause **tendon rupture.** This leads to the typical rheumatoid deformities.

Damage to **large** joints often dominates clinical picture.

Extra-articular manifestations:

Very common	Less common
Dry eyes (keratoconjunctivitis sicca)	Scleritis
	Spinal cord damage
Pleural effusions	Pericardial effusion
Nodules	Pulmonary nodules
	Pulmonary fibrosis
Lymphadenopathy	Splenomegaly
Carpal tunnel syndrome	Renal amyloidosis
Skin ulceration	
Vasculitis affecting fingers and toes	Peripheral neuropathies

Extra-articular manifestations cause many complications and occur more frequently in men than women.

Nearly all patients with RA have an **anaemia** proportional to their disease activity together with a **raised ESR** and **rheumatoid factor in** the blood (80%).

Typical X-ray changes of joints appear after about 6 months of disease activity.

Treatment:

RA is considered incurable and the sufferer may have a bewildering range of functional, social, emotional and medical problems. Possibilities (excluding alternative therapies!) include counselling, physiotherapy, occupational therapy, surgery for badly damaged joints (eg hip replacement) and drugs. The advice of specialist "pain clinics" is sometimes useful.

Orthodox drug therapy in RA is thought of in 3 "lines":

Line 1 $\rightarrow$ Attempts symptomatic control by use of the huge range of **non-steroidal anti-inflammatory drugs.**

Line 2 $\rightarrow$ Attempts modification of disease process by the use of **gold, d-penicillamine, sulphasalazine** and the **anti-malarials.**

Line 3 $\rightarrow$ Represents last ditch therapy and includes steroids and "cytotoxic" drugs.

Prognosis:

A small proportion of people with RA recover with few remedial problems. Some have disease which progresses to deformity and death within a few years. The majority suffer insidious progression punctuated by slight remissions.

Paradoxically, an "explosive" onset is associated with relatively good long term outcome.

OSTEOARTHRITIS

A very common degenerative disorder of joints characterized by loss of articular cartilage with thickening (sclerosis) of underlying bone. It occurs in nearly everyone over the age of 60!

Background:

Approx. 10% of the population have problems related to OA.
Mean onset age = 50 yrs.
Commoner in women.
Related to age, obesity, previous joint injury and previous joint deformity.

Pathology:

› Progressive changes in cartilage biochemistry lead to extensive loss of cartilage volume.
› Underlying bone is generally thickened but some areas become porous with formation of bone "cysts".
› Re-modelling of bone edges produces **osteophytes** (bony lumps).
› The joint capsules become fibrotic.

Clinical features:

Asymmetrical joint involvement with pain related to joint use (hence worse at the end of day). Varying degrees of immobility and deformity.
Morning stiffness tends to wear off after 15 minutes exercise.
Symptoms often weather sensitive.

Treatment:

Is non-specific and depends on the use of simple analgesics ± NSAIAs.*

Weight loss, a walking stick and gentle activity can be a great help. Orthopaedic surgery offers a variety of procedures to improve joint function or relieve pain.

*   non-steroidal anti-inflammatory agents.

COMPARISON OF THE MAIN CLINICAL FEATURES OF RA AND OA

	Rheumatoid Arthritis	**Osteoarthrosis**
Pathogenesis:	Inflammatory	Degenerative
Sex:	M:F = 1:3	M:F = 1:1
Age:	20-55	50$^+$
Joints:	MCP, PIP wrists, MIP	DIP, 1st CMC hips, knees
Other features:	rheumatoid nodules extra-articular manifestations	Heberden's nodes Bouchard's nodes
Blood tests:	anaemia ESR ↑ RF* 70-80% positive	Hb normal ESR normal RF negative
Synovial fluid:	cloudy ↑ viscosity white blood cells RF positive	clear ↓ viscosity cartilage fragments RF negative
Symptoms:	systemic disturbance with anorexia fever and weight loss EMS**>15 mins	no systemic disturbance EMS<15 mins

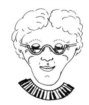

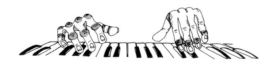

rheumatoid arthritis   osteoarthrosis

*   rheumatoid factor.
**   early morning stiffness.

SERONEGATIVE ARTHRITIDES

The "seronegative" arthritides are a group of inflammatory conditions that involve the spine and peripheral joints. They are called seronegative because the blood of sufferers contains no "rheumatoid factor" or other specific immunological "markers". They tend to run in families.

ANKYLOSINGSPONDYLITIS*

A relatively common condition affecting young adults (male/female = ~8/1)

Pathology:

Inflammation of the ligaments supporting spinal joints leading to healing by calcification. In other words, the supporting ligaments of the spine ossify. The sacro-iliac and spinal joints are usually affected first, but hips, knees, shoulders and ankles may also become involved.

Clinical features:

The common presentation is **early morning low backache and stiffness relieved by movement.** There may also be malaise, weight loss and low grade fever.

Inflammation of the Achilles tendon** or plantar fascia occasionally causes pain in the heel.

As the disease progresses and the spinal ligaments harden, the spine becomes stiff and abnormally bent*** leaving the patient doubled up.

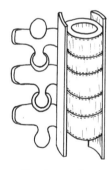

Restriction of respiratory movements can be an added complication. Iritis and urethritis may appear as "extra-articular" manifestations of the disease.

Bamboo spine

---

*   Ankylosis = hardening – Spondylitis = inflammation of spinal joints
**   Achilles, Greek hero and son of Peleus (a famous warrior) and Thetis (an immortal sea nymph). Famous for his part in the battle of Troja. Invulnerable, except for his ankle bone, by which his mother held him when she dipped him in the river Styx.
*** The x-ray appearance is referred to as a "bamboo spine"

Management:

Physiotherapy + exercise to maintain mobility plus NSAIAs for pain relief.

Prognosis:

Generally good with regard to life expectancy. In fact, the disease often becomes less active as the years go by. Nevertheless the constant pain and discomfort can be profoundly difficult to cope with.

REITER'S DISEASE

An arthritic condition that seems to be a complication of NSU* or infective diarrhoea (eg dysentery).

It is more common in young men.

Clinical features:

NSU or dysentery

Conjunctivitis/arthritis (usually lower limbs and asymmetrical)

Long history of remissions and relapses

When the disease is active, there may be iritis and lesions on the skin and mucous membranes, eg circinate balanitis (ulceration of glans penis) and keratoderma blenorrhagica (blisters on the soles of the feet).

Heel pain and low back pain (from Achilles tendinitis and sacroiliitis respectively) may also occur.

Management:

Symptomatic treatment of acute phases.

---

*   non-specific urethritis.

PSORIATIC ARTHRITIS (arthropathy)

Psoriasis is described in chapter 24.

About 1 in 10 psoriasis sufferers also develop arthritis, mainly affecting the fingers and toes.

The severity of the skin condition seems to bear little relation to the severity of the arthritis. It is even possible to have psoriatic arthropathy with **no** active skin lesions.

ARTHRITIS ASSOCIATED WITH INFLAMMATORY BOWEL DISEASE

Patients with Crohn's disease or ulcerative colitis (see chapter 13) some-times develop acute arthritis, usually asymmetrical and affecting the lower limbs.

They also appear to be more prone to developing ankylosing spondylitis.

NOTE:

A number of chronic arthritic conditions of children are described, the most famous being **Still's disease,**[*] a severe disorder characterized by arthritis, fever, skin rash, lymphadenopathy and enlarged liver and spleen.

---

[*]   Sir George Still (1818-1941), poet, classicist and eminent paediatrician of Great Ormond Street Hospital, London.

CRYSTAL DEPOSITION DISEASES

GOUT

Gout is the clinical condition produced by the deposition of uric acid crystals in joints. It is characterized by episodes of acute arthritis, usually affecting only one joint.

Aetiology:

There is a body "pool" of uric acid derived from the diet and from cellular metabolism. In normal circumstances, uric acid is eliminated via the kidneys and gut and thus the blood "level" of uric acid (urate) is kept within safe limits.

Should the blood urate level rise beyond a certain point, however, there is a tendency for small amounts of uric acid to crystallize out in the joints. This may produce a devastatingly painful attack of acute gout. Note, however, that hyperuricaemia* in itself will not **necessarily** lead to gout.

Rarely, after repeated attacks of gout, subcutaneous nodules of crystals may form around the big toe, Achilles tendon, elbows or in the pinna of the ear. The nodules are called "tophi" and the condition is then referred to as **chronic "tophaceous" gout**.

The main causes of gout are:

1) Overproduction of uric acid due to an inherited error of metabolism (usually in men and post-menopausal women) –

2) Overproduction of uric acid due to "myeloproliferative" disorders** or blood cancers and/or treatment with cytotoxic drugs –

3) Undersecretion of uric acid due to kidney failure or **treatment with diuretics** .

---

*   Too much acid in the blood.
**   See chapter 23.

Hyperuricaemia (and thus gout) is also associated with:

› high IQ
› obesity
› high alcohol intake
› hypertension
› high blood triglyceride levels

Attacks can be **precipitated** by trauma, surgery, dietary excess, alcohol and starvation.

Epidemiology:

Men with gout outnumber women with gout by 8:1.
Most women have diuretic induced ("secondary") gout and are older when they have their first attack.

Clinical features:

The condition is characterized by sudden onset of a red, hot, shiny, tender joint. The sufferer is febrile*, irritable and anorexic**.

75% of first attacks involve the big toe (1st MCP) (the other 25% usually involve the ankle or knee).

Gout may be complicated by kidney stones (made of urate crystals) and, sometimes, renal failure.

Management:

Involves correction of precipitating factors (where possible) plus indomethacin (or another NSAIA) or colchicine for the pain of an acute attack.

Allopurinol or probenecid seem to help prevent long term recurrence.

Prognosis:

Good, as long as associated problems (hypertension, hypertriglyceridaemia etc) are well managed.

---

* has a temperature.
** doesn't want to eat.

A CLASSIFICATION OF LOW BACK PAIN

ARISING FROM THE SPINE ITSELF:

Soft tissue

Disc lesions
Osteoarthrosis (spondylosis)
Muscle and ligaments strains
Sacro-iliac strain

Bony tissue

Inflammatory:

Ankylosing spondylitis
Infection
TB

Metabolic:

Osteoporosis (associated with Cushing's and post-menopausal hormonal changes)
Osteomalacia
Paget's disease

Neoplastic:

Primary: myeloma
Secondary: breast, prostate (lung, thyroid, kidney)

Structural:

Fractures
Spinal stenosis
Spondylolisthesis*

REFERRED FROM VISCERA:

Chest:

Heart
Lungs
Pleura

Abdomen:

Kidney
Aorta

FROM NERVE DAMAGE:

Herpes zoster
Neurofibromata

PSYCHOGENIC:

Tension

*   The slipping out of position of one vertebra in relation to another

CONDITIONS ASSOCIATED WITH ARTHRITIS AND CTDs

CARPAL TUNNEL SYNDROME

Caused by compression of the **median** nerve as it passes beneath the flexor retinaculum at the wrist. It is characterized by tingling and pain in the hand.

Aetiology:

Any soft tissue swelling around the wrist may produce carpal tunnel symptoms but the condition is commonly "idiopathic", occurring particularly in people who use their hands a lot and in middle aged women.
It can also be symptomatic of
› pregnancy
› oral contraceptives
› the menopause
› gout
› TB
› underactive thyroid
› acromegaly
› rheumatoid arthritis (in which it is frequently bilateral)

And, much more rarely,
› cervical spine disorders
› motor neurone disease

Clinical features include:

Pain (burning and tingling in the (approximate) distribution of the median nerve), worse at night and relieved by raising the arm or placing the hand in cold water.
Some sensory deficit may be found on examination.
Tapping the flexor retinaculum may reproduce the symptoms.

Treatment:

Various treatments are tried, eg rest, splints, diuretics and local steroid injections. Surgical "decompression" is a last resort.

19. Connective Tissue Disorders

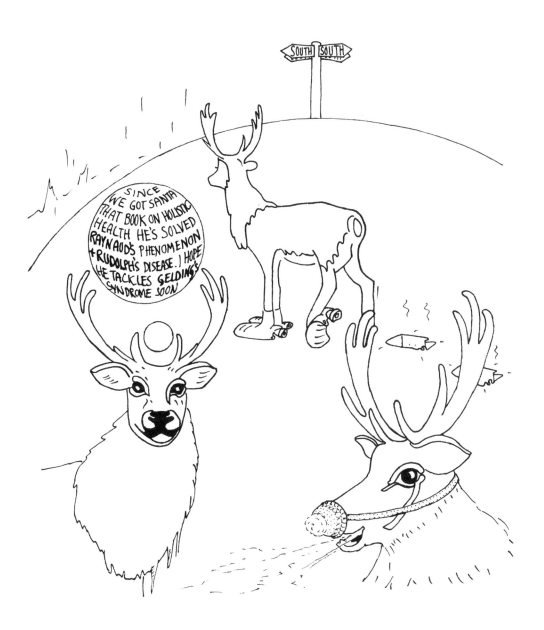

RAYNAUD'SPHENOMENON*

Defined as intermittent, cold-precipitated symmetrical attacks of pallor and/or blueness (cyanosis) of the digits **without** any evidence of obstructive arterial disease.

The fingers (± toes) are first white (arterial spasm), then blue (lack of oxygen locally) and finally red (reactive dilatation of arterioles).

The cause is obscure but the condition is often familial and commoner in young women (in whom it is called Raynaud's **disease**).

» Connective tissue disorders (see chapter 19), work involving vibrating tools, and certain drugs (including β-blockers and oral contraceptives) may all precipitate the syndrome.

Management:

Avoidance of injury to the hands, stopping smoking and very warm gloves all help.

Nifedipine is sometimes useful and surgical sympathectomy is available as a last resort.

---

* Maurice Raynaud (1834-1881), French physician who worked in Paris.

CONNECTIVE TISSUE DISORDERS

OVERVIEW

Introduction

Systemic Lupus Erythematosus

Polymyalgia Rheumatica

Polyarteritis Nodosa

Scleroderma

INTRODUCTION

In some people, the control mechanisms which prevent an immune response to "self" are deficient or absent. In others, antibodies produced against foreign antigens may **also** react with **normal** body tissue, thereby causing damage. The diseases produced by either mechanism are called **auto-immune**.

Examples of auto-immune conditions are:

> Thyroid disease (certain forms – see chapter 14)
> Hypoparathyroidism
> Pernicious anaemia
> Addison's disease
> Insulin dependent diabetes
> Myasthenia gravis
> Primary biliary cirrhosis
> Chronic active hepatitis
> Rheumatoid arthritis
> Systemic lupus erythematosus (SLE)
> Dermatomyositis

The last three are examples of connective tissue diseases. Other CTDs (including polymyalgia rheumatica, giant cell arteritis and poly-myositis) are also thought to be mediated by immune mechanisms.

Someone once said that the connective tissue diseases are rather like a range of mountains, all with the same uncanny air about them.
They have a habit of changing places with each other, sinking without trace and then cropping up in some new terrain.

However, the CTDs do exhibit some common features:

> Involvement of many organs
> Fever, malaise and joint pains
> Insidious onset
> Anaemia
> A raised ESR
> Good response to **steroids**

SYSTEMIC LUPUS ERYTHEMATOSUS

SLE is an archetypal and relatively common connective tissue disease. It is a multisystem illness characterized by widespread **vasculitis** associated with the production of auto-anti-bodies and immune complexes. It is most common in young women, blacks and people taking isoniazid (an anti-TB drug) or hydralazine (an anti-hypertensive drug). It primarily affects **joints, skin,** the **CNS** and the **kidney.**

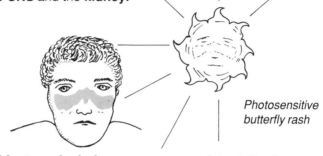

Photosensitive butterfly rash

The clinical features include some or many of the following:

› Joint pain
› Photosensitive butterfly shaped rash on face, often spreading to body
› Pleurisy
› Pericarditis
› Fits
› Psychosis
› Diplopia (double vision)
› Renal involvement producing oedema, proteinuria, hypertension and renal failure
› Raynaud's phenomenon
› Hair loss
› Oral ulceration
› Purpura (small bruises)
› Enlarged liver and spleen

» Various blood tests can be used to confirm the initial clinical impression.

Management:

A variety of drugs are used in management including NSAIAs, steroids, azathioprine, anti-malarials and cytotoxics. The skin rash is photosensitive, so avoiding strong sunlight is sensible.

Prognosis:

The prognosis is variable and drug therapy can often control symptoms quite effectively. Kidney involvement is associated with a poor prognosis.

POLYMYALGIA RHEUMATICA

A relatively common disease affecting elderly people and characterized by severe stiffness, shoulder and pelvic girdle pain and a **very high ESR.**

Clinical features:

The condition tends to develop slowly with muscle tenderness, hip and shoulder stiffness, weight loss, malaise, low grade fever and depression. The hip and shoulder stiffness may completely immobilize the patient from time to time.

There may also be an associated anaemia.

Management:

Systemic steroids bring dramatic relief and the disease often "burns itself out" after a few years.

VERY IMPORTANT NOTE

About 1 in 3 patients with polymyalgia rheumatica have **"giant cell arteritis"** (a particular type of inflammation affecting artery walls). This may cause no problems but, in some people, may produce **temporal arteritis**, a condition characterized by severe unilateral headache and scalp tenderness in the temporal region (sometimes noticed when combing the hair).

» *WITHOUT STEROID TREATMENT, THE ARTERITIS MAY SPREAD FROM THE TEMPORAL ARTERY TO INVOLVE THE BLOOD SUPPLY OF THE EYE PRODUCING SUDDEN, UNTREATABLE BLINDNESS –*

Never ignore an elderly person complaining of malaise, headache and temporal tenderness.

POLYARTERITIS NODOSA

A **rare** systemic connective tissue disease, usually affecting young men and characterized by chronic inflammation of the media of small and medium sized arteries.

Clinical features:

Malaise, fever and weight loss are accompanied by the symptoms and signs of damage to major organs (caused by the vasculitis).

Kidney damage, severe hypertension, joint and muscle pains (especially in the calf) and peripheral neuropathies are relatively common.

Management:

Steroids and/or cytotoxic drugs.

Prognosis:

Up to 50% mortality within a few months of diagnosis.
The 5 year survival improves with steroid therapy.

SCLERODERMA

Scleroderma, also known as systemic sclerosis, is another (less common) connective tissue disorder that causes progressive scarring (fibrosis) of different organs.

Incidence:

Females>males
Common onset 30-50 years.

Pathology:

The condition is thought to be related to **abnormalities of small blood vessels**.

Clinical features:

Systemic sclerosis can produce a bewildering array of symptoms and signs.

› Raynaud's phenomenon
› Stretching and thinning of the skin of the face and around the mouth
› Skin pigmentation changes
› Hair loss
› Problems swallowing (due to oesophageal muscle atrophy)

are all fairly common.

» Kidney damage occurs in up to 50% of cases and may prove fatal.

Management:

Symptomatic.

NOTE:

For descriptions of polymyositis and dermatomyositis, which are very rare, refer to a standard textbook of medicine.

20. Bone Disease

Stony and still though it seems,

bone quickens;

it flows.

It is never the same at any two moments .....

Richard Selzer

BONE DISEASE

OVERVIEW

Metabolic Bone Diseases

Osteoporosis
Osteomalacia
Paget's disease
Renal osteodystrophy

Calcium & Phosphate Levels in Common Bone Diseases

Acute Osteomyelitis

Osteogenic Sarcoma

METABOLIC BONE DISEASES

OSTEOPOROSIS

Osteoporosis means a decrease in bone **density** without abnormalities in blood calcium levels.

Population:

Bone density seems to decrease as a function of age. It is often exaggerated in post menopausal women.

Aetiology:

Not understood but   Steroids
                            RA
                            Prolonged immobilization
                            Hyperthyroidism

                  are all associated with osteoporosis.

Clinical features:

May be none, but can cause chronic backache, loss of height and spinal deformities.

Less dense bones break more easily and thus hip and wrist fractures following minor trauma (or sudden vertebral collapse causing acute severe backache) may result from osteoporosis.

Management:

There is no clear consensus on the best course of management but avoiding calcium and vitamin D deficiency would seem logical (especially in peri-menopausal women).

Sex hormone supplementation (though not necessarily desirable) may also help.

OSTEOMALACIA *

Osteomalacia means mineral (calcium) deficient bone.

Pathology:

Dietary vitamin D deficiency, inadequate exposure of skin to sunlight (vitamin D is partially produced in the skin under the influence of light), malabsorption of vitamin D and inherent defects in vitamin D metabolism will all produce abnormal bone mineralization.
Some drugs also interfere with vitamin D synthesis.

Population:

Asian children, the elderly and the chronically infirm are the groups most at risk in Brittain.

Clinical features:

Children: Bow legs – strange walk
               Lumpy costochondral junctions (so called "Rickety Rosary")
               Depression of chest wall over 6th rib
               Muscle flaccidity
               Muscle spasms
               Fits
               Softening of cranial bones

Adults: Proximal muscle weakness – strange walk
               Bone pain
               Bone deformities/fractures

Management:

Vitamin D supplementation.

* Rickets is osteomalacia of children.

PAGET'S DISEASE *

An unusual but (worldwide) fairly common bone disease characterized by a simultaneous increase in the production and reabsorption of bone. This produces deformed, highly vascular bones of uneven density. The tibia and skull are most frequently affected.

Clinical features:

> Bone pain
> Localized bone enlargements/deformities (eg a change in the circumference of skull producing a change in hat size) (although fewer people wear hats nowadays)
> Fractures through abnormal areas
> Blindness or deafness (from compression of the IInd or VIIIth nerves by enlarging skull)
> Heart failure (from the effort of supplying highly vascular, abnormal bones)
> Higher incidence of bone cancer

Management:

Symptomatic.
Calcitonin injections seem to halt progress of condition.

---

*   Sir James Paget (1814-1899), born in Norfolk, one of 17 children. Studied and worked at St. Bartholomew's Hospital. Eventually became President of the Royal College of Surgeons and surgeon to the Queen. Reputed to have had the largest private practice in London.

RENAL OSTEODYSTROPHY

Renal failure interferes with vitamin D metabolism and calcium homeostasis. It can thus produce metabolic bone diseases referred to collectively as "Renal Osteodystrophy".

Clinical features:

> › Bone pain
> › Bone deformity
> › Sore eyes (from "metastatic calcification" of conjunctiva)

Management:

Depends on the nature of the biochemical deficit.

If there is an osteomalacia type picture, cautious vitamin D supplementation may help.

CALCIUM AND PHOSPHATE LEVELS IN COMMON BONE DISEASES

In health, about 40% of plasma calcium travels in the blood bound to **albumin.** The UNbound portion is the clinically important part. Routine lab tests measure **total** plasma calcium. Thus patients with a **low** plasma albumin (eg those with liver disease or renal disease) will produce a laboratory plasma calcium reading **lower** than it actually is. Conversely, patients with $\uparrow$ plasma albumin (caused by dehydration, or by taking the blood sample with a tourniquet on), will produce a plasma calcium reading **higher** than it actually is.

So, assuming that plasma albumin level is normal, that the patient isn't dehydrated and that the blood sample was correctly taken:

> $\uparrow$ blood levels of PTH will increase Ca level and decrease PO_4 levels.*
>
> $\uparrow$ vitamin D levels** will $\uparrow$ Ca and decrease PO_4 by increasing calcium absorption in the **gut** and increasing phosphate excretion in the urine.
>
> $\uparrow$ thyroxine levels may produce $\downarrow$ serum calcium.
>
> Calcitonin (made in thyroid) decreases plasma Ca and PO_4 levels.

LOW CALCIUM:

> $\downarrow$ Ca + $\uparrow$ PO_4 suggests chronic renal failure or hypoparathyroidism.
>
> $\downarrow$ Ca + normal or $\downarrow$ PO_4 suggests osteomalacia, pancreatitis or overhydration.
>
> Thyroid and parathyroid surgery may produce hypocalcaemia.

---

*   By enhancing Ca reabsorption from the kidney, enhancing the action of vitamin D and decreasing PO_4 reabsorption by the kidney. The output of PTH is directly responsive to the NON-albumin bound level of plasma calcium.

** Vit D is absorbed from the diet and synthesized in the skin by the action of sunlight. Before exerting its effect it must be processed in the liver and converted to a more active form in the kidney.

Symptoms/signs of ↓ calcium include:

> Depression
> Muscle spasms
> Perioral pins and needles

HIGH CALCIUM:

↑Ca + ↓ or normal phosphate suggests primary or tertiary hyperparathyroidism.

↑ Ca + ↑ or normal phosphate suggests:

a) Myeloma or vitamin D excess in which plasma **alkaline phosphatase** levels will be **normal**

or

b) Bone secondaries in which plasma alkaline phosphatase may be **raised**.

or

c) Thyrotoxicosis or sarcoidosis, in which plasma alkaline may be normal or raised.

Symptoms and signs of ↑ Ca include:

> Abdominal pain
> Nausea
> Vomiting
> Constipation
> Depression
> Polyuria
> ↓ Appetite and weight loss
> Thirst
> Weakness
> Renal stones
> Renal failure
> Eye problems
> Sudden cardiac arrest

ACUTE OSTEOMYELITIS

Acute osteomyelitis used to be an acute life threatening disease of children.

A general improvement in health and nutrition is probably responsible for the ↓ incidence nowadays.

The common organism involved is staph. aureus which reaches bone via the bloodstream from some more or less obvious primary focus (eg a boil or infected cut).

Acute osteomyelitis usually starts in the metaphysis of a bone.

Clinical features:

The classic presentation is sudden onset of pain in a bone with acute tenderness in an ill, feverish, flushed child.

Tenderness over the metaphysis of a long bone in an ill person should be presumed to be acute osteomyelitis until proved otherwise.

Management:

X-rays, blood cultures and urgent antibiotic therapy, since treatment within the first 48 hours should produce complete resolution.
Delay may lead to abscess formation and the need for surgery to drain the collected pus.
Ineffective treatment may lead to **chronic osteomyelitis** with flare ups of pain and fever and discharge of pus through skin via sinuses connecting infected bone to the surface.

OSTEOGENIC SARCOMA

Most common between ages of 10 and 20 (also seen as a complication of Paget's disease in the elderly).

Common sites = lower femur (50%), upper tibia (20%), humerus (10%), other (20%).

Clinical features include:

> › Pain (worse at night)
> › Local swelling
> › Pathological fracture
> › The effects of metastases

Metastasis to the lungs (via the bloodstream) occurs very early.

Treatment:

Amputation (if early disease) plus radio- and chemotherapy.

Prognosis:

Very poor despite treatment.

21. Renal Medicine

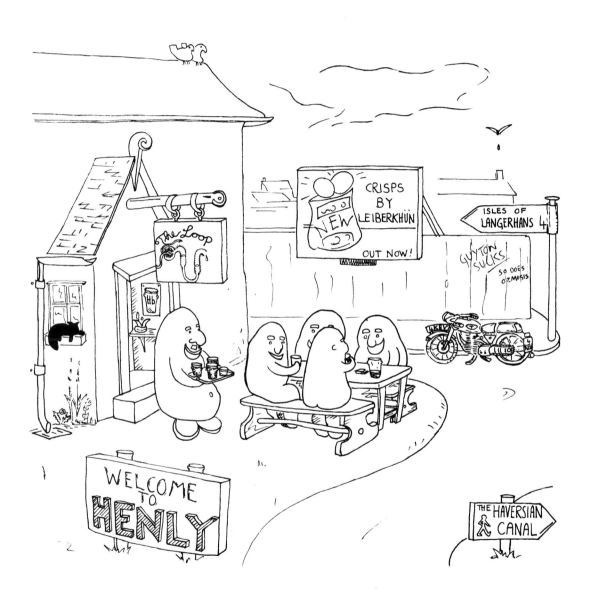

RENAL MEDICINE

including Urinary Tract Infections

OVERVIEW

Introduction

Medical Conditions Affecting the Kidney

Chronic pyelonephritis
Acute pyelonephritis
Glomerulonephritis
Systemic diseases associated with kidney damage
Congenital kidney diseases
Drug induced syndromes
Hypertension

Common Presentations of Kidney Disease

Proteinuria
Haematuria
Hypertension
Severe proteinuria (nephrotic syndrome)
Acute nephritis
Acute renal failure
Chronic renal failure

Cystitis

Asymptomatic Bacteriuria

Urethral Syndrome

INTRODUCTION

Renal medicine is one of the most complex topics in orthodox medical science. It is hard to gain an overview of the subject because much of the available literature blurs the distinction between common *presentations* of renal disease and common renal *pathologies*. There is also a clear demarcation between urinary tract conditions dealt with by physicians and those dealt with by surgeons, ie:

Medical:

> › Diseases of the kidney excluding stones and malignancy
> › Renal infection and most infections of the lower urinary tract

Surgical (urology):

> › Urinary tract stones
> › Urinary tract malignancies
> › Diseases of the prostate and testes
> › Mechanical problems affecting bladder/urethra (including incontinence)
> › Some lower urinary tract infections

Doctors with a special interest in dialysis/renal transplant develop a combination of medical and surgical skills and work in multidisciplinary teams.

The medical conditions mentioned above are dealt with in this section, and most of the surgical topics are described in chapter 22. Incontinence is dealt with briefly in chapter 26. Renal transplant is outside the scope of this book.

MEDICAL CONDITIONS AFFECTING THE KIDNEY

The following conditions may cause **any** of the presentations described later in this chapter.

CHRONIC PYELONEPHRITIS (reflux nephropathy)

Chronic inflammation of the kidneys possibly related to abnormal back-flow of infected urine up the ureters. Affected kidneys become scarred and shrunken.

ACUTE PYELONEPHRITIS

Bacterial infection of the kidney substance. This causes severe malaise, high fever and intense loin pain ± symptoms and signs of cystitis.

GLOMERULONEPHRITIS

The term glomerulonephritis is used to describe both clinical* and patho-logical entities.

The pathological classification of glomerulonephritis is complicated. Different specialist centres often use different language to describe the same thing. Suffice it to say that glomerulonephritis may be **primary** (eg post streptococcal glomerulonephritis) or **secondary** to systemic disease.

In both situations, damage to glomeruli is caused by immune mechanisms eg either the production of immune complexes which jam up the glomerular capillaries or direct damage to glomerular capillary basement membranes by antibodies.

Glomerulonephritis is serious because it often results in renal failure.

SYSTEMIC DISEASES ASSOCIATED WITH KIDNEY DAMAGE

Diabetes
Connective tissue disorders
Gout
Amyloid

---

*   See "acute nephritis" below.

CONGENITAL KIDNEY DISEASES

Polycystic disease is the most well known.

DRUG INDUCED SYNDROMES

Analgesic abuse in particular.

HYPERTENSION

High blood pressure can both cause and result from kidney damage.

COMMON PRESENTATIONS OF KIDNEY DISEASE

> › Proteinuria
> › Haematuria
> › Hypertension
> › Severe proteinuria (the NEPHROTIC syndrome)
> › Acute nephritis
> › Acute renal failure
> › Chronic renal failure

PROTEINURIA

Proteinuria means protein in the urine.
It is easily detected by "dipstick" testing.
It suggests either severe urinary tract infection or leakage of protein from glomeruli or tubules secondary to another disease process.
Protein in sterile urine would suggest kidney damage.
Dipsticks may produce a "false" reading if the urine specimen is "contaminated " with vaginal mucus, menstrual blood etc.

Common causes:

> › Urinary tract infection
> › Diabetic kidney damage
> › Glomerulonephritis
> › The nephrotic syndrome (see below)
> › "Postural proteinuria." This is a benign condition of young adults who just happen to have proteinuria when they have been standing up for some time. The early morning urine is normal. Persistence of the condition for longer than 10 years would require more thorough investigation.
> › Severe hypertension, congestive heart failure and any pyrexial illness *may* produce proteinuria.

Initial management:

Take a careful history (? recent sore throats, previous UTIs, drugs etc).
On examination, look for evidence of the nephrotic syndrome, renal failure, heart failure and hypertension.
See if the kidneys are palpable.

HAEMATURIA

Haematuria means blood in the urine. If not be visible to the naked eye, it is called microscopic haematuria.

Causes:

Haematuria suggests either **UTI, nephritis** or **urinary tract tumours**. Careful history taking and examination will usually narrow down the possibilities, eg:

Young men –
gonorrhoea
renal or urethral trauma
urinary tract stones
jogging (trauma)

Women –
cystitis
pyelonephritis
cervical carcinoma
urinary tract stones

The elderly –
prostatic disease
urinary tract stones
bladder tumours
renal TB
radiotherapy

Haematuria + urinary frequency + dysuria suggests infection.
Haematuria + urinary tract pain may suggest stones, infection or trauma.
Painless haematuria should raise the suspicion of malignancy.
Haematuria + deteriorating renal function suggests nephritis.
Bleeding disorders, schistosomiasis, infective endocarditis and chemotherapy drugs may also cause haematuria.

Initial management:

Make sure that red coloured urine is not caused by eating beetroot or red sweets or by taking phenolphthalein, phenindione or rifampicin.

Take a careful history and examine the patient.

Consider urine tests, blood tests and the various "imaging" procedures (abdo X-ray, IVU, ultrasound, CT scan and cystoscopy) to help confirm the diagnosis.

HYPERTENSION

Renal disease can cause hypertension and hypertension can cause renal disease. Thus chronic renal disease has an inexorable tendency to get worse. Renal disease only accounts for about 5% of recognized cases of hypertension.

Most cases of renal hypertension are assumed to be due to a disturbance of the renin/angiotensin mechanism. Some support for this idea comes from the condition known as **renal artery stenosis*** in which a fairly sudden onset of hypertension is associated with shrinking of one kidney and increased plasma renin levels. The problem may be corrected by surgery but nephrectomy is sometimes necessary to control hypertension.

SEVERE PROTEINURIA (nephrotic syndrome)

Severe proteinuria associated with **lowered blood albumin** concentration, **peripheral oedema** and (sometimes) hypercholesterolaemia. It is a relatively rare condition seen in both children and adults.

Causes include:

› Glomerulonephritis
› Diabetes
› SLE
› Drug therapy (especially gold and penicillamine)
› Severe allergic reactions
› Amyloid
› Myeloma (see chapter 23)

Initial management:

General management includes ↑ protein, ↓ salt diet, diuretics and treatment of any coexisting illness. Consider kidney biopsy to confirm diagnosis. The majority of children with the nephrotic syndrome are found to have a relatively benign form of glomerulonephritis ("minimal change glomerulonephritis") which sometimes responds well to a short course of steroids.

---

*   Mainly a problem of male smokers with widespread atheroma.

ACUTE NEPHRITIS (acute glomerulonephritis)

This is an expression used to describe the combination of **haematuria, proteinuria, oliguria, hypertension** and transitory **uraemia** (see below) in an acutely ill patient.

Causes:

Although rare nowadays, acute nephritis is the classical expression of immune complex glomerulonephritis associated with **streptococcal infection**. SLE, polyarteritis nodosa and Henoch Schönlein purpura* (see chapter 23) may also present as acute nephritis.

Initial management plan:

> Fluid restriction, low protein diet if kidney failure, bed rest
> May need dialysis in acute phase
> Treat hypertension and heart failure if present
> Penicillin if streptococcal infection implicated in aetiology

COMPARISON OF OEDEMA IN ACUTE NEPHRITIS AND THE NEPHROTIC SYNDROME

	ACUTE NEPHRITIS	NEPHROTIC SYNDROME
Oedema:	Slight	Marked
Distribution:	Around eyes, ankles	Generalized
Protein in urine:	Moderate	Marked
Plasma osm. press.:	Normal	Decreased
Cause of oedema:	Fluid retention	Reduced plasma osmotic pressure

Note:

You may come across an hereditary condition of childhood (boys more than girls) called **Alport's syndrome.** This is the combination of nephritis with eye defects and nerve deafness. It may lead to chronic renal failure and hypertension.

---

*   i) Edvard Henoch (1820-1910), professor of paediatrics, Berlin. Romberg's nephew.
    ii) Johann Schönlein (1793-1864), Bavarian physician and pathologist.

ACUTE RENAL FAILURE (acute uraemia)

Acute Renal Failure – ARF – means rapidly rising serum urea and potassium levels associated with a urine output of less than about 15mls/hour. High potassium levels may lead to cardiac arrest so ARF is a **MEDICAL EMERGENCY** (see also chapter 28).

Causes:

The clinical features of acute renal failure make more sense when you understand the underlying mechanisms, ie:

"PRE-RENAL" (incipient) FAILURE:

This occurs when renal blood flow is reduced 1) by depletion of blood volume (haemorrhage, dehydration, shock etc), 2) by cardiac failure or 3) by bilateral partial renal artery occlusion.

Since (by definition) there is no structural damage to the kidney in "pre-renal" failure, the **situation can be reversed by replenishing the circulating volume.** Clinical features of pre-renal failure include thirst, dry mouth, weak rapid pulse, low blood pressure, cold extremities, dry tongue, inelastic skin and oliguria.* Failure to act promptly may lead to **established renal failure**.

ESTABLISHED ACUTE RENAL FAILURE:

This results from **structural damage** to the kidney (more often necrosis of tubules rather than glomeruli). The commonest cause is misdiagnosed/untreated pre-renal failure.

Many drugs and poisons are "nephrotoxic" and may thus cause acute established renal failure (especially in overdose). Acute glomerulonephritis, pyelonephritis and interstitial nephritis may also result in ARF as may acute haemolysis (eg blood transfusion mismatch – see chapter 23). For some reason, jaundiced patients are particularly prone to develop ARF. The signs of established renal failure include those of **overhydration** (pulmonary oedema, ↑ JVP), hypercalcaemia (arrhythmias) and **uraemia** (anaemia, bleeding from mucous membranes, vomiting, hiccup and drowsiness).

---

*   Diminished urine output.

POST-RENAL FAILURE:

This means acute **obstruction** of the flow of urine from the kidneys to the bladder. Stones, blood and tumours are possible causes and the characteristic clinical feature is **complete anuria** (± other signs of established renal failure). Renal pain, renal tenderness and palpable kidneys may reflect the underlying obstruction.

Initial management plan:

The management of renal failure is a specialized skill. It involves correcting obvious underlying lesions and maintenance of homeostasis until the patient recovers or chronic renal failure develops. In the most serious cases, **renal dialysis** may be the only hope of maintaining life. **Never forget, however, that pre-renal failure is reversible and can be avoided by replacing fluid volume.**

CHRONIC RENAL FAILURE (uraemia)

It is notoriously hard to diagnose chronic renal failure from history and examination alone (unless a past history of renal problems provides the clue). In the early stages, diagnosis is dependent on laboratory tests of renal function (such as plasma urea and creatinine concentrations).
By definition, CRF is an irreversible slow decline towards end-stage renal failure (the "uraemic syndrome"). It may result from chronic pyelonephritis or chronic glomerulonephritis. Other causes include diabetic nephropathy, drugs, hypertension, hereditary polycystic disease and gout.

Clinical features of chronic renal failure (uraemia):

> › Anaemia
> › Bedwetting
> › Bone pain
> › Calcium deficiency
> › Coma
> › Convulsions
> › Diarrhoea
> › Dry, pigmented skin
> › Failing vision (from hypertensive retinopathy)
> › Foetid breath
> › Fractures
> › Growth disturbance
> › Gynaecomastia
> › Headache

> Heart failure
> Hiccup
> Hypertension
> Impotence
> Ischaemic heart disease
> Itching
> Loss of appetite
> Menstrual disturbance
> Nausea
> Nocturia
> Nosebleeds
> Oedema
> Pericarditis
> Peripheral neuropathy
> Polyuria
> Pulmonary oedema
> Purpura
> Red eye
> Restless legs
> Rickets
> Secondary gout
> Secondary hyperparathyroidism
> Thirst
> Tiredness
> Tremor
> Vomiting

Management:

1) Attempt to preserve remaining kidney function by controlling hypertension, treating heart failure, avoiding UTIs, avoiding/treating any urinary tract obstruction, maintaining good fluid/salt balance, avoiding nephrotoxic drugs and restriction of dietary protein.
2) Attempt to control uraemic syndrome by lowering serum uric acid levels to avoid gout, treating calcium deficiency,* maintaining acid/base homeostasis, using aluminium hydroxide to reduce intestinal phosphate absorption thus delaying bone demineralization and careful monitoring of protein and potassium intake.
3) Consider dialysis or renal transplant.

---

* A failing kidney is unable to convert vitamin D to the active form 1,25 Dihydroxycholecalciferol. Intestinal calcium absorption is thus impaired.

CYSTITIS/ASYMPTOMATIC BACTERIURIA/URETHRAL SYNDROME

Background:

In orthodox medicine, you are not allowed to have a urinary tract infection unless a urine sample sent for microbiological investigation contains more than 10^5 bacteria per ml of urine.

However, some people with "significant" numbers of bacteria in the urine have no symptoms of urinary tract infection.

Others, with apparently "sterile" urine, suffer perpetual misery from the symptoms of urethritis/cystitis,* and are said to have the "urethral syndrome."

Allergies to nylon, washing powders and bubble baths (plus sensitivity to the effects of sexual intercourse, cold etc) doubtless explain some cases of urethral syndrome but certainly not all.

Recurrent cystitis/urethritis "unresponsive" to antibiotics is an important problem in general practice (and a much more important problem to those – mostly women – who suffer from them).

Clinical features:

The symptoms of **urethritis** are dysuria, urgency, frequency and a feeling that the bladder isn't being emptied properly.

Fishy smelling, cloudy urine with haematuria and supra-pubic pain/tenderness *in addition* to the symptoms of urethritis would suggest **cystitis**.

Management:

Many patients presenting with the above certainly produce urine samples containing significant numbers of pathogenic bacteria and respond well to the classic orthodox strategy of high fluid intake, regular bladder emptying, scrupulous perineal hygiene and antibiotics. Many, however, do not and repeated or long term use of antibiotics produces its own spectrum of problems (candidiasis, intestinal dysbiosis etc).

Non-orthodox approaches focusing on improving the ***general*** health of the patient whilst promoting healing of urinary tract epithelia are often markedly successful in those cases lost or abandoned by orthodox medicine.

---

*   There is, however, some evidence that "sterile" urine may contain "significant" numbers of non-bacterial organisms, such as Chlamydia and viruses.

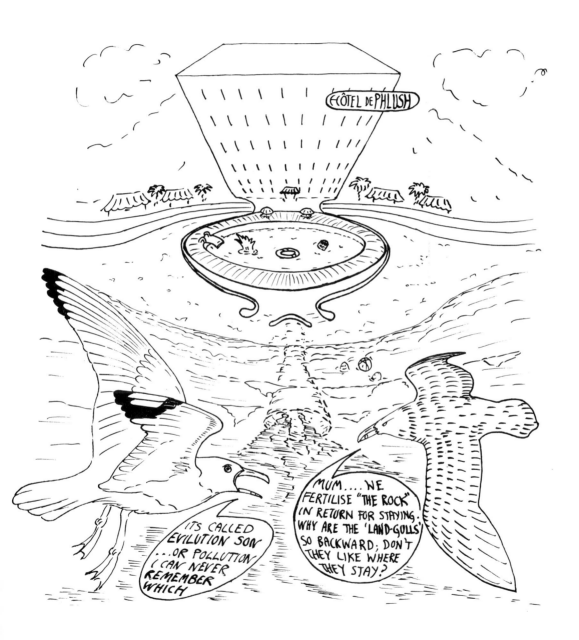

UROLOGY

OVERVIEW

Urinary Tract Stones (urolithiasis)

Urinary Tract Malignancy

> Kidney
> Bladder
> Prostate
> Testis

Benign Prostatic Hypertrophy

Prostatitis

Benign Testicular Tumours

Orchitis

Epididymitis

Testicular Torsion

Glossary of Urinary Tract Investigations

URINARY TRACT STONES (urolithiasis)

Stones (calculi) can form anywhere in the urinary tract and may cause **obstruction** or **infection**. Most urinary tract stones are made of **calcium** compounds. Idiopathic kidney calcium stones are the commonest type of urolithiasis.

Aetiologicalfactors:

Kidney stones:

> › Urinary tract infection
> › Dehydration
> › Being male
> › Meat eating
> › Sedentary lifestyle
> › ↑ blood calcium levels
> › Analgesic drugs

Bladder stones:

> › Poor diet/malnutrition
> › General poor health
> › Urinary tract infection

Types of stone:

Calcium salts:	90% (10% being ammonium salts formed in infected, alkaline urine)
Uric acid stones:	5% (see chapter 18)
Miscellaneous:	5%

» Calcium stones show up on x-ray, uric acid stones don't.

Situations in which blood calcium may be raised, favouring the formation of calcium stones:

Excess Ca **absorbed** from gut:

> › Vitamin D excess
> › Too much milk + antacids taken in the attempt to ease the symptoms of peptic ulcer disease

Excess Ca **resorbed** from bone:

> Hyperparathyroidism
> Bone secondaries
> Myeloma
> Cushing's disease
> Steroids
> Immobility

High blood calcium levels lead to high urinary calcium levels (hypercalcuria). However, the commonest cause of hypercalcuria is an **idiopathic** tendency for the kidney to *excrete* too much calcium into the urine.

Clinical features:

The clinical features of urolithiasis depend on where the stones are, whether they are causing obstruction and whether the urine is infected.

Thus many urinary tract stones cause no symptoms or signs and are discovered by chance on routine x-rays.

Stones in kidney:

> Unilateral loin pain
> Possibly loin tenderness
> Haematuria ± slight proteinuria

Stone jammed in ureter:

> Severe colic (may be severe enough to provoke shock)
> Tenderness/guarding over the course of the ureter
> Enlarged kidney (from backflow of urine)
> If the kidney with blocked outflow happens to be the only one working correctly, a ureteric stone could produce complete anuria.

Bladder stones:

> Frequency
> Haematuria/slight proteinuria
> "Gravel" in the urine

If the urine becomes infected in any of the above, the patient will develop frequency and dysuria.
The urine may contain blood, proteins and organisms.

Complications of kidney stones:

> › Recurrent urinary tract infection
> › Acute "post renal" failure
> › Chronic renal failure

Management:

Abdominal x-rays, urography (see glossary) and blood tests for calcium, PTH and uric acid levels (plus urine microbiological tests as appropriate) usually to produce a diagnosis.

Thereafter, the aim is to manage the following as they arise:

Renal colic: ↑ fluid intake
                                      Strong painkillers
                                      Smooth muscle relaxants

Urinary tract infection: Antibiotics

Stone obstructing ureter: High fluid intake + general support.
                                      Stones > 6mm in diameter are unlikely to
                                      be passed spontaneously and usually
                                      require surgery. More recently, the use of
                                      lithotripter* machines (using high energy
                                      sound waves) has enabled some stones
                                      to be shattered in situ.

It goes without saying** that any known underlying aetiological factors must be dealt with.

NOTE:

Nephrocalcinosis means calcification of kidney tissue. Some individuals with hypercalcuria (for one of the reasons already mentioned) develop patches of nephrocalcinosis rather than distinct renal stones. Fortunately, people with nephrocalcinosis usually have no symptoms or signs and are not prone to serious kidney dysfunction.

---

*   Stone smasher.
** But we're going to say it anyway.

URINARY TRACT MALIGNANCY

KIDNEY

About 90% of primary kidney cancers are adenocarcinomas. Renal cell adenocarcinomas are sometimes referred to as "hypernephromas".

Background:

Males > females
Age 40-60
Relatively common – 2% of all UK cancer deaths

Pathology:

Renal cancers usually develop in the top or bottom pole of kidney. They may spread to surrounding tissues directly and/or via bloodstream to lung, bone and brain.

Clinical features:

About 1 in 3 sufferers present with **painless haematuria**. Unexplained low grade fever is another classic presentation.

Other features include anaemia, weight loss, palpable abdominal lump, loin pain and hypercalcaemia. Since hypernephromas secrete erythropoietin, some patients also develop polycythaemia (see chapter 23).

Management:

Surgical removal + post operative radiotherapy produce an overall 5 year survival of between 35 and 50%.

BLADDER

Bladder tumours occur most commonly in elderly male smokers. Industrial exposure to aniline + β naphthaline is also linked with bladder cancer.

Pathology:

Most bladder cancers are "transitional cell" tumours and are not as aggressive as many other malignancies. They tend to arise at the bladder base and often form cauliflower like masses.

Clinical features:

Once again, **painless haematuria** is a relatively common presentation but nocturia, frequency, urgency and hesitancy may all occur.

Pain and weight loss are relatively late features.

Management:

Bladder endoscopy ("cystoscopy") plus biopsy via the urethra helps to determine the grade and stage of the tumour.

Less advanced growths can be burnt off using a special type of cystoscope. More advanced lesions are subjected to pre-operative radiotherapy followed by bladder removal (cystectomy)*. Very advanced cases are treated with radiotherapy and chemotherapy to help control pain etc.

Prognosis:

Prompt treatment of early lesions produces up to 80% 5 year survival. More advanced cases have less than a 30% chance of surviving 5 years, despite treatment.

---

*   Urine is removed from the body via an "ileal conduit" = a small portion of ileum (with its blood supply attached) removed from the small intestine (which is joined up again). One end of the conduit is opened on the abdominal wall as an ileostomy – the ureters are implanted into the conduit.

PROSTATE

Prostatic cancer is the **3rd commonest malignancy of males** and is particularly common in the very elderly (so common, in fact, that it is often found as an "incidental" finding at autopsies for death from another cause).

Pathology:

Most prostatic malignancies are adenocarcinomas arising in the posterior lobe of the prostate (making them easy to feel on rectal examination). Local spread to bladder or bowel and metastasis to **bone** are common.

Clinical features:

The clinical features of prostatic malignancy make sense when you remember that the prostate surrounds the urethra and is very close to the bladder in front and rectum behind, ie:

› Frequency
› Nocturia
› Hesitancy
› Dribbling
› Inability to pass urine ("acute retention")
› A lump palpable per rectum
› Bone pain (from metastases)

High blood levels of an enzyme called "acid phosphatase" reflect disease activity.

Management:

Orthodox management depends on whether metastases are present at the time of diagnosis. In reasonably fit men with no metastases, the tumour is either removed (prostatectomy) or irradiated. Since most prostatic cancers only grow in the presence of testosterone, metastatic tumours are treated by removal of the testes (bilateral orchidectomy) or by oestrogen therapy. Radiotherapy helps to control bone pain.

Prognosis:

Overall about 25% 5 year survival. About 10% die within 6 months of diagnosis and another 10% are alive and well 10 years later. The rest fall somewhere in between.

TESTIS

Testicular malignancies are the commonest cancers of young men (accounting for about 0.5% of all male cancers). The aetiological factors are not understood (although testicular tumours are 30 times more likely to occur in "undescended" testes).

Pathology:

The two most important testicular malignancies are:

Seminomas: Arise from seminiferous tubules.
                    Age of onset 30-40 years.
                    Not fast growing.
                    Lymphatic spread to para-aortic lymph nodes.

Teratomas: Arise from germ cells.
                    Occur in younger age group (20-30 years).
                    Relatively aggressive.
                    Early metastasis to liver and lungs.

Clinical features:

Painless enlargement of the testis. There may also be an accumulation of fluid (hydrocoele).* Later case show general features of malignancy and signs of metastases.

Management:

Surgical removal of testes (orchidectomy) via an inguinal incision ± radiotherapy. Some centres use chemotherapy.

Prognosis:

Seminomas: Very good indeed if no metastases at diagnosis.

Teratomas: 80% 5 year survival if no metastases.
                    Relatively poor otherwise.

---

*   See page 500.

BENIGN PROSTATIC HYPERTROPHY

Benign, idiopathic enlargement of the prostate gland is common in elderly males. It causes partial bladder neck obstruction and urinary retention.

Background:

Bladder neck obstruction by an enlarged prostate causes bladder muscle hypertrophy as the bladder works to "overcome" the blockage. Urinary reflux may lead to dilation of the ureters and renal calyces and even, eventually, to renal failure. The tendency for urine to be retained in the bladder predisposes to urinary tract infections and stones.

Complete obstruction to urine outflow (*acute* retention) is an emergency (see below).

Clinical features:

›   Difficulty starting/stopping urination
›   Poor stream
›   Hesitant flow
›   Frequency
›   Nocturia
›   Occasional haematuria (at the end of urination)
›   Prostate palpable on PR examination

Management:

A variety of surgical approaches are available to relieve obstruction to the flow of urine. By far the most popular these days is the **trans-urethral** (ie using a cystoscope) **resection of the prostate** (TURP for short). This procedure shaves away prostatic tissue from the *inside* of the urethra. It does not involve an abdominal or perineal incision and doesn't affect "potency".* However, infection, haemorrhage, incontinence and stricture formation are possible post-operative complications.

---

*   In most ages.

NOTE:

Acute retention of urine:

If faced with an unwell elderly male patient complaining of an inability to pass any urine, most practitioners immediately think of prostatic disease. It is, however, important to consider the following points:

i) Is the problem retention or anuria (in retention, a distended bladder can be felt rising out of the pelvis on abdominal examination)?

ii) Does the past history suggest prostatic disease?

iii) Is there a history of previous surgery or neurological disorder that might affect the urination mechanism?

iv) Is there any evidence of renal failure?

Most orthodox GPs would immediately refer any case of acute retention for hospital management. Usually, an injection of morphine plus a hot bath are sufficient to enable the patient to pass water. Otherwise urethral or supra-pubic* catheterization is necessary to avoid the possibility of a ruptured bladder.

---

*   Through the skin and abdominal wall directly into the bladder.

PROSTATITIS

Acute or chronic inflammation of the prostate, usually associated with gonococcal, E.coli, staphylococcal or streptococcal infection.

Clinical features:

Acute:

> › Frequency
> › Dysuria
> › Nocturia
> › Urgency
> › Urethral discharge
> › Prostate tender on PR examination

Untreated prostatitis may lead to acute retention, abscess formation or infection spreading to kidney or epididymis.

Chronic:

May be mild symptoms of low back pain, perineal pain and dysuria with (possibly) mild fever. The prostate may feel hard (from scarring) on PR examination. May lead to acute retention.

Management:

Acute:

Bed rest + antibiotics.

Chronic:

Chronic prostatitis is hard to treat. Antibiotics sometimes help but TURP is often the most effective approach.

BENIGN TESTICULAR TUMOURS

> › Epididymal cyst (spermatocoele)
> › Hydrocoele
> › Varicocoele

These three benign conditions all present as "a lump in the testis" or "a swollen testis". The problem is to differentiate them from each other and from testicular malignancy.

EPIDIDYMAL CYSTS:

Small painless masses, separate from the main body of the testis, containing sperm. They do not require any particular treatment, but can be "aspirated" (sucked out) or removed via a scrotal incision.

HYDROCOELE:

A hydrocoele is a collection of fluid within the tunica vaginalis around the testis. It is usually a **secondary** phenomenon (to orchitis, epididymitis, trauma, cancer or TB) so the problem is to discover the underlying cause. The fluid can be drawn off with a needle and sent for microbiological and cytological investigation. Surgical investigation of the testis is sometimes necessary.

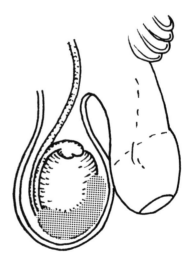

VARICOCOELE:

A varicocoele is a collection of varicose veins from the pampiniform plexus of veins draining the testis. They are relatively common in young men and seem to occur more often around the left testis than the right. The swelling (which feels like a "bag of worms") tends to disappear when the owner lies down.

The problem can be solved (if necessary) by surgically tying off the internal spermatic vein (via an inguinal incision). *Very* occasionally, varicocoeles are associated with **renal cancer,** so most patients with them are screened appropriately.

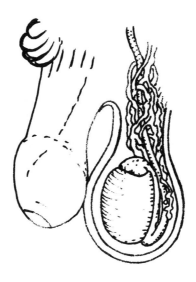

ORCHITIS

Acute (usually infective) inflammation of the testes.

Aetiology:

Usually viral, eg **mumps**, Coxsackie.

Clinical features:

Testicular pain and swelling with red, tender scrotum plus fever and malaise.

No urinary symptoms.

Management:

Bed rest (sometimes antibiotics).

Complications:

May (rarely) lead to sterility.

EPIDIDYMITIS

Inflammation of the epididymis secondary to prostatic surgery or prostatitis.

Clinical features:

> › Fever
> › Scrotal tenderness and swelling
> › Urethral discharge (not always)
> › May be cystitis or hydrocoele plus symptoms of underlying prostatic disease

Management:

> › Bedrest
> › Pain relief
> › Antibiotics

TESTICULAR TORSION

A **surgical emergency** caused by sudden (usually spontaneous) twisting of the testis within the tunica vaginalis. This causes venous obstruction → oedema → arterial obstruction → infarction. It is most commonly seen around puberty but may occur at any age.

Clinical features:

Sudden onset of pain in one testis, so severe that the patient is unable to walk.

The scrotum appears red and hot and the testis is incredibly tender.

Management:

Immediate surgery to untwist the spermatic cord and, if the testis is infarcted, removal of the testis.

Viable testes can be fixed to the scrotum to stop the same thing happening again in the future.

GLOSSARY OF URINARY TRACT INVESTIGATIONS

Urine for M, C + S:

Urine sample taken for **M**icroscopic examination, microbiological **C**ulture and testing of the antibiotic **S**ensitivities of any organisms found.

Simple microscopic examination may reveal white blood cells (infection), crystals (urolithiasis) or red blood cells (various; ? malignancy, ? nephritis).

FBC:

Full blood count.
Shows up anaemia.
Also shows any abnormal increase in the numbers of white cells (which would reflect infection).

U + E, creatinine:

Urea, electrolytes (including Na, K) and creatinine levels in the blood reflect i) the kidney's ability to excrete the waste products of protein metabolism, + ii) the state of salt/water homeostatic mechanisms in the body.

IVU (IVP):

Intravenous urography/pyelography.
A special sort of abdominal X-ray in which a radio-opaque dye is injected into a vein so that it can be excreted via the kidneys.
By taking X-ray pictures at short intervals after the injection, the ability of the kidneys to excrete the dye into the tubules, down the ureters and into the bladder can be observed. Shows up abnormalities in kidney shape, size and function and also helps locate site of any urinary tract obstruction. **The archetypal investigation in renal medicine/urology.**

Cystoscopy:

Endoscopic examination of the urethra and bladder.

Micturating cystogram:

The bladder is filled with radio opaque fluid (via a catheter passed through the urethra) and successive X-rays are taken as the patient passes water. An efficient (if uncomfortable) way of diagnosing **ureteric reflux** of urine.

Ultrasound:

A useful non-invasive investigation in a patient not passing urine since it will show any swelling of the kidney duct system – caused by obstructing stones, tumours etc.

Retrograde pyelogram:

Radio-opaque fluid is injected into the kidney via a catheter passed into the ureters.

X-rays are then taken to show the outline of the kidney.

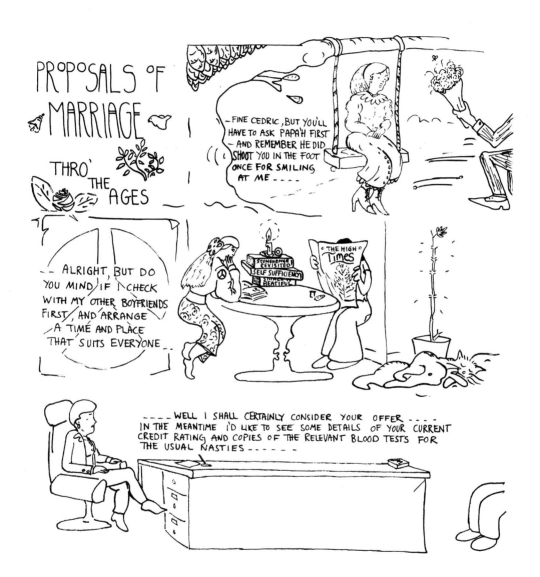

HAEMATOLOGY

OVERVIEW

Introduction to Anaemia

Anaemias Caused by Impaired Red Cell Formation

> Background
> Iron deficiency anaemia
> Sideroblastic anaemia
> B12 and folic acid deficiency anaemias

Anaemias Caused by Loss or Destruction of Red Cells

> Background
> Sickle cell disease
> Thalassaemia
> Auto-immune haemolytic anaemias

Miscellaneous Anaemias

Bleeding Disorders

> Henoch Schönlein purpura
> Idiopathic thrombocytopenic purpura
> Haemophilia

Haematological Malignancy and Proliferative Disorders

> Myeloproliferative disorders
> Leukaemias
> Lymphomas
> Myelomatosis

INTRODUCTION TO ANAEMIA

DEFINITION

Anaemia is defined as abnormally low blood haemoglobin concentration. The "normal range" for blood haemoglobin concentration (in g/dl) is:

Men: 15 ± 2.5 Women: 14 ± 2.5

Anaemia can also be thought of as the inability to deliver oxygen to the tissues in appropriate amounts. The *number* of circulating red blood cells is not necessarily diminished in anaemia; the important thing is whether each red cell contains enough normal haemoglobin.

Pathological consequences of anaemia:

Decreased haemoglobin $\rightarrow$ tissue hypoxia $\rightarrow$ body compensates by increasing heart rate, dilating arterioles, increasing marrow activity and reducing affinity of Hb for oxygen to try and improve oxygen delivery to the tissues. Anaemia exaggerates the effects of atheroma and may lead to fatty degeneration of heart muscle and liver tissue.

Clinical features:

Symptoms include:

> › Fatigue
> › Lassitude
> › Shortness of breath (esp. on exertion)
> › Palpitations
> › Angina
> › Intermittent claudication
> › Fainting/dizziness and (if heart failure develops) ankle oedema

Signs include:

> › Pallor (especially noticeable on mucous membranes)*
> › Rapid, full bounding pulse
> › Signs of heart failure (possibly)

* Pallor is not a reliable sign of anaemia.

ANAEMIAS CAUSED BY IMPAIRED RED CELL FORMATION

BACKGROUND

Red cell formation (haemopoiesis):

Red cells are manufactured in the bone marrow of the ribs, sternum, pelvis, vertebral bodies and ends of long bones.

The hormone erythropoietin* helps regulate the rate of red cell production and stimulates the bone marrow to produce more red blood cells if arterial oxygen levels fall. The efficient production of red cells depends on the presence of

> a sufficient number of stem cells ("normoblasts") in the marrow
> sufficient supplies of essential nutrients (iron, vitamin B12, folic acid)
> a balanced hormonal environment (thyroxine, androgens, etc).

Thus the following may interfere with red cell formation:

Renal failure

Causes decreased erythropoietin production

Bone marrow damage
[drugs, blood cancers]

Destroys stem cells

Essential factor deficiency
[iron, vitamin C, general disruption of nutritional homeostasis by cancer, endocrine disease or malnutrition]

Causes impaired haemoglobin synthesis

Vitamin B12 + folate deficiency

Disrupts DNA synthesis and causes defective maturation of RBCs

---

*   Produced by the kidneys.

IRON DEFICIENCY ANAEMIA

Iron metabolism:

The body is very efficient at conserving iron. The small (but inevitable) daily loss from dead skin cells, menstrual flow and body secretions is replaced by absorption of dietary iron from the duodenum and upper jejunum. The intestinal mucosal cells have a mechanism to ensure that only as much iron as is needed to maintain body iron "stores" is actually absorbed into the blood. Total body iron content is about 5 grams of which about 80% is "functional" (in haemoglobin, myoglobin and enzyme systems) and 20% is stored in the liver, spleen and bone marrow in the form of ferritin or haemosiderin. Average daily iron loss is about 1 mg (plus an extra 0.5mg/day during menstruation). This is replaced by absorption of 1mg/day from the 15mg or so ingested in an average diet.

Pathology:

Iron deficiency has 3 causes:

1) Blood loss,* eg menstrual bleeding or bleeding from the gastrointestinal tract, including ulcers, hiatus hernia, haemorrhoids, oesophageal varices, NSAIA therapy and cancer.
2) Decreased iron input (poor diet, malabsorption).
3) Increased body requirement (childhood rapid growth, pregnancy).

Iron deficiency anaemia usually develops slowly since iron stores have to be depleted before clinical signs develop.

Clinical features:

As well as the general features of anaemia, iron deficiency is also associated with angular stomatitis, atrophic glossitis (smooth red tongue), gastritis (associated with ↓ gastric acid secretion and mucosal atrophy), brittle, spoon shaped nails (koilonychia), pins and needles, difficulty swallowing and even oesophageal cancer.

---

*   Note that even minor blood loss can cause anaemia if it goes on long enough. 1ml of blood contains 0.5mg of iron.

SIDEROBLASTIC ANAEMIA

Sideroblastic anaemias are a group of anaemias caused by failure to incorporate iron into haem because of a defect in the relevant enzyme systems. They may be idiopathic or induced by drugs, alcoholism, lead poisoning or malnutrition. They are sometimes a prelude to leukaemia.

B12 AND FOLIC ACID* DEFICIENCY ANAEMIAS

Aetiology:

B12 deficiency may be caused by poor diet, malabsorption due to damage to the terminal ileum (coeliac disease, Crohn's, etc) or malabsorption due to lack of intrinsic factor (**pernicious anaemia**).

Folate deficiency may result from malnutrition, malabsorption, excess demands (malignancy, pregnancy, serious skin conditions) and drugs (phenytoin, alcohol, oral contraceptives, septrin).

Pathology:

B12 and folate are necessary for DNA synthesis. If there is deficiency of either, some red blood cells will fail to mature properly and may be larger than normal.** Moreover, other rapidly dividing cells (eg mucous membrane epithelial cells) will be affected and may atrophy. B12 has a particular function in maintaining the integrity of myelin sheaths in nerves and its deficiency may lead to neuropathies and even spinal cord degeneration (so called **subacute combined degeneration of the cord**).

Clinical features:

The general symptoms and signs of anaemia.
In addition B12 deficiency may cause painful swelling of the tongue and CNS symptoms.
Pernicious anaemia may also be associated with vitiligo, spleen enlargement, mild fever, premature greying and neurological abnormalities. (Beware of grey haired, blue eyed men over 40 with anaemia and a family history of blood problems; they probably have pernicious anaemia.)

---

*   Folic acid = folate.
**   Hence the terms macrocytic (big cells) and megaloblastic (big immature cells) which are also used to describe B12/folate deficiency anaemias.

ANAEMIAS CAUSED BY DESTRUCTION OF RED CELLS

Haemolytic anaemias occur when red cells are destroyed faster than the bone marrow can replace them.

Pathological destruction of red cells may be due to deficiencies in the structure of red cells or to external factors (drugs, infections, etc).

Causes of haemolysis:

Congenital: Defects in red cell membranes,
                       enzyme systems or
                       haemoglobin structure.

Acquired: Auto-immune haemolysis
                       Infections (eg malaria)
                       Drugs
                       Enlarged spleen (the organ in which most red
                       cell destruction normally takes place).
                       Miscellaneous conditions such as liver disease,
                       cancer etc.

› The most important **congenital** defects are **sickle cell anaemia** and **thalassaemia**.

› The most common **acquired** haemolytic anaemias are those caused by auto-immunity, **malaria** and drugs.

Clinical features common to all haemolytic anaemias:

› General symptoms and signs of anaemia
› Jaundice (see chapter 13 for description of haemolytic jaundice)
› Haemoglobin in the urine
› Gallstones
› Enlarged spleen

SICKLE CELL DISEASE

Caused by a congenital defect of haemoglobin in which the red cells contain mostly abnormal Hb"S" rather than normal Hb"A". The presence of HbS tends to make red cells assume an unusual "sickle" shape.* Sickle cells cannot carry as much oxygen as normal RBC's.

Background:

Autosomal dominant inheritance.
Common in Africa, India, the Middle East and the Mediterranean (possibly because the abnormal haemoglobin seems to offer some protection against the effects of falciparum malaria).
Heterozygotes with sickle cell "trait" (who have some red cells containing normal HbA and some containing abnormal HbS) are not usually troubled by symptoms unless they find themselves in a low oxygen environment (eg up a mountain, under anaesthesia or with a severe chest infection).
Homozygotes with the full blown condition are sensitive to even minor reductions in oxygen levels.

Clinical features:

Sickle cell disease usually makes itself apparent early in life in the form of acute **haemolytic crises.** These are characterized by bone pain (from infarcting bone), swollen fingers and toes, abdominal pain, blood in the urine and cerebrovascular accident. Death may occur from infarction of a major organ.

Children that survive into adulthood are plagued by ill health and suffer anaemia, leg ulcers, infections and haemolytic crises. Life expectancy is rarely greater than 40 years.

Management:

Since there is no treatment for the condition. It is important to prevent severe exacerbations by avoiding "low oxygen" situations such as chest infections. Blood transfusion is used as a last resort (although they occasionally make the situation worse). Frequent transfusions seem beneficial in pregnancy. Genetic counselling is obviously important in families known to carry the HbS gene.

* instead of

THALASSAEMIA

A group of hereditary defects of haemoglobin α- or β-chain synthesis.

The most common and most important condition is β-Thalassaemia Major, in which abnormal β-chain production causes a lack of normal adult haemoglobin. The body compensates for this by continuing to produce foetal type haemoglobin (HbF).

Clinical features (β-Thalassaemia Major):

Children appear normal at birth but eventually develop severe anaemia with enlarged spleen/liver, gallstones, leg ulcers, fragile bones and slightly odd shaped skulls.

Management:

Repeated blood transfusions (± splenectomy) help to maintain blood haemoglobin at more or less normal levels.

Frequent transfusions early in life can greatly reduce the risk of skeletal abnormalities (although it is sometimes difficult to avoid iron overload which, amongst other things, can damage the heart).

AUTOIMMUNE HAEMOLYTIC ANAEMIAS

Caused by auto-antibodies destroying red cells. There are several different types of AHAs but most are idiopathic.

Others are associated with haematological malignancies, SLE, infections and drugs (eg methyldopa).

The symptoms and signs are those common to all haemolytic anaemias.

MISCELLANEOUS ANAEMIAS

Anaemia may also be associated with:

URAEMIA:

Bone marrow function is suppressed; the resulting anaemia is made worse by decreased erythropoietin production.

LIVER DISEASE:

Multifactorial; involves bone marrow depression, haemolysis, iron/folate deficiency. Worse if spleen is enlarged.

HYPOTHYROIDISM:

Marrow depression; treatment with thyroxine will improve the anaemia.

CHRONIC DISEASE:

Chronic infection, chronic inflammation and malignancy will all produce anaemia for reasons that are poorly understood but possibly relate to defects in iron transport.

BLEEDING DISORDERS

Several causes of abnormal bleeding are listed in chapter 6 and we suggest you review this information before reading further. The following three conditions represent three different classes of bleeding disorder, ie:

1) BLOOD VESSEL ABNORMALITY
2) PLATELET DEFECT
3) CLOTTING FACTOR DEFICIENCY

1) HENOCH SCHÖNLEIN PURPURA

A disease caused by widespread vasculitis provoked by immune complex deposition in blood vessel walls. It is characterized by purpura, arthritis, kidney damage and abdominal pain. It mainly affects **children** and may be precipitated by streptococcal infection or drugs (eg aspirin, thiazide diuretics, sulphonamides and tetracycline).

Clinical features:

Itchy purpuric skin rash on the buttocks and lower limbs, brief but painful arthritis of the knees and ankles, long lasting colicky abdominal pain and haematuria. The blood pressure may also be raised.

Management:

Bed rest, simple pain killers and hope that the symptoms will not recur too often. Progressive renal disease complicates about 2% of cases and may be fatal.

2) IDIOPATHIC THROMBOCYTOPENIC PURPURA

A disorder of decreased platelet numbers caused by the production of anti-platelet antibodies. The aetiology is unknown but there may be some relationship to previous viral infection (especially in children).

Clinical features:

A typical story would be of a child, recently recovered from a simple febrile illness, who presents with purpura of sudden onset and, possibly, bleeding from mucous membranes. There are no other physical signs. Spontaneous recovery is usual although the condition may become chronic in adults. Very occasionally, the platelet count may drop so low that there is a risk of intracerebral bleeding or retinal haemorrhage.

Treatment:

A short course of steroids may help and, in very severe cases, splenectomy may be needed to stabilize the platelet count. Usually, however, the condition resolves spontaneously and without complication.

NOTE:

The progress of the condition can only really be monitored by measuring the platelet count. SLE* sometimes presents as immune based thrombocytopenia.

3) HAEMOPHILIA

Strictly speaking, haemophilia means a clotting defect caused by Factor VIII deficiency. However, the term is often used as a general label for congenital coagulation disorders that produce clinical features very similar to classical haemophilia, eg Factor IX deficiency ("Christmas Disease") and Von Willebrand's Disease.**

Inheritance:

Sex-linked recessive.

Clinical features:

Spontaneous bleeding (or bleeding after relatively minor trauma) may produce haemarthrosis (blood in joints, especially knee), bruises, haematuria or brain haemorrhage.

Treatment:

Apart from symptomatic treatment and bed rest, the only solution to the problem is Factor VIII replacement. Factor VIII can now be produced "artificially", thereby reducing the risk of transmission of AIDS or hepatitis B etc from donor blood products.

---

*   See chapter 19.
**   E.A. von Willebrand (1870-1947), Swedish physician.

HAEMATOLOGICAL MALIGNANCY AND PROLIFERATIVE DISORDERS

Broadly speaking, haematological malignancy can be considered under 4 headings:

1) MYELOPROLIFERATIVE DISORDERS

In which various marrow cells proliferate in a purposeless way reminiscent of cancer but without all the features of malignancy.

2) LEUKAEMIAS

Which are true primary malignancies of bone marrow. The name derives from the fact that many people with leukaemia have vastly increased numbers of white blood cells in their circulation.

3) LYMPHOMAS

A group of conditions in which neoplastic proliferation of lymphoid tissue causes solid tumours in lymph nodes which may spread to spleen and bone marrow and then "spill over" into the blood producing a "leukaemic" type of blood picture.

4) PLASMA CELL TUMOURS

The commonest is **multiple myeloma** (myelomatosis) in which **plasma cells** proliferate and crowd out the bone marrow.

We will now consider the pathology and clinical features of each of these groups.

MYELOPROLIFERATIVE DISORDERS*

MYELOFIBROSIS:

Bone marrow is replaced with fibrous tissue. The spleen, liver and lymph nodes try to take over haemopoietic function.

Clinical features include anaemia, bleeding, enlarged spleen, sweating, weight loss (from raised metabolic rate) and gout. Myelofibrosis may appear as the terminal stage of "silent" polycythaemia rubra vera or thrombocythaemia.

POLYCYTHAEMIA RUBRA VERA:

Caused by the overproduction of red cells, granulocytes and platelets.

Increased blood viscosity may produce headache, dizziness, thrombosis and heart failure. There is also a tendency to itchy skin (made worse by baths) and peptic ulcer.

Abnormal platelet function may produce bleeding (strokes, GI bleeds, anaemia etc).

Increased cell turnover may produce gout.

NOTE:

SECONDARY polycythaemia may occur in response to hypoxia (high altitudes, chronic lung disease and congenital heart disease) or erythropoietin secreting tumours.

ESSENTIAL THROMBOCYTHAEMIA:

Excessive production of incompetent platelets.

Clinical features result from a combined tendency to bleeding and thrombosis. Thus, at first sight, the condition may resemble peripheral arterial disease (see chapter 11).

---

*   "Myelo" refers to any cell in the granulocyte series ie granulocytes, red cells and platelets.

LEUKAEMIAS

The cause of leukaemia is unknown: viruses, genetic defects, radiation and drugs have all been implicated.

Leukaemias can be classified as:

a) **Myeloid** (malignant cells of granulocyte series) or **lymphocytic** (malignant cells of lymphoid series)

and

b) **Acute** or **chronic**

Acute leukaemias are characterized by the malignant proliferation of **immature** "blast" cells.

Chronic leukaemias produce malignant proliferation of **more mature** blood cells.

The chemotherapeutic treatment of leukaemia depends on the fact that the malignant cell line proliferates at a greater rate than normal marrow cells.

ACUTE LYMPHOBLASTIC LEUKAEMIA (ALL):

Rare but more common in children and characterized by proliferation of immature blast cells of the lymphoid series.

ACUTE MYELOID LEUKAEMIA (AML):

Rare but more common in adults; proliferation of various immature forms of granulocyte series.

CHRONIC MYELOID LEUKAEMIA (CML):

Peak incidence in middle age, excessive production of granulocytes; may deteriorate into acute leukaemia.

CHRONIC LYMPHATIC LEUKAEMIA (CLL):

A common form of leukaemia in the middle-aged/elderly characterized by proliferation of lymphocytes (often B cells).

The **clinical features** of all leukaemias may be explained when it is understood that the neoplastic cells –

i) are functionally incompetent and

ii) crowd out the bone marrow and disrupt the production of other cell lines.

Hence:

↓ red cell production	→	**anaemia**
↓ platelet production	→	**bleeding tendency** from mucous membranes under skin etc.
↓ granulocyte function	→	**susceptibility to infection** with fever, sore throat, mouth ulceration and skin rashes.
↑ turnover of cells	→	**gout**

"Metastasis" of abnormal cells in liver, spleen and lymph nodes may produce **hepatomegaly, splenomegaly** and **lymphadenopathy.**

Non-specific features include weight loss, anorexia and weakness.

Treatment of all forms is based on the use of cytotoxic drugs to eradicate or reduce the abnormal cell population followed by the use of blood transfusions, antibiotics and (in certain carefully selected cases) bone marrow transplants to keep the patient alive until normal bone marrow function is re-established.

Leukaemia may recur in the central nervous system after apparently successful treatment and cause headaches and signs of raised intracranial pressure.

Prognosis:

ALL is a major orthodox success story with 50% alive and well 5 years after treatment. CNS recurrence can be prevented by prophylactic radiotherapy.

AML is much less responsive to current treatment protocols and very few patients are alive one year after treatment. Bone marrow transplant (where available) offers a better prognosis. Even so, current treatment requires long stays in hospitals and can be unpleasant for the patient.

CLL can be very benign (especially in the elderly) and may respond well to minimal treatment (although prompt treatment of infection is very important). Overall 5 year survival = 50%.

CML treatment is unsatisfactory, with average survival less than 4 years after diagnosis. The terminal stage for many patients is the development of acute leukaemia (usually myeloid).

LYMPHOMAS

Lymphomas are of unknown aetiology (although the EB virus is known to be associated with Burkitt's lymphoma*).

They are classified as **Hodgkin's or non-Hodgkin's**** on the basis of the histological appearance of the neoplastic tissue and may arise from either lymphocytes or histiocytes (macrophages) within lymph nodes.

Lymph nodes, liver, spleen, bone marrow, tonsils and Peyer's patches*** may all be involved and advanced disease may spread to involve the skin and CNS.

Lymphomas are more common amongst people who are immunocompromised (eg AIDS sufferers).

HODGKIN'S LYMPHOMA:

This condition is considered separately from the other B cell, T cell and histiocytic lymphomas because of the distinct histological appearance of the involved tissue. It also has characteristic clinical features and is more amenable to orthodox treatment than other lymphomas.

Clinical features:

The main feature is lymphadenopathy (typically **painless** enlargement of some lymph glands in the neck). Other clinical features include fever, night sweats, malaise, weakness, weight loss, itching, anaemia and worsening

---

*   Denis Burkitt (1911-), FRS, member of External Scientific Staff of the Medical Research Council.

**   Thomas Hodgkin (1798-1866), Quaker physician at Guy's hospital who eventually gave up medicine to become a missionary.

*** Johann Peyer (1653-1712), Swiss nobleman and professor of Logic, Rhetoric and Medicine.

of symptoms after drinking alcohol. Opportunistic infection, jaundice, liver enlargement and spleen enlargement may also occur.

Hodgkin's has a large differential diagnosis including AIDS, CLL, sarcoid and TB. The orthodox "rule" is that any painless lymph node persisting longer than 6 weeks in the absence of an obvious cause should be biopsied in case it is Hodgkin's. Chest X-rays may show bone involvement and hilar lymphadenopathy. Simple blood tests help to exclude other haematological malignancies.

Treatment:

This depends on the extent of disease at diagnosis. Early, localized disease is treated by radiotherapy; advanced disease by repeated courses of chemotherapy followed by radiotherapy.

Prognosis:

Despite the high incidence of side effects from the treatment, 5 year survival is over 70% even in advanced disease; without treatment, Hodgkin's is nearly always fatal.

Discussion of the large number of non-Hodgkin's lymphomas is outside the scope of this book but you may find it interesting to read about them in a standard medical textbook.

MYELOMATOSIS

Is a malignant proliferation of plasma cells* in the bone marrow, usually affecting people over 50.

The clinical features relate to:

1) The production of large amounts of abnormal immunoglobulin leading to a very high ESR, kidney failure and susceptibility to infection.

2) Damage to bone from proliferation of cells in marrow producing bone pain, osteolytic lesions in the skull and long bones with characteristic X-ray appearance, fractures and **high blood calcium** (→anorexia, nausea, vomiting, thirst, polyuria, constipation, muscle weakness, peptic ulceration, depression, cardiac arrest etc).

---

*   The immunoglobulin producers of the immune system.

3) Marrow replacement by malignant cells causing anaemia and susceptibility to infection.

Treatment:

Radiotherapy to bone lesions, chemotherapy for malignant plasma cells,
steroids to lower blood calcium and urgent treatment of infections if they
arise.

Prognosis:

Average survival with treatment is about 3-4 years.

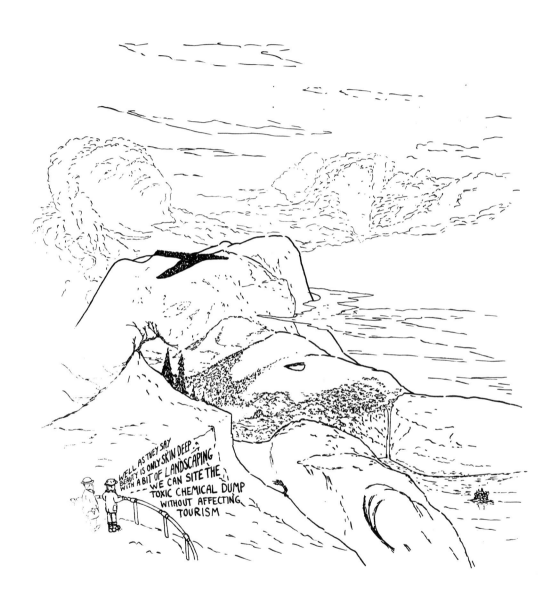

SKIN DISEASE

OVERVIEW

Introduction

Dermatitis/Eczema

Scaly Skin Conditions

> Psoriasis
> Lichen planus
> Pityriasis rosea

Acne

> Acne vulgaris
> Acne rosacea

Urticaria

Infective Skin Conditions

Bacterial:	Impetigo
	Erysipelas
	Cellulitis
Viral:	Herpes simplex
	Herpes zoster
	Warts
	Molluscum contagiosum
	Pityriasis rosea
Fungal:	Candida albicans
	Dermatophyte infections
	Pityriasis versicolor
Infestations:	Scabies
	Pediculosis

Cutaneous Malignancy

BCC (basal cell carcinoma)
SCC (squamous cell carcinoma)
Melanoma

Blistering Skin Diseases

Pemphigus vulgaris
Pemphigoid
Dermatitis herpetiformis
Erythema multiforme

Cutaneous Reactions to Orthodox Drugs

Skin Manifestations of Systemic Disease

Glossary

INTRODUCTION

If an elephant walked into the room right now, you would probably have no difficulty in diagnosing that it was, in fact, an elephant.

Even if you had never seen one before, if a second one arrived you would quickly come to the conclusion that it was another one of whatever the first one was.

In a similar way, dermatologists are skilled in diagnosing skin rashes, lumps and bumps because they have seen so many before.

Thus, as so often in other branches of medicine, reading about diseases of the skin is virtually useless unless you also see the conditions in a living person. For this reason, the descriptions that follow are fairly brief; we would encourage you to go out of your way to see real-life examples of the conditions mentioned.

DERMATITIS/ECZEMA

Eczema and dermatitis are synonyms for inflammation of the skin. All eczematous skin conditions are characterized by red, itchy, weeping (ie oedematous) skin patches which are prone to secondary infection and which become progressively drier and harder ("lichenified") as time goes by because of repeated scratching. Eczema (in its various forms) is very common.

Classification:

Perhaps the most useful classification of eczema/dermatitis is:

Endogenous: Atopic eczema
                   Seborrhoeic eczema

Exogenous: Direct irritant dermatitis
                   Allergic contact dermatitis

Clinical features:

Atopic eczema:

> › Runs in families.
> › Common in infants.
> › May be associated with hayfever and asthma.
> › Itchy, sometimes weeping and ultimately scaly rash on face and in flexures.

Seborrhoeic eczema:

> › Crusty rash ("dandruff") affecting hairy skin (which contains many sebaceous glands).
> › Scalp, face (in males), axillae and groin creases are often affected.
> › Seborrheic eczema of the scalp in babies is known as "cradle cap".

Direct irritant dermatitis:

> › Caused by direct action of strong chemicals.
> › Develops soon after first exposure to irritant (usually within 24 hours).
> › Characterized by redness, blisters and cracks in skin.
> › Does not spread beyond area directly in contact with chemical.

Allergic contact dermatitis:

> › Eczematous rash develops after **second** exposure to "allergic" substance (eg lanolin, dyes, preservatives in skin creams, antibiotic ointments, nickel in jewellery/bra straps etc).
> › Rash most marked over area of initial contact but can spread all over body.

Management:

In most cases of eczema/dermatitis, symptomatic relief can be achieved by using steroid creams of varying strength and, in severe cases, by taking oral prednisolone. However, as discussed in chapter 8, topical and oral steroids produce serious side effects after prolonged use (eg steroid creams can produce irreversible thinning of the skin).

Oily ointments and bath preparations can ease the dry discomfort of chronic eczema. Barrier creams and gloves can help prevent contact and direct irritant dermatitis. However, the key to the management of eczema lies in the discovery of the *underlying* allergic or irritant factor (eg food – especially dairy products – in atopic eczema).

Secondary infection of eczematous patches can be avoided if the lesions aren't scratched but should be treated if it occurs.

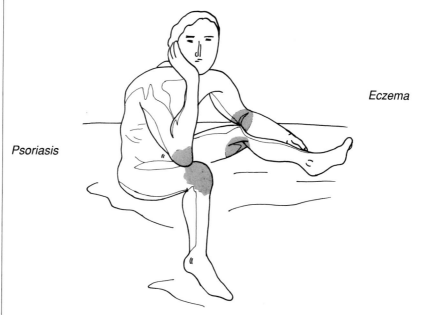

Eczema

Psoriasis

Distribution of eczema and psoriasis on flexor and extensor surfaces.

SCALY SKIN CONDITIONS

PSORIASIS

Is a relatively common skin condition (affecting up to 2% of Caucasians, males = females) that runs in families. It is characterized by thick scaly plaques on **extensor** surfaces (especially knees, elbows and scalp).

Background:

In psoriatic skin, epidermal cells seem to proliferate at an abnormally high rate and the surface cells are poorly keratinized. Some dermatologists think that these abnormal cells have abnormal surface antigens which, if the skin is exposed to minor trauma (eg scratching) get into the circulation and provoke antibody formation. When these antibodies react with the surface antigens of the faulty "keratinocytes" at the dermo-epidermal junction, immune complexes are formed. This produces inflammation of the skin and, ultimately, a classic patch of psoriasis.

Clinical features:

May present acutely as small scaly patches on a red base (widely distributed over the body) or as a chronic problem with **symmetrical, silvery, scaly plaques** (mostly on extensor surfaces and scalp).
Sometimes itchy. Up to 1 in 10 cases develop a seronegative arthritis ("psoriatic arthropathy") associated with pitting of the finger nails. The arthritis can be disabling, particularly when it affects the sacro–iliac joints or the small joints of the hands.
In some cases of psoriasis, called "erythrodermic psoriasis" the inflamed plaques join up to cover the whole body. At its worst, this can present the patient with problems similar to those suffered by a person with wide-spread burns (ie problems of maintaining fluid balance and temperature homeostasis, pain etc).

Management:

Pastes and ointments containing either coal tar or dithranol are the mainstay of orthodox management. Treatment with ultraviolet light is sometimes very effective. Steroids and even cytotoxic drugs are used in the worst cases.

Some cases get better spontaneously, others get worse inexorably.

LICHEN PLANUS

Acute or chronic itchy rash, of unknown aetiology, affecting the flexor surface of the wrists and ankles. It may also affect the trunk and mucous membranes.

Population:

Adults. Rare in children.

Clinical features:

Itchy, shiny, small, flat topped lumps with fine white lines passing through them ("Wickham's striae"). Patches of lichen planus often occur where the skin has been scratched or injured (this is known as Koebner's phenomenon). On mucous membranes, lesions form white patches resembling "leukoplakia" (see chapter 13). Mucous membrane lichen planus is sometimes pre-malignant.

The condition usually resolves of its own accord after a few months (although it sometimes recurs).

Treatment:

Nothing specific, but topical steroids are thought by some to promote healing.

PITYRIASIS ROSEA

An itchy skin condition of unknown cause (? viral) and short duration.

Population:

Children and teenagers.

Clinical features:

A few days before the main rash erupts, a "herald" patch* appears on the abdomen or upper back. This is followed by an itchy, pink, maculo-papular rash on the trunk, upper thighs and upper arms which appears to follow the lines of skin creases. The rash has usually gone within 6 weeks.

Treatment:

Nothing specific. Various approaches (antihistamines, calamine lotion etc) are used to relieve the itchIness.

*   A single, scaly, red macule.

ACNE

ACNE VULGARIS

A skin condition affecting mostly young people and characterized by blackheads and pustules on the face, shoulders and upper chest.

Background:

Problems start at puberty when androgenic hormones stimulate sebaceous glands to produce more sebum (grease). For some reason (possibly to do with the colonisation of sebaceous glands by the organism *corynebacterium acnes*), the sebaceous glands become blocked by lumps of keratin, sebum and bacteria. This causes retention of sebum within the glands producing the typical "blackheads" (comedones). If blackheads become secondarily infected, they may turn into pustules and heal by scarring.

Clinical features:

Most adolescents have some blackheads or pimples at one time or another and even those affected by more severe acne are usually free of the condition by the time they reach their early twenties. However, for the teenager with widespread blackheads and pimples on the face, shoulders and upper thorax, life can be profoundly miserable.
Stress, a sugary diet and the premenstrual hormonal state can all exacerbate the condition. Sunlight usually improves it.

Treatment:

All sorts of topical creams and lotions (often containing benzoyl peroxide, sulphur or salicylic acid) are available from chemists and do help some people. Low dose tetracycline (an antibiotic) taken for up to 6 months is sometimes prescribed and is often quite effective in the short term.

Nevertheless, many cases seem profoundly resistant to medical intervention.*

---

*   It is worth mentioning, however, that some cases of acne can be substantially improved by adopting a vegan diet, taking moderate exercise, increasing water intake and living in a more or less sunny and stress free environment. It is probably also worth pointing out that many "diseases" wouldn't develop in the first place if human beings lived this type of existence .....)

ACNE ROSACEA

This is a strange condition (not directly related to Acne vulgaris) characterized by redness of **facial** skin (sometimes complicated by papules and pustules) in people who have always "blushed" easily.

Background:

The cause is unknown (although exposure to infrared/UV radiation or infection with a mite called Dermodex folliculorum are sometimes suggested as aetiological factors).

Clinical features:

Mild rosacea is quite common.
The raised red rash is usually seen on the cheeks and nose but it may spread over the rest of the face.
Affected skin often looks tight and shiny since there is oedema in the upper dermis.

Unlike acne vulgaris, any pustules that form heal without scarring. The condition is made worse by exposure to sunlight.

Complications:

Some people with rosacea develop eye problems (eg blepharitis and conjunctivitis) and some go on to develop an enlarged, red, pitted nose (rhinophyma) covered with multiple small broken blood vessels (telangiectases).

Management:

The use of steroids on affected skin can make the condition **worse.** Orthodox treatment is long term low dose tetracycline therapy. The cosmetic problem of rhinophyma can be dealt with surgically.

URTICARIA

Urticaria is the medical name for "nettle rash" – weals on a red background – and may be precipitated by numerous external and internal factors. The important thing distinguishing allergic urticarial eruptions from other skin rashes is that **urticaria comes and goes**.

Background:

Urticaria is a hypersensitivity reaction mediated by histamine release (see chapter 2).

Precipitating factors:

> Drugs (eg penicillin and aspirin)
> Food (eg shell fish and egg)
> Chemicals
> Environmental conditions (eg heat, cold, sunlight)
> Pressure (eg tight clothes)
> Exercise
> Mite and flea bites

Many cases of chronic urticaria are unexplained.

Management:

Avoiding precipitating factors is the most efficient way of managing the problem, but not necessarily the most practical. Modern antihistamines* are often quite effective and are less sedating than old fashioned piriton.

---

*   eg terfenadine (Triludan).

INFECTIVE SKIN CONDITIONS

BACTERIAL

IMPETIGO and **ERYSIPELAS** see chapter 7.

CELLULITIS:

Spreading streptococcal infection of the subcutaneous tissues.
Intravenous "drips" are a common cause of cellulitis in hospital medicine.
Orthodox treatment is with penicillin.

VIRAL

HERPES SIMPLEX (cold sores):

Vesicular lesions on skin and mucous membranes.
Face and fingers are common sites of superficial herpes simplex infection.
The regional lymph nodes are often enlarged.
Treatment is with anti-viral solutions, eg idoxuridine.
See chapter 13 for oral herpes simplex.
See chapter 7 for genital herpes simplex.

HERPES ZOSTER (shingles):

See chapter 7.

WARTS:

The wart virus produces lesions on the fingers, soles of feet and genitalia (although small, flat warts are sometimes seen on the face or backs of hands).
In the majority of cases, warts will disappear of their own accord (given time) but can be removed by freezing, strong chemical lotions or minor surgery.

MOLLUSCUM CONTAGIOSUM:

A viral skin condition characterized by small crops of raised, "umbilicated"* lumps. They tend to resolve spontaneously but can be removed by pricking with a (sterile) cocktail stick dipped in phenol.

PITYRIASIS ROSEA:

See under scaly skin conditions.

FUNGAL

CANDIDA ALBICANS (thrush):

See chapter 13 for oral candidiasis, chapter 26 for vaginal candidiasis.

Skin candidiasis tends to affect warm, damp creases and produces clearly demarcated, irritating, dark red patches with a few smaller lesions scattered around. It is a frequent complication of simple nappy rash. Immunodeficiency, diabetes, poor nutrition, malignancy and general ill-health all make candida infection more likely.
The edges of finger and toe nails can sometimes become infected with candida, producing a chronic inflammation ("chronic paronychia").
Orthodox treatment is with **nystatin** formulations.

DERMATOPHYTE INFECTIONS:

Dermatophytes are a family of filamentous fungi causing superficial infections of skin, nails and hair. There are four common patterns of infection:

Tinea corporis (of the body) – ringworm:

Characterized by enlarging, scaly, red patches which become pale in the centre. The resulting raised, scaly circles look as if they could have been made by a burrowing worm.

---

*   With a dent in the middle.

Tinea pedis (of the foot) – athlete's foot:

Commonly starts between the fourth and fifth toes. The affected skin becomes itchy, pale, damp, flaky and mushy as the condition spreads to the other toes and onto the foot.

Tinea capitis (of the head) – ringworm affecting the scalp:

Similar appearance to tinea corporis. Can cause bald patches.

Tinea cruris (of the creases):*

Itchy, moist rash affecting the groin crease and upper thigh, usually in men.

Tinea of fingernails:

Tinea infection produces thick, brownish finger nails.

Management:

A variety of topical preparations (eg miconazole), available without prescription, are effective against tinea infection.
Resistant cases (nail bed infections in particular) are sometimes managed with the antifungal drug griseofulvin (taken orally).

PITYRIASIS VERSICOLOR:

A fungal infection of young adults caused by the organism Pityrosporum ovale. It produces brownish, scaly patches on the trunk which look pale in dark skinned people and dark in light skinned people.
Selenium sulphide preparations get rid of it, but it can be quite persistent, recurring from time to time.

---

*   The names given to this condition by rugby players are beyond the scope of this book.

INFESTATIONS

SCABIES:

Is an exquisitely itchy, highly contagious skin condition caused by the mite Sarcoptes scabei.

Transmission:

Direct body contact.

Clinical features:

Intense itching (worse at night) often on the wrists or between the fingers (sometimes on the penis or round the nipples). Close examination reveals small burrows under the skin (where the mite has laid eggs). There may be scratch marks or urticarial weals resulting from an allergic reaction to mite protein.

Treatment:

Painting the whole body from the neck down with an anti-mite solution (eg Lindane 1%), leaving it for 24 hours before washing it off and repeating the process at least twice, usually solves the problem. All close contacts should be treated and bed linen, clothes etc thoroughly washed in the normal way.

PEDICULOSIS (lice/crabs/nits):

There are different species of blood sucking lice which prefer either the head, the body or the pubic area. "Nits" are the egg capsules which the lice stick to hair shafts or clothing seams. Head lice are common amongst school children, pubic lice amongst sexually active adults. Body lice are rare these days.

Lice infestation causes itching. Scratching may cause secondary bacterial infection and associated regional lymphadenopathy.

Treatment with malathion preparations removes the lice; fine tooth combing removes the nits.

CUTANEOUS MALIGNANCY

Skin cancers together account for up to 10% of all cases of malignancy.
There are three 3 main types:

> › Basal cell carcinoma
> › Squamous cell carcinoma
> › Malignant melanoma

BASAL CELL CARCINOMA (rodent ulcer)

Population:

> › 60/80 age group
> › Males more than females
> › People living in sunny climates

Aetiology:

> UV light. Radiation. Prolonged contact with arsenical compounds.

Pathology:

> The malignant change occurs in the basal cells of hair follicles. Spread is by direct infiltration; metastasis is very rare.

Clinical features:

> Rodent ulcers tend to occur around the nose and inner canthus (ie above an imaginary line joining the mouth to the ear); they start as reddish, dome shaped pearly nodules and progress to form ulcers with raised, rolled, pearly edges. Growth is slow but inexorable and, untreated, may cause gross disfigurement.

Investigations:

> Biopsy.

Management:

> Surgical excision. If excision really is total, surgery offers **cure.** However, 15% cases have recurrence at the original site after operation.

SQUAMOUS CELL CARCINOMA

Population:

> › The elderly
> › Outdoor workers
> › Chemical and X-ray workers
> › People living in sunny climates

Aetiology:

> › Leukoplakia
> › Sun damaged skin
> › Pitch, tar, soot, paraffin, creosote, arsenic exposure over long periods
> › Radiation
> › Chronic ulceration

Pathology:

Malignant tumour of keratinocytes* which may spread locally or metastasize via blood.

Clinical features:

Ulcers with scab at centre and raised, rolled, hard, everted edges; commonly on exposed areas of face, neck and hands esp. in fair skinned people; may grow very rapidly.

Investigations:

Biopsy.

Management:

Surgical excision ± radiotherapy.

Prognosis:

Up to 80% 5 year survival after orthodox treatment; early diagnosis improves prognosis; outlook worse if metastases.

---

*   Keratin forming cells.

MALIGNANT MELANOMA

A pigmented skin cancer responsible for 1 in 200 British cancer deaths.

Population:

> › Mostly the over 30s but can affect younger age group
> › Female/male = 2:1
> › People in sunny climates more at risk

Aetiology:

Exposure to sunlight.

Pathology:

Malignant proliferation of melanocytes at the dermo-epidermal junction.

Clinical features:

Deeply but variably pigmented lesions, sometimes ulcerated, often on hands, feet, neck or face.

Some authorities suggest that pre-existing moles on palms, soles and genitalia are more likely to undergo malignant change.

» Any naevus* is suspicious if it exhibits the following features:

> › rapid growth
> › itching
> › bleeding
> › ulceration
> › variable pigmentation
> › "satellite" lesions (other pigmented patches around the main patch)

Hairy moles are thought never to turn malignant.

Malignant melanomas spread remarkably rapidly – always look for local lymphadenopathy. Bloodborne metastasis to lung, liver and brain and bone occur early on.

---

*   Naevus = mole.

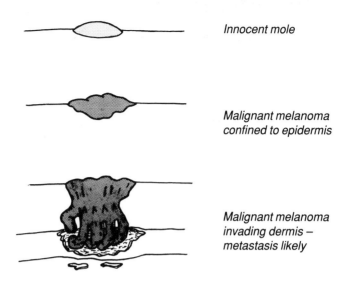

Innocent mole

*Malignant melanoma
confined to epidermis*

*Malignant melanoma
invading dermis –
metastasis likely*

Management:

The clinical suspicion of malignant melanoma always leads to surgical excision (often on the same day as the dermatology outpatient appointment). Removed tissue is examined to determine *depth* of penetration into underlying tissue.
Skin grafting may be necessary over excision site.
Chemotherapy is sometimes tried.
Radiotherapy is rarely helpful.

Side effects:

Early removal of a thin tumour has few (if any) side effects. Skin grafting, chemotherapy and radiotherapy each produce a variety of problems.

Prognosis:

Early removal of thin tumours (with no evidence of metastasis) produces 90% 5 year survival. Thicker tumours have worse than 40% five year survival and the incidence of metastasis carries an awful prognosis (<6% 5 year survival). Careful follow-up is essential since melanomata can recur years after original operation.

BLISTERING SKIN CONDITIONS

There are four well recognized but rare blistering ("bullous") skin diseases:

> › Pemphigus vulgaris
> › Pemphigoid
> › Dermatitis herpetiformis
> › Erythema multiforme

Before the introduction of steroid therapy, pemphigus vulgaris frequently proved fatal.

PEMPHIGUS VULGARIS

Population:

> › Middle aged men and women
> › More frequent in Jews

Aetiology:

> Auto-immune.

Pathology:

> IgG antibody destroys the intracellular "cement" of the "Malpighian" layer in the epidermis. The epidermis therefore splits above basal layer with the formation of **"intra-epidermal" blisters.**

Clinical features:

> Starts insidiously with the development of raw areas on mucous membranes (mouth, genitalia) which are painful but not itchy. Blisters may then start to form on the skin (limbs and trunk) but are easily broken by friction and pressure leaving painful, raw areas. The surrounding skin looks normal. The patient feels very unwell and has a fever. **Without treatment, secondary bacterial infection and protein, fluid and electrolyte loss from weeping skin may be fatal.**

Management:

> High dose oral prednisolone is usually necessary to bring pemphigus under control. Once new blisters have ceased to form, the dose is grad-

ually reduced. However, many patients require life long "maintenance" therapy. From time to time cases get better spontaneously. Local treatment of the skin is similar to the management of burns: the primary aim is to protect raw areas and avoid secondary infection.

Prognosis:

Better than it was in the short term but the overall prognosis is still poor because of the difficulty in juggling disease activity with steroid side effects.

PEMPHIGOID

Similar to pemphigus but

> › Sudden onset
> › Patients older
> › Blisters deeper and **less** likely to break
> › Patient not so ill
> › Skin around blisters may be red and itchy
> › Mouth ulcers uncommon

Management:

Steroids. It is often possible to stop therapy after a couple of years.

DERMATITIS HERPETIFORMIS

Relates to gluten enteropathy (Coeliac disease)* and, possibly, to other immune disorders. Causes clusters of **intensely** itchy vesicles on the extensor aspects of the elbows and knees (+ between scapulae and on buttocks).
No fever, no mouth ulcers. Starts suddenly and may go just as suddenly. Secondary bacterial infection is common.

Management:

A gluten free diet is usually curative. The anti-leprosy drug, **Dapsone,** helps to control the skin lesions.

*   See chapter 13.

ERYTHEMA MULTIFORME

A skin condition of **unknown aetiology.** It is, however, **associated with** allergic reactions to **certain drugs** (eg sulphonamides, aspirin and penicillin) and herpes simplex infection.

Clinical features:

› General systemic disturbance (fever, sore throat, headache, joint pains and diarrhoea) is followed by eruption of a pleomorphic* red rash that may blister.
› Forearms, legs and mouth are often involved.
› Skin lesions may resemble archery targets (they have concentric rings of different colours).
› The condition usually gets better of its own accord in about five weeks.

Management:

Stop drugs.
Topical treatment for itching.

Complications:

Severe erythema multiforme – known as the Stevens-Johnson syndrome** – may need steroid therapy.

---

* Many forms.
** Albert Stevens (1884-1945), New York paediatrician.
Frank Johnson (1894-1934) New York paediatrician.

CUTANEOUS REACTIONS TO ORTHODOX DRUGS

Many orthodox drugs cause allergic reactions, particularly skin rashes.

Measles-like rashes and urticarial reactions are common, but almost any type of skin rash can occur (blistering, acne-like, purpuric etc).

"Fixed drug eruptions" are those in which the same rash appears in the same place when the same drug is given. Some drug reactions (particularly those provoked by penicillin) can last for some time after the drug has been withdrawn.

NOTE:

A classic example of a drug reaction is that of ampicillin which, if prescribed inappropriately in a case of infectious mononucleosis, can cause a widespread erythematous rash.

SKIN MANIFESTATIONS OF SYSTEMIC DISEASES

Acromegaly:

Seborrhoeic eczema.

Addison's disease:

Increased skin pigmentation.

Coeliac disease:

Dermatitis herpetiformis.

Cushing's syndrome:

Acne.

Diabetes:

Necrobiosis lipoidica diabeticorum.*
Fungal infections.

Lupus erythematosus:

Photosensitive butterfly rash on cheeks. Also "discoid" lupus erythemato-sus – a skin condition characterized by well demarcated red patches that have a characteristic histological appearance.

Malignancy:

Secondary deposits. Pigmentation changes.
Itching.
Acanthosis nigricans.**

Systemic sclerosis:

Hardening and "shrinking" of the skin of the face/hands. This produces an appearance of early aging, beaked nose, lined face, ischaemic fingers etc.

Thyroid disease:

Hair loss.

---

*   Literally "fatty looking skin death of diabetics."
** Brown plaques over armpits/groin.

GLOSSARY

Bulla (big blister):

> Same as a vesicle but bigger.

Lichenification:

> Epidermal thickening caused by continued scratching/rubbing.

Macule:

> A flat, clearly demarcated area of different skin colour.

Nodule:

> A firm lump, some of which projects above the skin surface but with the greater part below the skin surface.

Papule:

> A small raised area of skin.

Plaque:

> A flat topped lesion in the skin which can be felt but not necessarily clearly seen.

Purpura:

> Blood under the skin.

Pustule:

> A pus filled lesion.

Telangiectasis:

> Dilated visible capillaries.

Vesicle (small blister):

> A fluid filled raised lesion smaller than 5mm in diameter.

Weal:

> A slightly raised skin lesion with pink edges and a pale centre.

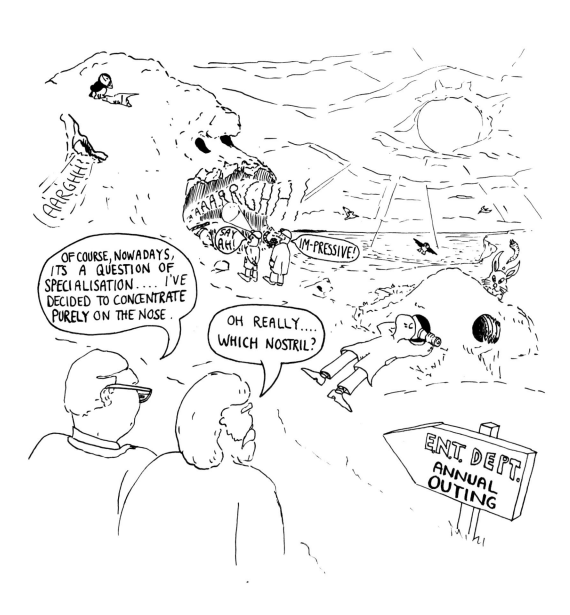

OVERVIEW

EYE DISEASE

Introduction

The Assessment of Eye Problems

Common Clinical Presentations of Eye Disease and Their Significance

The red eye
Sudden loss of sight in a non-red eye
Gradual loss of sight in a non-red eye
Blurred vision
Double vision
Floaters
Nystagmus
Watering eyes
Headache
Painful eyes
Sore eyelids

Four Important Eye Diseases

Acute conjunctivitis
Acute iritis
Acute glaucoma
Cataract

ENT

Introduction

Common Pathologies in ENT

Ear: Otitis externa
Otitis media – acute, chronic, secretory, complications
(incl mastoiditis)
Injury to the eardrum
Otosclerosis

Nose: Sinusitis
             Hayfever
             Nasal polyps
Throat: Tonsillitis – quinsy, adenoiditis etc
             Laryngitis
             Malignant tumours of the larynx and pharynx

Common Presentations of ENT Disease

Ear: Earache
             Tinnitus
             Vertigo
             Deafness
Nose: Catarrh
             Nosebleed
Throat: Hoarseness
             Stridor
             Dysphagia

EYE DISEASE

INTRODUCTION

Most primary care practitioners are very wary of eye problems and have no hesitation in referring to a specialist if there is **any suggestion of diminished visual acuity** without a simple explanation.

We would urge similar caution on readers of this section, which is only a brief introduction to a highly complex specialty.

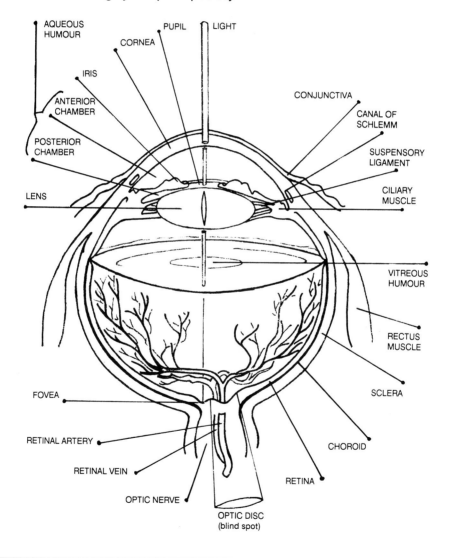

THE ASSESSMENT OF EYE PROBLEMS

The following is a *very* basic guide to the clinical assessment of a patient presenting with eye problems.

History:

? history of trauma

? previous eye disease

? systemic disease with eye complications

? on drugs

? blurred vision or ↓ visual acuity

? pain in eye or photophobia

? discharge from eye

? problem unilateral or bilateral

Examination:

Eyelids	– look for:	Swelling Closure Discharge
Redness	– is it:	Localized Diffuse Circumcorneal
Cornea	– is there:	Transparency Bright light reflex
Anterior chamber	– assess: – is there:	Depth Hypopyon (pus in anterior chamber) Hyphaema (blood in anterior chamber)
Pupil	– assess:	Size Shape Outline Reactivity
Fundus:		Examine as usual
Visual acuity	– assess:	If diminished, see if correctable by looking through pinhole. If yes, probably refractive error. If no, consider specialist referral.

COMMON CLINICAL PRESENTATIONS OF EYE DISEASE

– and their significance

THE RED EYE

There are four major causes (other than trauma) for an acutely painful red eye:

Inflammation of the outer eye:	Conjunctivitis
Inflammation of the cornea:	Keratitis
Inflammation of the inner eye:	Iritis
Acute increase in intra-ocular pressure:	Glaucoma

Three of these are dealt with below. Keratitis will briefly be considered here.

ACUTE KERATITIS:

The cornea is very vulnerable to external damage. Inflammation/infection of the cornea usually presents as a **corneal ulcer**.

Corneal ulcers may result from severe untreated conjunctivitis, from bacterial infection after injury or from the spread of herpes simplex infection from a cold sore. (Herpes simplex corneal ulcers are referred to as "dendritic ulcers" because of their branching appearance.) Some skin diseases (eg acne rosacea) can cause keratitis, as can overexposure of the eye (eg in hyperthyroid exophthalmos or eyelid damage).

Congenital syphilis is also associated with keratitis.

Clinical features:

> › Sore red eye.
> › Cloudy corneal opacity.
> › Visual loss if severe.

Management:

Treat underlying infection.
Treat any associated condition.
Don't use steroid drops if dendritic ulcer suspected.
Corneal grafting may be necessary in severe cases.

SUDDEN LOSS OF SIGHT IN NON-RED EYE

VASCULAR CAUSES:

Retinal arteriosclerosis, malignant hypertension (which causes retinal necrosis), retinal artery or vein occlusion, temporal arteritis and retinal haemorrhage (associated with diabetes, retinal vein thrombosis, hypertension, ↑ ICP, trauma etc).

Vitreous haemorrhage also causes sudden blindness and is associated with diabetes and bleeding disorders.

RETINAL DETACHMENT:

Associated with short sight (+ trauma, diabetes and arteriosclerosis).

Clinical features:

Flashes of light.
Floaters.
Partial loss of vision.

Management:

Laser treatment.

GRADUAL LOSS OF SIGHT IN NON-RED EYE

CATARACT:

Cataract means loss of transparency of the lens. There are various types; **senile cataracts** are the most common. They tend to develop slowly (over age 55) and produce a distortion of vision that is like looking through glass that is gradually frosting. In diabetics, cataracts form earlier and progress more rapidly. Surgery to remove the lens (or suck out its nucleus) is the orthodox management. Strong glasses, contact lenses and prosthetic lens implants can be used to correct the resulting visual deficit after surgery. Surgery will not usually be offered unless the retina is healthy.

SIMPLE GLAUCOMA:

Slow increase in intra-ocular pressure causing gradual visual failure.

Clinical features:

Suspect glaucoma if a long sighted patient complains of rainbows/haloes around lights and has a **family history** of glaucoma. Other features include blurred vision, visual field defects and a "cupped" optic disc seen through an ophthalmoscope.

Management:

Eye drops to constrict pupil, acetazolamide to ↓ aqueous production. Possibly surgery.

DIABETIC RETINOPATHY:

See chapter 15.

BLURRED VISION

Young healthy person	→	Suspect refractive error, try pinhole test
Older person	→	Distance vision – ? cataract
	→	Near vision – ? retinal circulatory problem
	→	Both – ? glaucoma
Episodic blurring	→	? Glaucoma, carotid artery insufficiency or migraine

DOUBLE VISION

1) Paralysis or weakness of extra-ocular muscles (causes include trauma, strokes, neuropathy associated with MS, diabetes, myasthenia and thyroid disease).

2) Poor eye co-ordination (needs glasses and orthoptic advice).

3) Change of angle of a longstanding squint. Needs orthoptic advice.

FLOATERS

Floaters* associated with flashes and sparks may indicate **detached retina.** (Beware the patient with short sight and diabetes or arteriosclerosis.)

NYSTAGMUS

Congenital nystagmus usually produces few complaints except some ↓ in distance vision. Acquired nystagmus (MS, vestibular disease) is usually associated with giddiness (see chapter 16).

WATERING EYES

Watering in a white, painless eye is not sight threatening BUT is often hard to treat. If watering + discharge, needs local antibacterial treatment. If persistent, may need specialist referral (? syringing of tear duct). Eyelid spasm and ingrowing eyelashes may also cause persistent watering. **Watering plus pain or photophobia may suggest corneal damage and is thus much more serious.**

HEADACHE

Headache plus **visual symptoms** would suggest the possibility of migraine, temporal arteritis or glaucoma.

PAINFUL EYES

Visual disturbance + pain in the eye is always potentially serious – eg:
› Iritis
› Glaucoma
› Shingles
› MS
› Temporal arteritis

Trauma (eg ingrowing eyelash) causes pain associated with redness and watering. Trigeminal neuralgia may produce pain in a white eye with no visual disturbance.

---

*   Black blobs floating through the visual field.

SORE EYELIDS

Internal styes (infection of meibomian gland = chalazion) are common and often resolve spontaneously. Some need surgical incision to relieve.

External styes (infection of lash follicle = hordeolum) usually resolve spontaneously (local bathing with clean hot water may help). A rodent ulcer of eyelid may be mistaken for a stye.

Blepharitis (infection of eyelid margin) may cause lid deformity and corneal damage from secondary infection if not treated.

Entropion or ectropion (in- or out-turning of the lid) may cause discomfort, watering and corneal damage etc. Treatment is by plastic surgery.

FOUR IMPORTANT EYE DISEASES

ACUTE CONJUNCTIVITIS

Inflammation of the conjunctiva.

Aetiology:

> Bacterial infection (especially Staphylococcus aureus)
> Viral infection (eg Herpes simplex)
> Trauma
> Association with systemic disease (eg the sicca (dry eyes) syndrome in connective tissue disorders)

Clinical features:

> Red eyes (usually **bilateral**)*
> **Vision not affected**
> Gritty feeling + watering
> Sticky eyelids (worse first thing in the morning)
> Swollen eyelids
> Discharge + crusting

Management:

A swab taken for microbiological investigation is desirable but not often done. Antibiotic eye drops (particularly chloramphenicol – trade name Chloromycetin) are the mainstays of orthodox management.

Gentle bathing to remove crusting from lids is soothing. Dark glasses relieve mild photophobia.

ACUTE IRITIS

Inflammation of the iris, ciliary body and choroid (which together are sometimes referred to as the **uveal tract**). Although acute iritis is sometimes seen as a complication of eye infection, most cases seem to be the result of antigen/antibody interaction affecting a previously sensitised iris.

---

*   Remember, the conjunctiva covers the inside of the eyelids as well as the outer parts of the whites of the eyes.

Acute iritis is thus associated with a number of autoimmune connective tissue disorders and chronic inflammatory diseases, eg:

› Reiter's disease
› Ankylosing spondylitis
› Juvenile RA
› Sarcoidosis
› TB
› Syphilis
› Leprosy

Clinical features:

› **Blurred vision** (which may develop *extremely* rapidly)
› Red eye (with the redness concentrated around the cornea – so called "circumcorneal injection")
› Very painful ache in eye
› Watering
› Photophobia
› **Visual acuity** ↓
› Pupil **constricted** (inflammation causes spasm of sphincter muscle)
› Inflammatory exudate in the anterior chamber of eye. The white cells may stick in clumps to the back of the cornea forming "keratic precipitates", visible sometimes to the naked eye*. There may even be a collection of pus in the anterior chamber (an "hypopyon") which produces a characteristic appearance
› If adhesions form between the inflamed iris and the lens ("posterior synechias"), the pupil can't move freely and takes on an irregular outline
› Eyeball tender

Management:

Specific management of underlying condition (if possible). Drops to dilate pupil will avoid development of synechias and relieve the pain of iris spasm. Steroid drops to reduce inflammation.

---

* As well as a torch, magnifying glass and ophthalmoscope, ophthalmologists also use a "slit lamp" microscope which allows detailed examination of different layers of the eye. Some of the early inflammatory signs of acute iritis are only visible using a slit lamp.

ACUTE GLAUCOMA

An acute eye condition in which the pressure within the eyeball increases to a level where:

1) the blood supply to the neural tissue of the retina is impaired and
2) the transparency of the cornea is diminished.

These two pathologies may cause blindness.

» The term glaucoma actually refers to a group of conditions — "closed angle glaucoma" is the acute type.

About 1 person in a hundred develops glaucoma (in one of its forms) over the age of 40 and the incidence then increases with increasing age.

Pathology:

Aqueous humour is the clear fluid that fills the anterior and posterior chambers of the eyeball. It is secreted from the ciliary body and enters the posterior chamber before flowing through the pupil into the anterior chamber. It then drains into a venous sinus through gaps at the angle between the iris and cornea. If this angle is blocked, drainage is prevented and the intra-ocular pressure rises. People who are long sighted have narrow anterior chambers and are particularly at risk. Inflammatory exudates (eg from acute iritis), blood etc may also block the drainage angle and may produce **secondary glaucoma.**

» Dilation of the pupil also narrows the drainage angle and so glaucoma may be precipitated by a visit to the cinema.

Over 50 **drugs** are known to precipitate glaucoma, including **steroids** and some of the common orthodox treatments for Parkinson's disease and depression.

Clinical features:

Very painful eye (sometimes both eyes) in a sick person. There may be a previous history of brief attacks of seeing **coloured haloes around lights** associated with temporal headache and blurring of vision. Perhaps also a family history of "eye trouble".

A typical case presents as severe headache plus nausea and vomiting with red, painful eye and severe visual loss of more or less rapid onset.

There may be a watery discharge. Any redness of the eye is most noticeable around the rim of the cornea (which overlies the iris) and the cornea itself becomes oedematous giving a cloudy, "bathroom glass" effect. The pupil appears **dilated** and sluggish in its response to light. It eventually becomes fixed in dilation. It may also appear slightly elongated in the vertical plane.

Management:

As we have said, most orthodox doctors are (correctly) very wary of serious eye disease and will rapidly refer eye problems to an ophthalmologist. Of all possible symptoms/signs, **visual disturbance of any kind should never be dismissed as unimportant.** Expert treatment of acute glaucoma involves the use of eye drops to constrict the pupil plus the drug acetazolamide (given orally) to ↓aqueous production. Some cases will need surgery ("iridectomy") to relieve the obstruction to aqueous flow.

Prognosis:

Untreated glaucoma causes blindness. The earlier definitive treatment is given, the higher the chance that vision will be preserved.

CATARACT

A cataract is an opacity in the lens of the eye. Since the lens is avascular and most lens cells have no nuclei (and thus cannot divide), there is no capacity for the **repair** of lens damage (from whatever cause). An "insulted" lens simply goes cloudy.

Cataract is the commonest cause of blindness in the UK (about 1/4 of all cases; glaucoma comes 2nd).

Background:

Minor changes in lens transparency do not usually affect vision and are a common accompaniment of increasing age.

Most significant cataracts are the result of **"senile" change** but some are the result of **developmental abnormalities** (eg in association with congenital syphilis, Down's syndrome etc).

Some are **secondary** to injury, inflammatory eye disease (eg prolonged iritis), or metabolic and endocrine defects (there is a particular association between **diabetes** and cataract).

Clinical features:

Progressive, slow, painless $\downarrow$ in visual acuity ($\pm$ dark spots in visual field). Double images may be seen through one eye.

On examination, an advanced cataract appears as a white opacity within the pupil. An early one is seen through the ophthalmoscope as a black shadow obscuring the red reflex.

Management:

Operative removal of some or all of the lens tissue (these operations are done with beautifully delicate instruments using an operating microscope) followed by prescription of thick convex lens glasses.

Alternatively, the opaque natural lens can be replaced by small acrylic "artificial" lenses. Lens implants cannot, obviously, accommodate to near/far changes of vision, but are often very effective at restoring a patient's general quality of life.

ENT – DISEASES OF THE EAR, NOSE AND THROAT

INTRODUCTION

All practitioners involved in primary care spend quite a large proportion of their time dealing with conditions relating to the ear, nose or throat (particularly sore throat, earache and "sinusitis").

The surgical discipline of ENT (oto-rhino-laryngology!) is nowadays, however, a skilled, technical and specialist field and deals with many thousands of referrals each year.

A detailed study of hospital based ENT practice is thus outside the scope of this book. What follows is a limited discussion of common pathologies and presentations*.

---

*   It is easier to understand the pathology of ENT disease when you remember that all the cavities and recesses of the ear, nose and throat are i) very close together ii) connected by a labyrinth of tubes and passages.

EAR

OTITIS EXTERNA

› Inflammation of the skin of the external ear canal.
› Usually caused by bacterial or fungal infection (often introduced by the twisted corner of a dirty towel).

Clinical features:

Itching, discomfort exacerbated by jaw movement and (possibly) a slight discharge from the ear. Otoscopic examination reveals mucky, inflamed, oedematous skin in the external ear canal.

Management:

Gentle cleaning away of muck and debris plus use of antibiotic drops or antiseptic dressings in the ear. Occasionally, systemic antibiotics and painkillers are required. It obviously helps if the patient doesn't scratch their ears.

ACUTE OTITIS MEDIA

› **Bacterial infection of the middle ear cavity**, common in children.
› Often follows colds, flu, tonsillitis and childhood exanthema such as measles.
› May also follow traumatic damage to the tympanic membrane or exposure to sudden, extreme changes in atmospheric pressure.
› The inflammation involves the middle ear cavity, the Eustachian tube* and the passages connecting to the mastoid air cells so accumulating pus cannot escape. This leads to increasing pressure on the eardrum which may burst, thus allowing pus to drain and the infection to resolve.

Clinical features:

Severe, throbbing earache, and a conductive deafness ± tinnitus. There is usually fever. The tympanic membrane appears dull, reddened and (maybe) bulging.

---

* Bartolomeo Eustachi (1513-1574), Italian nobleman and physician to the Pope – also professor of anatomy at Rome.

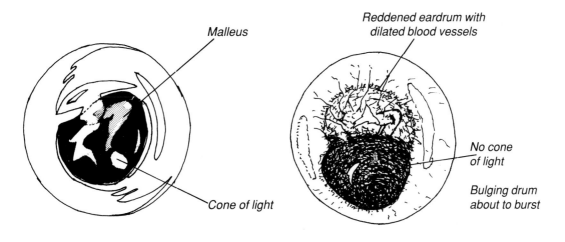

Normal eardrum   *Acute otitis media*

If the TM bursts, there will be a purulent discharge from the ear and an obvious hole visible via the otoscope.

Management:

Orthodox management involves the use of antibiotics (penicillins) to avoid a burst TM plus appropriate general nursing.

CHRONIC OTITIS MEDIA

› Acute OM that is either partially or ineffectively managed may persist as **chronic suppurative otitis media** with a perforated eardrum that won't heal properly.

In cases where the TM perforation is **central** and the discharge is **not purulent**, there is little risk of serious complications.

However, if the TM perforation is on the **posterior edge or at the top**, there is a risk that the tympanic ring, ossicles and mastoid air cells (ie the *bony* structures) may become infected with the eventual formation of a **cholesteatoma**. This is an accumulation of infected muck trapped in the attic (upper part) of the tympanic cavity which may, as it increases in size, destroy the ossicles and even the thin bone separating the cranial cavity from the middle ear (which could lead to meningitis/encephalitis).

Clinical features:

Dangerous chronic OM presents with purulent, smelly discharge from an upper or postero-marginal perforation in the tympanic membrane in a patient still suffering intermittent fever after their original acute OM.

Management:

Management of "safe" CSOM involves treatment of any underlying upper respiratory tract infection plus the use of antiseptic ear drops.

Dangerous (bony infection) chronic OM may require surgery to suck out infected material and drain debris from the mastoid air cell system (mastoidectomy). Mastoidectomy procedures result in deafness, so the alternative is to drain the middle ear/mastoid cavity and then to try and reconstruct the eardrum/ossicles mechanism (tympanoplasty).

SECRETORY OTITIS MEDIA ("glue ear")

A common condition, seen in children, in which repeated bouts of acute OM, mostly without burst eardrums (and usually treated with antibiotics), lead to more or less permanent blockage of the Eustachian tubes and an accumulation of thick, sticky mucus in the middle ear cavity. This produces deafness, a bunged up feeling in the ear and, sometimes, tinnitus and discomfort. These in turn may lead to problems at school, eg in the development of co-ordinated skills such as reading and writing.

Otoscopic examination shows fluid behind the TM. Deafness is "conductive".

Orthodox management (once repeated doses of antibiotics are accepted as ineffective and assuming the child hasn't "grown out of" the problem) often involves the insertion of a "grommet" into the TM (myringotomy). This allows fluid to drain from the middle ear. The grommets eventually fall out of their own accord and the eardrum heals.

Glue ear frequently responds to the sort of dietary intervention used by non-orthodox practitioners in the management of childhood allergies.

COMPLICATIONS OF OTITIS MEDIA

Unresolved or spreading infection/inflammation may produce:

> › Mastoiditis
> › Meningitis
> › Brain abscess
> › Facial paralysis
> › Inflammation of the "labyrinth"
>
> **Acute mastoiditis** should always be looked for in any patient with otitis media. It requires emergency management since it could lead to meningitis.

The clinical features of acute mastoiditis are:

> › Pain and tenderness over the mastoid process
> › High fever + pulse rate
> › Obvious unwellness
> › Profuse discharge through perforated eardrum
> › Increasing deafness

Management:

> Maximum dose antibiotics ± surgical drainage of mastoid processes where necessary.

INJURY TO THE EARDRUM

Aetiology:

> Trauma (cotton buds etc). Very loud noises. Very severe pressure changes (rapid aircraft descent, a "clip round the ear").

Clinical features:

> › Pain as TM bursts
> › Tinnitus
> › Deafness
> › Sometimes a little bleeding from ear
> › TM tear visible through otoscope

Management:

Do nothing unless symptoms and signs of infection appear.

OTOSCLEROSIS

Thickening of the bone at the footplate of the stapes, reducing its mobility and thus inhibiting conduction of vibration from TM to cochlea.

Background:

Problem usually starts in young adults, often with a family history of early deafness.

Aetiology unknown.

Clinical features:

› Bilateral progressive deafness ± tinnitus
› Paradoxically, sufferers often find it easier to hear conversation when in noisy surroundings ("paracusis")
› TM looks normal
› Bone conduction better than air conduction

Management:

Surgical replacement of stapes by a prosthesis (stapedectomy) is usually curative **if done early enough.**

NOSE

SINUSITIS

Acute or chronic infection of the maxillary, frontal, ethmoidal or sphenoidal air sinuses.

Background:

Acute sinusitis is usually the result of bacterial infection secondary to colds, flu or childhood exanthema.
It may also result from trauma, dental infection, anatomical abnormality of the air passages preventing free drainage of mucus or tumours developing within the sinuses.

Chronic sinusitis usually relates to persistent low grade infection and poor drainage of the sinus cavities.
It is also seen as part of an "allergic" clinical picture.

Clinical features:

› Pain + tenderness over affected sinuses (supra-orbital pain first thing in the morning is common in frontal sinusitis)
› Blocked nose (maxillary and ethmoidal) — may be discharge from the nose or down the back of the throat (post-nasal drip)
› Chronic sinusitis may produce headache, night-time cough (associated with post-nasal drip) and a tendency to breath through the mouth. It is obviously a predisposing factor for the development of otitis media

Management:

Acute sinusitis is managed in orthodox medicine with antibiotics plus surgical drainage of pus if absolutely necessary.

Chronic sinusitis (especially maxillary) sometimes responds to vasoconstrictor nasal sprays (ephedrine), but is often managed by surgical drainage procedures (eg washout of the maxillary sinuses). A number of techniques can be used to **permanently** improve the drainage from the affected sinuses (eg the Caldwell-Luc* "radical antrostomy" for chronic maxillary sinusitis, in which some of the medial wall of the sinus is removed to provide free drainage into the nose).

Complications:

> › Spread to other sinuses.
> › Spread to other parts of respiratory tract and middle ear .
> › Spread to surrounding bone.**

HAYFEVER (allergic rhinitis)

Allergic inflammation of the mucous membranes lining the nasal cavity.

Aetiological factors:

"Atopic" family history.
Exposure to inhaled allergens (dust, pollen, moulds, mites etc).
Exposure to ingested allergens (dairy products, drugs etc).

Clinical features:

Watery, profuse discharge from nose (rhinorrhoea) with tears, sneezing fits, blocked nose and (sometimes) conjunctivitis.

Management:

Avoid contact with precipitating allergens.
Topical antihistamines, steroids etc (in orthodox practice).
Desensitisation.

---

*   George Caldwell (1834-1918) – American ENT surgeon
       Henri Luc (1853-1923) – Paris ENT surgeon
**   Acute frontal sinusitis may spread to involve the orbit and surrounding tissues. It may also lead
       to meningitis or intracranial abscess.

NASAL POLYPS

Oedematous mucosa from the ethmoidal or maxillary sinuses forming pedunculated polyps (polyps on stalks) that protrude into the nasal cavity.

Aetiology:

Normally an expression of allergy.
Nasal polyps in children are sometimes associated with cystic fibrosis.
Occasionally, nasal polyps turn out to be neoplastic.

Clinical features:

› Blocked nose.
› Poor sense of smell.
› Runny nose.
› Sneezing fits.
› Polyps visible on examination of nasal cavity (requires expert use of head mirror, post nasal mirror and nasal speculum).

Management:

Removal under local or general anaesthesia.

THROAT

TONSILLITIS

Acute tonsillitis is usually viral or bacterial (see chapter 7).

Clinical features:

> Infection of the tonsils in children causes fever, malaise, sore throat and difficulty swallowing.
> The tonsils appear inflamed and may be coated with exudate. Cervical lymph nodes may be enlarged.
> Infection may spread to other parts of the upper respiratory tract.

Management:

Orthodox management is bed rest, simple pain killers and antibiotics (if bacterial infection suspected).

Tonsillectomy may be advised in recurrent cases (especially if associated with persistent middle ear infection).

QUINSY (peritonsillar abscess)

A quinsy is a collection of pus around the upper part of the tonsils. It is a complication of acute tonsillitis.

Clinical features:

> About a week after tonsillitis starts there may be a deterioration in general condition, a rise in temperature and acute discomfort on swallowing (± referred pain in the ear).
> Examination of the throat reveals a large bulge pushing downward and medially.
> The uvula may be pale and swollen.

Management:

Antibiotics plus immediate drainage of the pus through a small incision midway between the base of the uvula and the upper wisdom teeth on the affected side (using local anaesthetic – eg cocaine spray).

The tonsils are often removed a few weeks later to avoid recurrence.

ADENOIDITIS

Repeated upper respiratory tract infections in children often causes hypertrophy of the lymphoid tissue (adenoids) on the back wall of the pharynx behind the nose.

This causes mouth breathing and sleep disturbance and increases the tendency to respiratory infections, otitis media and sinusitis.

Adenoidectomy is often performed along with tonsillectomy in "catarrhal" children.

LARYNGITIS

Acute laryngitis is inflammation of the larynx (usually secondary to colds, influenza, smoking or talking too much) producing loss of voice ± fever and malaise.

Not talking, treatment of any underlying infection and no smoking usually resolves the condition in a few days.

Continual overuse or misuse of the voice (eg singers, teachers) may lead to chronic laryngitis/hoarseness which may be associated with the forma-tion of polyps on the vocal cords. These can be removed surgically.

Acute laryngo-tracheo-bronchitis and epiglottitis in children were dealt with in chapter 12.

MALIGNANT TUMOURS OF THE LARYNX AND PHARYNX

Malignant tumours of the head and neck are more common than is generally realised. ENT surgeons have to deal with salivary gland tu-mours, malignant disease of the middle ear, carcinoma of the maxillary, frontal and ethmoidal sinuses, malignant tumours of the nasopharynx, malignant disease of the tongue and cheek, carcinoma of the tonsils, supra-glottic, glottic and sub-glottic tumours of the larynx and malignan-cies of the hypopharynx* called **post-cricoid** tumours.

---

*   The beginning of the oesophagus.

Detailed discussion of these topics is beyond the scope of this chapter but you should note that

› Persistent or increasing hoarseness
› Persistent or increasing dysphagia
› Cervical lymphadenopathy
› General signs of malignancy including weight loss, malaise etc

should raise the suspicion of pharyngeal or laryngeal malignancies, especially in high risk groups (smokers, the socially disadvantaged, the elderly etc).

Note that long standing **iron deficiency in middle aged women** is a risk factor for the development of "post-cricoid" carcinomas.

COMMON PRESENTATIONS OF ENT DISEASE

EAR

Earache:

Directly related to the ear:	Otitis externa Otitis media Mastoiditis External/middle ear malignancies	
Referred earache:	IXth nerve: Vth nerve: IX/Xth nerves:	Post-tonsillectomy Dental problems Temporo-mandibular joint strain* (TMJ or Costen's syndrome) Malignant disease of the posterior tongue, pharynx or larynx**

Tinnitus:

Ear:	All ear conditions, including wax in ears, *may* cause tinnitus. Remember Meniere's disease (see chapter 16).
Head/Neck:	Dental problems TMJ problems Cervical spine displacements
Systemic:	Fever Hypotension Atherosclerosis Anaemia Drugs (eg aspirin, quinine) Alcohol

*   Earache + tinnitus associated with a faulty bite.
**   Earache + dysphagia is a VERY sinister combination

Vertigo:

Meniere's disease ⎫
Vestibular neuronitis ⎬   see chapter 16
Benign postural vertigo ⎭
Vertebro-basilar ischaemia
Drugs, such as streptomycin
Inflammation or neoplasm affecting the labyrinth
VIIIth nerve tumour
Blockage of the Eustachian tube
Wax in the ear

Deafness:

"Conductive" deafness: Wax
                                Otitis media
                                Injuries to the eardrum
                                Pressure trauma
                                Otosclerosis

"Sensory-neural":   "Senile" deafness (presbyacusis)
                                Complications of infections (eg meningitis)
                                Congenital (eg rubella)
                                Blast injury
                                Drugs (like streptomycin)
                                Meniere's disease

Sudden deafness requires immediate specialist attention.

Slowly progressive sensory-neural deafness may be the first sign of a rare (but potentially curable) tumour of the VIIIth nerve called "acoustic neuroma".

NOSE

Catarrh:

> Vasomotor rhinitis (a tendency for vessels of the nasal mucosa to dilate for unknown reasons)
> Sinusitis
> Allergy
> Nasal polyps
> Anatomical abnormalities of nasal septum
>
> Vasoconstrictor nose drops often make things *worse* in the long run.

Nosebleed (epistaxis):

> Nose: "Spontaneous"
>   Trauma (picking, a punch on the nose etc)
>   Nasal/sinus tumours
>
> Systemic: Hypertension
>   Bleeding disorders (see chapter 23)
>   Anaemia
>   Haematological malignancy
>
> The anterior part of the nasal septum contains an area – "Little's area"* – where several blood vessels join. This is a common site of "spontaneous" bleeding.

NOTE:

> If direct pressure on the nose with head downwards and mouth open fails to stop a nose bleed in reasonable time, the nasal cavity may need packing with gauze – a procedure best carried out in hospital.

---

*   James Little (1836-1885) – American professor of surgery.

THROAT

Hoarseness:

Pharynx:	Malignancy of oro-pharynx or laryngo-pharynx "Pharyngeal pouches"*
Larynx:	Laryngitis Laryngeal tumours
Systemic:	Myxoedema

Stridor:

Laryngitis
Epiglottitis
Croup
Diphtheria
Foreign body in throat

Dysphagia:

Within the pharynx/oesophagus:	Foreign bodies Tonsillitis Quinsy Pharyngeal tumours
Outside pharynx/oesophagus:	Cancer of neck, lung or mediastinum ↓ thyroid
Nervous problems:	Motor neurone disease MS Myasthenia Stroke etc

Conditions of the oesophagus are dealt with in chapter 13.

---

* A pharyngeal pouch is a herniation of pharyngeal mucosa through the muscles that form the hypopharynx, usually on the left side. Food tends to get trapped in such pouches and is regurgitated undigested (and sometimes noisily!).

26. Gynaecology

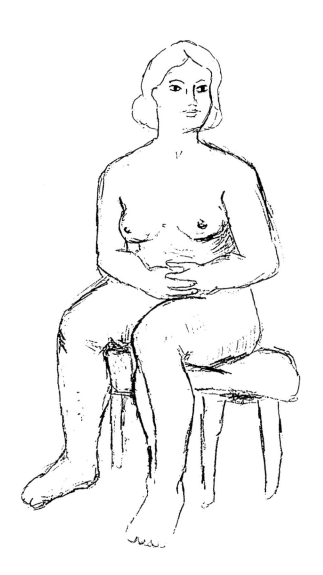

GYNAECOLOGY

OVERVIEW

Menstrual Disturbance

    Increased bleeding
    Decreased bleeding
    Painful periods
    Premenstrual syndrome

The Menopause

    Post-menopausal bleeding

Inflammatory Conditions of the Vulva, Vagina and Upper Genital Tract

    Candidiasis
    Bartholinitis
    Trichomoniasis
    Cervical erosions
    Acute and chronic pelvic inflammatory disease

Fibroids

Benign Ovarian Tumours

Endometriosis

Gynaecological Malignancy

    Cervical carcinoma
    Smear tests
    Uterine carcinoma
    Ovarian carcinoma
    Carcinoma of the breast

Prolapse and Incontinence

Contraception

Infertility

Important Gynaecological Symptoms

    Pain
    Bleeding
    Vaginal discharge
    Urinary symptoms
    Painful intercourse

MENSTRUAL DISTURBANCE

INCREASED BLEEDING

There are many old fashioned terms used to describe irregularities of menstrual rhythm and flow, all of which may lead to confusion. It is much better to use simple English when describing menstrual disorders.

Menstrual bleeding may be excessive in a variety of ways:

› Too frequent but otherwise normal
› Regular cycle but bleeding heavy, prolonged or both
› Irregular cycle* with heavy and possibly prolonged bleeding

Cervical and uterine carcinomas also cause vaginal bleeding; menstrual bleeding is characterized by its **cyclical** nature.

Increased menstrual bleeding may be thought of as:

› **dysfunctional** (presumed to be of hormonal origin)
  or
› **secondary** to other disease, particularly fibroids

DYSFUNCTIONAL BLEEDING:

This results from arrhythmic production of ovarian hormones and disturbance of pituitary feedback mechanisms. In practice, the precise nature of the underlying hormonal imbalance is rarely understood** but emotional disturbance is sometimes a precipitating factor. Heavy periods for a few cycles after the menarche are not uncommon and usually lighten spontaneously after a few months.

---

*   Menstruation normally occurs 14 days after ovulation; the length of the secretory phase of the cycle doesn't change much and thus irregular menstruation suggests variation in the proliferative phase of the cycle.

** A particular version of dysfunctional uterine bleeding known as **cystic glandular hyperplasia** (metropathia haemorrhagica) is quite well understood, however. In this condition, failure of ovulation leads to oestrogen stimulation of the endometrium lasting 6 to 8 weeks. This causes excessive endometrial proliferation. When oestrogen levels finally fall, menstrual loss will be unusually heavy and may last for 3 or 4 weeks. This picture is usually seen around the menarche or the menopause.

Heavy menstruation near the menopause may be due gradual failure of ovarian function but **malignant disease of the uterus must always be excluded** (in orthodox practice by dilatation of the cervix and curettage of the uterine lining – D&C – so that uterine tissue may be examined by a histopathologist).

INCREASED BLEEDING SECONDARY TO OTHER DISEASE:

This is usually due to fibroids, in which case bleeding will be heavy but the cycle length will be normal. Cervical polyps, endometriosis, pelvic sepsis, IUDs, thyroid dysfunction and carcinomas of the uterine body, cervix and ovary may all present as menstrual disturbance. "Dysfunctional" bleeding may coexist with any of these ....

Management of increased bleeding:

This depends on the severity and duration of the complaint. A mild to moderate disturbance can be "watched" for 2 or 3 months (make sure your patient is not pregnant) after which you should consider specialist referral. Correction of anaemia (if present) may be all that is needed. **Severe** blood loss (even of short duration) needs immediate expert help. The orthodox approach is, as always, to use clinical examination and diagnostic tests (eg D&C and pelvic ultrasound) to confirm or exclude "serious organic pathology". Further management depends on the diagnosis. Dysfunctional uterine bleeding may resolve with a short courses of an oestrogen/progesterone preparation ("the pill"). Persistent bleeding around the time of the menopause is sometimes treated by hysterectomy.

NOTE:

Intermenstrual (between period) bleeding is usually due to a local cause or to "break through" bleeding in the middle of the cycle associated with ovulation. Break through bleeding only lasts a few hours. Other causes include cervical erosions (see below), cervical polyps, carcinoma of the cervix, uterine polyps and endometrial cancer. Local cervical lesions may bleed after intercourse. Unless you are sure that the bleeding is associated with ovulation, it would seem unwise not to seek further diagnostic help. Speculum examination is usually all that is required to exclude serious, treatable pathology.

DECREASED BLEEDING (amenorrhoea or oligomenorrhoea)

Amenorrhoea (absent menstruation) is normal before the menarche, after the menopause, during pregnancy and after delivery (for a time). "Pathological" amenorrhoea may be **primary** (patient has never menstruated) or **secondary** (periods cease for some non-physiological reason). Oligomenorrhoea means infrequent menstruation and presents a clinical problem similar to secondary amenorrhoea.

PRIMARY AMENORRHOEA:

Breast growth and sexual hair growth precede menstruation. The suspicion of pathological primary amenorrhoea should only be raised if –

1) Breast growth has not started by age 14.
2) Absent secondary sexual development at age 14 is associated with short stature.
3) Menstruation has not started by age 16.
4) Signs of ambiguous sexual development coexist with amenorrhoea.

If, on the basis of the above, a definite abnormality is suspected, the patient may need sophisticated endocrinological investigation. Generally speaking, the abnormality is likely to be either an anatomical malformation of the genital tract (imperforate hymen, absent vagina etc), a failure of pituitary/ovarian development, a masculinizing tumour of the ovary (or adrenal gland) or a genetic difference between phenotype and genotype.

SECONDARY AMENORRHOEA:

Caused by pregnancy until proved otherwise. Single missed periods are common and usually "correct themselves." Amenorrhoea lasting longer than 3 months suggests the need for clinical examination to exclude pregnancy (even if the possibility is denied). If pregnancy is excluded, then expert opinion is needed.

Secondary amenorrhoea implies either disturbance of hypothalamic/pituitary/ovarian function or failure of the uterus to respond to oestrogen and progesterone.

Apart from pregnancy, the common causes are:

› emotional disturbance
› weight loss
› hyperprolactinaemia (too much prolactin in the blood)

› post-pill amenorrhoea

Endocrine causes (especially thyroid dysfunction) and other "small print" conditions (including ovarian tumours, adrenal hyperplasia, premature menopause and genetic abnormalities) account for about 5% of cases.

Treatment depends on diagnosis but failure to menstruate per se does no harm and spontaneous "recovery" is common. Taking the pill to produce a "fake" bleed each month will, in the end, just make matters worse.

OLIGOMENORRHOEA:

Presents the same clinical problem as secondary amenorrhoea and has the same causes. A condition called the **polycystic ovarian syndrome,** in which abnormal ovarian function is associated with obesity, hirsutism and infertility, may present as oligomenorrhoea. Treatment of the infertility aspect is often possible with an ovarian stimulator drug called **clomiphene**; the hirsutism is harder to manage.

PAINFUL PERIODS (dysmenorrhoea)

Painful periods can be classified as primary (spasmodic) or secondary (congestive).

The **primary** type is more common and is characterized by menstrual pain that starts soon after puberty (the first few anovulatory cycles are often painless). Dragging discomfort just before the period turns to colicky pelvic pain (caused by uterine contraction) ± backache. The underlying mechanism is unclear but it may be that prostaglandins from disintegrating endometrium cause uterine spasm and hence ischaemic pain. Orthodox management involves the use of pain killers (eg paracetamol or mefenamic acid – trade name Ponstan) that block prostaglandin production. In severe cases, "the pill" is often prescribed to inhibit ovulation. Childbirth sometimes puts an end to spasmodic dysmenorrhoea (as does surgical dilatation of the cervix, in some cases).

Secondary dysmenorrhoea occurs after some years of relatively painless periods and may be related to fibroids, endometriosis or pelvic inflammatory disease. Management involves treatment of the underlying cause.

NOTE:

Some women experience mid-cycle pain which may be related to ovulation.

PREMENSTRUAL SYNDROME

The premenstrual syndrome is a topic that creates strong feelings amongst orthodox health care professionals and its management is hampered by orthodox attempts to try and define a single cure. Some quite up to date textbooks do not even refer to the subject, but a recent example of an orthodox description goes like this:

More sufferers in over 35 age group. Affects about 10% females. May be due to relative progesterone deficiency.*

Clinical features: Symptoms start up to 12 days before period and are relieved by its onset. Include lower abdo swelling, anxiety, irritability, depression, lassitude, emotional lability, constipation, weight gain, sore breasts and headaches.

Management: Reassurance, diuretics if severe fluid retention, tranquillizers may be of occasional benefit, ergotamine for migraine, progesterone given from days 12 to 26 may help; severe breast pain may be relieved by bromocriptine.

This account is relatively enlightened; another popular student text states *"Strong claims have been made of the effectiveness of oral progesterone but tranquillizers and psychotherapy appear to be equally effective."*.......

The use of vitamin B6 supplementation and Evening Primrose oil has filtered into the consciousness of some gynaecology departments but it is still very difficult for women to get comprehensive nutritional and general therapeutic advice tailored specifically to the expression of the syndrome in their particular case. Possibly *all* the treatments that have been tried have *some* place in the management of *some* cases.

Details of a more integrated approach to treatment are beyond the scope of this chapter but the various PMS advisory services developed in recent years have produced excellent literature on the subject.**

---

*   and who knows how many males.

**   One leading centre involved in the nutritional approach to PMS includes the following additional symptoms in its definition of the syndrome: craving for sweets, palpitations, dizziness or fainting, forgetfulness, confusion, insomnia, loss of sexual interest, disorientation, clumsiness, tremors/shake, suicidal thoughts, agoraphobia, generalized aches, increase in physical activity, excessive thirst, bad breath, sensitivity to light and sound.

THE MENOPAUSE

Menopause means cessation of menstruation. The period around the menopause is referred to as the climacteric. Climacteric problems relate – 1) to changes in menstruation itself and 2) to the effects of the hormonal change on the body, mind and spirit.

The average age of menopause in the UK = 50 years.

Some menstrual disturbance is almost inevitable before periods finally cease and, in itself, is not necessarily a cause for concern unless there is very heavy or prolonged bleeding (or unless bleeding starts again after a period of amenorrhoea of 3 months or more). Just remember that most serious pathologies of the female genital tract become more common as age increases.

The general problems of the menopause are considered by the orthodox under 5 headings –

› ENDOCRINE
› GENITAL
› CARDIOVASCULAR
› BONY
› EMOTIONAL

Endocrine changes include:

› Decreased oestrogen production by ovary
› Raised levels of FSH and LH
› Decreased thyroid function

When oestrogenic influence is withdrawn, the uterus shrinks, the vaginal epithelium becomes thin and loses some of its protective acid secretion, vulval tissue shrinks and a variety of other symptoms related to endocrine disturbance occur including:

› atrophic vaginitis
› hot flushes
› sweats (which may appear some months after the actual menopause)
› poor sleep
› tiredness
› loss of concentration
› joint pains

Cardiovascular changes include:

Increased liability to cardiovascular disease and alteration in blood lipid levels.

Bony changes include:

A certain degree of "demineralization" of bone which makes them more brittle.

NOTE:

The emotional and spiritual changes of the menopause are complex and, for some, relate to a perceived loss of femininity.

Some orthodox physicians regard the menopause as an endocrine deficiency disorder and certainly many of the distressing features can be relieved by short term oestrogen therapy. However, patients on long term hormone replacement need meticulous follow up because of the predisposition to pelvic cancer as a result of the therapy.

Oestrogen pessaries are often very effective in relieving the symptoms of **atrophic vaginitis** (= chronic vaginal infection with vaginal discharge, discomfort and painful intercourse). It is interesting to note that the vaginal epithelium (during reproductive years) is many layers thick and rich in glycogen which the resident lactobacilli convert to lactic acid thereby providing considerable resistance to infection. It may, therefore, be possible to maintain the microflora of the post-menopausal vagina by the use of one of the recently introduced lactobacillus preparations in pessary form. (These already seem to be of considerable benefit in the treatment of Candida albicans infection.)

POST-MENOPAUSAL BLEEDING

Defined as bleeding from the genital tract 1 year or more after periods have ceased. (This is not a rigid definition. Any post-menopausal bleeding following a period of amenorrhoea deserves full investigation.)

PMB is usually due to **carcinoma** of the cervix, vagina, vulva, uterine body or ovary.

Benign causes include:

› uterine or cervical polyps
› fibroids
› vaginitis
› urethral "caruncle" (a small, tender, bright red swelling at the urethral orifice; probably result of chronic infection; removed surgically)
› trauma
› foreign bodies
› withdrawal of oestrogen therapy
› confusion with rectal bleeding or haematuria
› atrophic "endometritis" (inflammation of lining of uterus)

» ***ALL CASES OF PMB DESERVE IMMEDIATE, THOROUGH, EXPERT EXAMINATION AND FURTHER INVESTIGATION IF NECESSARY.***

Treatment is of the underlying cause.

INFLAMMATORY CONDITIONS

The following inflammatory conditions affect the female genital tract –

VULVA:

- › Sexually transmitted disease (see chapter 7)
- › Streptococcal or staphylococcal infections (boils and impetigo) (see chapter 7)
- › **Candida**
- › Vulval warts
- › Secondary vulvitis (from scratching, profuse vaginal discharge, incontinence or diabetes)
- › **Bartholinitis** (infection of the vestibular glands)
- › Atrophic conditions

VAGINA:

- › **Trichomonas vaginalis**
- › **Candida**
- › Atrophic vaginitis (see above)
- › Secondary vaginitis (foreign body, irritant pessaries, douches, fistulae between vagina and bladder or bowel)

CERVIX:

- › Acute gonococcal cervicitis (see chapter 7)
- › Acute cervicitis associated with childbirth
- › Chronic cervicitis
- › **Cervical erosions**
- › Nabothian cysts

UTERUS:

- › Acute gonococcal endometritis
- › Acute endometritis associated with childbirth
- › Uterine TB
- › Atrophic endometritis

OVARIES, Fallopian TUBES:

- › **Acute salpingo-oophoritis**
- › **Chronic salpingo-oophoritis**
- › TB
- › Pelvic cellulitis/peritonitis

Discussion of all the above is beyond the scope of this book. Only the conditions in bold type will be considered further.

CANDIDIASIS

Candida albicans (also known as Monilia or **thrush**) is a common fungal infection of the lower genital tract. It is one of the commonest causes of non-physiological vaginal discharge.

Aetiology:

Common precipitants include:
› Antibiotic therapy
› Pregnancy
› Diabetes
› Immunodeficiency
› Steroids (notably the oral contraceptive)

Clinical features:

Vaginal discharge + irritation and soreness (intercourse may be painful).
White patches may be seen on the vulva and vagina.
Partner may complain of irritation/soreness.

Diagnosis:

Swabs for microbiological investigation.

Management:

Antifungal pessaries.
Treatment of both partners.
Redress the balance of vaginal + gut microflora by the use of lactobacillus preparations and avoidance of yeast containing foods.

BARTHOLINITIS*

Acute infection of vestibular glands, often associated with gonorrhoea.

Clinical features:

Tender swelling under bottom part of the labium minus with pain and, early on, pus coming from the duct of a Bartholin's gland.

Management:

Usually involves surgery to drain pus and prevent recurrence.

TRICHOMONIASIS

A sexually transmitted infection with the protozoon Trichomonas vaginalis.

Aetiology:

Often found as an accompaniment to gonorrhoea.

Clinical features:

Fishy, thin, profuse, yellowish, slightly bubbly vaginal discharge plus vulval/vaginal irritation.

Diagnosis:

Highly mobile, flagellated (with a tail) organisms can be seen if discharge is examined under a microscope.

Management:

Treat both partners.
Orthodox approach is to use the antibiotic metronidazole ("Flagyl").

---

* Casper Bartholin, 1655-1738, Danish professor of philosophy, medicine, anatomy and physics at the University of Copenhagen. He later went into politics .....

CERVICAL EROSIONS

Despite the name, cervical erosions are not ulcers and are regarded as a normal variation in the appearance of the cervix.

An outgrowth of columnar epithelium from the endocervix onto the squamous epithelium of the ectocervix causes an irregular red, velvety area around the external opening of the cervix.

Pregnancy, oral contraceptives and puberty all tend to produce cervical erosions and the only symptom is likely to be an increase in the amount of "normal" vaginal discharge (although they may sometimes cause slightly blood stained discharge or post-coital bleeding).

They do not, in themselves, predispose to cervical cancer.

ACUTE AND CHRONIC PELVIC INFLAMMATORY DISEASE (salpingo-oophoritis)

PID (inflammation of Fallopian* tubes and ovaries) is a relatively common problem and usually results from "ascending" bacterial infection from the vagina or uterus.

Microbiology:

Common infecting organisms include

› Gonococcus
› Chlamydia
› Staphylococcus
› Streptococcus

Gut organisms (eg E. coli) may cause "secondary" PID in acute appendicitis. TB may also infect the tubes and ovaries.

Risk factors:

› Multiple sexual partners
› Abortion
› Postpartum (after childbirth) infection

---

* Gabrielle Fallopio, 1523-1563, Italian theologian, professor of surgery, anatomy and botany.

Clinical features:

Acute:

> › Fever
> › Recent menstrual disturbance
> › Vaginal discharge (from associated cervicitis)
> › Lower abdominal pain
> › Extreme tenderness on vaginal examination

Untreated may lead to abscess formation.
Treated or untreated, PID may lead to scarring/blockage of tubes and hence to **infertility**.

Chronic:

Chronic salpingitis may follow an acute attack or may develop slowly (eg after abortion). It tends to ebb and flow in intensity.

Clinical features include general ill health, lower abdominal pain, backache, painful intercourse, heavy, painful periods, vaginal discharge, and infertility.

Pelvic examination reveals tenderness and Fallopian tubes filled with pus or fluid ("pyosalpinx" or "hydrosalpinx").

Management:

Acute:

After microbiological investigation of vaginal swabs, orthodox management involves antibiotics, bed rest and general nursing care. "Resistance" to this regime leads to surgical investigation (**laparoscopy** – looking into the pelvis via a fibre-optic tube inserted through the abdominal wall – or **laparotomy** – opening up the abdomen to see what's going on).

Infected tissue is removed which usually means removing the uterus, tubes and often one – but hopefully not both – ovaries.

Chronic:

Long term antibiotic therapy or, if this fails, surgical removal of uterus, tubes and (if necessary) ovaries.

FIBROIDS (fibromyomata)

Fibroids are extremely common, benign, slow growing, fibrous tumours of uterine muscle. They vary in size from very small to dramatically large.

All fibroids start their growth within the substance of the uterine wall (ie they are interstitial). As they grow, some remain interstitial, some project out of the peritoneal surface of the uterus (and are known as subserous) and some project into the uterine cavity (and are known as submucous or subendometrial). Subendometrial and subserous fibroids may continue their inward and outward projection to become polyps hanging on narrow stalks ("pedunculated" polyps).

Fibroids

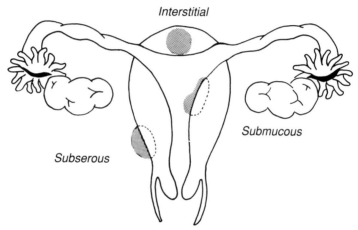

Fibroids have a striking and characteristic naked eye appearance with a pale, silky, whorled arrangement of tissue bundles. They originate from smooth muscle cells and their development may relate to the action of oestrogens.

Fibroids are associated with nulliparity (having no children) and are three times commoner in black women. They do not arise as new tumours after the menopause. About 2% of fibroids found in in the cervix.

Once developed, fibroids may lead to infertility or miscarriage. Pregnancy and "the pill" cause fibroids to hypertrophy and become softer and more vascular. Like other tumours, fibroids may undergo a variety of "secondary changes", often as the result of diminished blood supply; they may degenerate, calcify, atrophy, become infected, undergo torsion if pedunculated and, *very* rarely, may turn malignant.

Symptoms include:

> › Firm, non-tender abdominal swelling plus heavy sensation in lower abdomen.
> › Heavy periods (± clots); may lead to anaemia (tiredness, palpitations, shortness of breath etc).
> › Urinary "frequency" or retention of urine (sometimes related to menstruation when pelvic structures are more engorged with blood) suggesting local pressure from fibroid.
> › More rarely: pain (suggests some complication eg torsion), painful periods, vaginal discharge.

Signs include:

> › Asymmetrical, non-tender uterine enlargement which may be palpable on abdominal examination.
> › Uterine enlargement and displacement of the cervix on vaginal examination.

Management:

Treatment is surgical if fibroids are very large or if they are causing heavy bleeding, urinary retention or obstructed labour. Any suspicion of malignancy (eg fibroids continuing to grow after the menopause) is also an indication for surgery. The choice is between myomectomy (shelling out the tumours intact) or (more common) hysterectomy. These procedures are usually carried out via abdominal incisions but may occasionally be performed vaginally. Operative mortality is about 1 in 200; myomectomy is slightly more risky if tumours are multiple.

NOTE:

Complications of a "fibroid pregnancy":

> › Submucous tumours may cause infertility.
> › Submucous and interstitial tumours may cause abortion.
> › Any fibroid may obstruct labour.
> › Fibroids sometimes undergo "red degeneration" during pregnancy which presents as pain, tenderness, fever and vomiting. It will usually resolve in about a week with no specific management other than bed rest and pain relief.

BENIGN OVARIAN TUMOURS

94% of ovarian tumours are benign.

There are six types:

> › Simple "functional" cysts
> › Serous cystadenomas
> › Pseudomucinous cystadenomas
> › Teratomas
> › Fibromas
> › Endometriomas

> Benign ovarian tumours may be solid or form cysts; some secrete excessive amounts of sex hormone (androgens and oestrogens). Large tumours may twist, rupture or bleed, producing a more acute clinical problem.

Clinical features:

> › Abdominal swelling
> › Vague abdominal discomfort
> › Urinary frequency
> › Ankle oedema (very large tumours only obstructing inferior vena cava)
> › Menstrual disturbance (uncommon – more likely to happen with ovarian **carcinomas**)

> Some small tumours cause no symptoms and are found by chance during "routine" vaginal examination.

Clinical features of common complications:

> Torsion:
>
> Tumour twists on the stalk attaching it to the ovary. This causes venous blockage and, ultimately, arterial obstruction.
> This produces severe abdominal pain + vomiting (± shock) and a very ill patient.
>
> Rupture:
>
> May be spontaneous or follow injury.
> Rupture of a very large cyst may precipitate shock but small cysts often rupture without symptoms.
>
> Haemorrhage:
>
> The presentation is very similar to torsion.

Management:

Having established the presence of an ovarian "cyst" (ultrasound is a useful investigation), the orthodox management is to surgically remove all tumours larger than 5 cm in diameter (removing the ovary as well if necessary) on the principle that 6% of ovarian cysts turn out to be malignant and not benign. Both ovaries are checked for tumours during the operation.

Torsion, haemorrhage and rupture also usually need an operation.

ENDOMETRIOSIS

Endometriosis means the occurrence of endometrial tissue in places other than the lining of the uterus.

Wherever it occurs, it undergoes cyclical proliferative changes reflecting the menstrual cycle and thus may cause symptoms and signs that come and go over the course of a month. It tends to affect women between the age of 30 and the menopause. Although, in principle, endometriosis may affect any organ or tissue, common sites include the walls of the uterus (this is called adenomyosis), the ovaries, the round ligaments, the recto-vaginal septum and the pelvic peritoneum. It is also sometimes found in lower abdominal scars and in the umbilicus.

The aetiology of endometriosis is not understood.

Clinical features:

Very variable, but premenstrual pain of some sort is common. Other features include:

> Painful periods
> Painful intercourse
> Heavy periods
> Irregular bleeding
> Infertility (ovarian malfunction or tube blockage)

Bowel endometriosis can present as bowel obstruction. Vaginal and rectal examination may reveal masses that feel like carcinomas. The uterus is often retroverted. Laparoscopy reveals "chocolate" cysts (cysts filled with the old blood produced by the ectopic endometrial tissue).

Management:

"Conservative":   Hormonal treatment with progesterone type drugs to suppress ovulation (and thus cyclical hormonal changes).

"Surgical":   Removal of cysts or, if necessary, uterus, tubes and ovaries.

Note that the symptoms of endometriosis often improve during pregnancy.

GYNAECOLOGICAL MALIGNANCY

"ANATOMICAL" CLASSIFICATION:

Trophoblast:*	Hydatidiform mole Choriocarcinoma
Vulva:	Vulval carcinoma
Vagina:	1° vaginal carcinoma 2° vaginal carcinoma
Cervix (~2000 deaths/year):	Cervical intra-epithelial neoplasia stages I, II and III Invasive carcinoma
Uterus (~1000 deaths/year):	Endometrial carcinoma
Ovaries (~4000 deaths/year):**	Malignant cystadenomas and pseudomucinous cystadenomas Granulosa/theca cell malignancies Malignant teratomas Secondary tumours

Breast

Only cervical, uterine, ovarian and breast cancer will be dealt with here. In orthodox practice, breast cancer is dealt with by general surgeons rather than gynaecologists.

---

*   Developing placental tissue.

**   Remember, 94% of ovarian tumours are benign

CERVICAL CARCINOMA

Epidemiology:

Responsible for 3% of female cancer deaths (= ~2000 deaths per year in England + Wales).
The death rate increases with increasing age.
The majority of deaths occur in the 45-75 age group.
The number of younger women affected seems to be increasing.

Risk factors:

› Young age at first intercourse
› Number of sexual partners
› Number of sexual partners of partners
› Sexually transmitted diseases, especially genital herpes
› Partners with genital warts (papilloma virus infection)
› Having more children at a young age
› Smoking
› The oral contraceptive pill
› Lower social "class"

Natural history:

Invasive carcinoma of the cervix is thought to be preceded by a long period of "dysplastic" change in the cervical epithelium around the squamo-columnar junction (where the columnar epithelium of the endocervix meets the squamous epithelium of the ectocervix). Mild dysplasia develops into severe dysplasia ("carcinoma in situ") which then becomes invasive carcinoma. This may spread locally or via the lymph and (later on) the blood. Advanced (stage IV) carcinoma of the cervix invariably involves the bladder and rectum.

In some people, the change from mild dysplasia to invasive carcinoma occurs rapidly. In others, the dysplastic cell changes undergo spontaneous regression.

Clinical features:

Blood stained vaginal discharge or slight irregular bleeding (especially post-coital).
Advanced cases may cause infected bloody discharge, pain, weight loss, anaemia and bladder and bowel disturbance (from fistula formation).

Management:

Colposcopy (examination of the cervix with a binocular microscope) – performed in outpatients with the patient awake – allows a skilled clinician to judge which areas of cervix are normal and which are not.

Small biopsies ("punch" biopsies) can be taken during colposcopy to try and establish whether the abnormal cells represent pre-invasive or invasive carcinoma. Pre-invasive lesions can be directly destroyed using heat, cold or laser.

If a wide area of cervix shows dysplastic change and it is not clear whether there could be invasive carcinoma within the dysplastic areas, a "cone" biopsy is performed in which the whole squamo-columnar junction is removed and examined by the histopathologists. (This procedure, though not as disruptive to the woman as an hysterectomy, is nevertheless fairly "invasive" and can lead to (solvable) problems in maintaining a future pregnancy.)

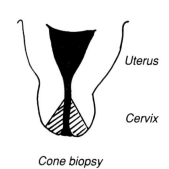

Uterus

Cervix

Cone biopsy

If invasive carcinoma is found, the options are:

Early disease: External and/or intra-vaginal radiotherapy ± hysterectomy (more or less radical, depending on the habit of the gynaecologist concerned .....).

Late disease: Radiotherapy, general support and pain relief. Occasionally chemotherapy

Prognosis (radiotherapy treatment only):

5 year survival: Stage I   —   up to 90%
                     Stage II   —   up to 65%
                     Stage III   —   up to 35%
                     Stage IV   —   less than 15%

SMEAR TESTS

There is no doubt that the organized, intensive cervical screening pro-grammes introduced in Finland, Iceland, British Columbia and Aberdeen have dramatically reduced both the incidence of and the mortality from invasive cervical carcinoma.

It is unfortunate that the introduction of screening services in England and Wales has been so haphazard and patchy – the greatest uptake has been amongst social classes I + II (rather than the most at risk IV and V) and the mortality rate has remained virtually unchanged for the past 20 years.

At present, in many areas, 55% of smears taken relate to the lowest risk group (those under 35) but, hopefully, the situation is changing (although laboratory resources and finances remain severely stretched).

The Committee on Gynaecological Cytology suggests that the "priority" groups should be:

› Women over 35
› Women who have been pregnant more than 3 times
› Women who have been sexually active the first time they seek profes-sional contraceptive advice

The recommended screening interval is every 5 years but, after age 65, smears need not be taken if 2 consecutive routine smears have proved negative.

The up to date method of describing pre-cancerous changes in the cervix is the **CIN classification** (cervical intra-epithelial neoplasia):

CIN I = Mild dysplasia
CIN II = Moderate dysplasia
CIN III = Carcinoma in situ
⇓
Invasive carcinoma

UTERINE CARCINOMA

Epidemiology:

Most cases occur after the menopause, commonly between ages 55 and 65.

Aetiology:

› About half the sufferers have no children.
› There is some association with obesity and diabetes.
› Post-menopausal oestrogen replacement may be a risk factor.
› Endometrial cancers are often found in uteruses containing fibroids.

Any woman complaining of post-menopausal bleeding should be investigated on the assumption that she may have endometrial carcinoma.

Other symptoms and signs, such as slight pain or abdominal enlarge-ment, are likely to pass unnoticed in the early stages. Infected discharge, pain and weight loss may occur in advanced disease.

Management:

Diagnosis of uterine cancer depends on histological examination of en-dometrial tissue obtained during a D&C.

Early treatment of early disease involves hysterectomy + salpingo-oopho-rectomy ± radiotherapy (internal and/or external). This gives 5 year survival rates of over 60%.

Late disease is treated with radiotherapy and large doses of progesto-gens (which cause some tumours to shrink).

As with all cancers, the outcome of treatment depends a good deal on the age, fitness and attitude of the patient.

OVARIAN CARCINOMA

Epidemiology:

Although only 6% of ovarian tumours turn out to be malignant, these account for around 4000 deaths a year in the UK.
Most cases occur between 50 and 70 years of age.

Clinical features:

The symptoms are usually vague and slow to develop and, unfortunately, many women have widely disseminated disease before they seek advice.

Pain, weight loss and post-menopausal bleeding may occur and examination may reveal hard, fixed ovarian tumours, secondaries in the recto-vaginal pouch and ascites.

Management:

Definitive diagnosis and assessment of the stage of the disease isn't made until the operation, during which as much tumour as possible is removed.

Chemotherapy (and sometimes radiotherapy) is usually combined with surgery.

Prognosis:

5 year survival	$\rightarrow$	early disease	>50%
	$\rightarrow$	late disease	<5%

CARCINOMA OF THE BREAST

Epidemiology:

The commonest malignancy in women, causing 20% of all female cancer deaths, ie 10,000 deaths per year. 1 in 17 females develop the disease. The peak incidence is between 45 and 55 years of age.

Risk factors include:

> › Living in the west (Wales in GB)
> › Family history
> › Low socio-economic grouping
> › Poor nutrition
> › Nulliparity (no children)
> › Early menarche
> › Late menopause
> › Elderly primigravidae (having your first baby from mid-thirties onwards)
> › ? the pill

Pathology:

Various pathological types. Spreads locally, via lymphatics and via bloodstream. Eventual metastasis to lung, liver, bones, brain, ovaries, adrenals. May spread to other breast.

Clinical features:

The usual presentation is of hard, painless lump, possibly tethered to skin, ± axillary lymphadenopathy. May be peau d'orange,* nipple retraction and blood stained discharge from nipple.

Investigation:

Biopsy plus X-rays and scans to determine degree of metastatic spread.

---

*   Blockage of superficial lymphatics giving the skin of the breast a pock-marked appearance reminiscent of orange skin.

Treatment:

There is no clear consensus on treatment. Options range from radiotherapy through radiotherapy plus lumpectomy to mastectomy plus axillary node removal. "Radical mastectomy" is getting less popular. All treatments work better if cancer is diagnosed early. Some tumours are "hormone dependent" and may respond to drugs such as tamoxifen (an anti-oestrogen). All sorts of other endocrine manipulations have been tried including the removal of ovaries and adrenal glands, the administration of androgens and (paradoxically) the administration of oestrogens.

Prognosis:

5 year survival after treatment of early disease = 70%.
Very poor prognosis if advanced.
As yet, there is no unequivocal evidence for the overall effectiveness of screening or orthodox treatment in terms of incidence or survival.

PROLAPSE AND INCONTINENCE

PROLAPSE

Uterine and vaginal prolapse involves the uterus or vaginal walls falling downwards and possibly protruding outside the body.

99% of cases occur in women who have had children and in whom the pelvic supporting ligaments and pelvic floor muscles become lax. Atrophic changes after the menopause exaggerate the problem. The symptoms and signs of prolapse depend on which structure has descended and how far. "Dragging" sensations, tiredness, urinary frequency, stress incontinence and backache are all common.

Types of prolapse:

Vaginal:

› Anterior wall
(cystocoele)
› Posterior wall
(rectocoele)
› Rectovaginal pouch
(enterocoele)

Cystocoele

Rectocoele

bladder

rectum

bladder

rectum

prolapse

prolapse

Uterine:

› Uterus retroverts, cervix moves down but stays within vagina (1st degree prolapse).
› Cervix protrudes from vagina (when standing, straining or coughing (=2nd degree prolapse).
› Uterus stays outside vulva with vagina turned inside out, pulling bladder, peritoneal pouches and loops of gut down as well (3rd degree prolapse or "procidentia").

1st degree

2nd degree

3rd degree

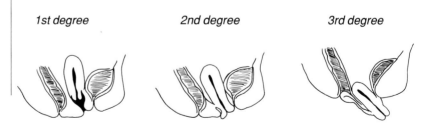

Management:

A number of ingenious operations have been devised to repair vaginal and uterine prolapses and are most successful in younger, fitter patients (although the procedures would be unsuitable for a younger woman with prolapse who wished to become pregnant again).

In cases unsuitable for surgery, the worst of the symptoms and signs can sometimes be relieved by wearing a plastic ring pessary (which must be changed every 3–4 months to avoid ulceration of surrounding tissue).

INCONTINENCE

Incontinence can be divided into 3 categories:

> Stress incontinence
> Urge incontinence
> "True" incontinence

STRESS INCONTINENCE:

Means leaking small quantities of urine when coughing, sneezing, laughing or straining.

It occurs when the pelvic floor support of the bladder neck is weakened and is therefore common in women who have had children.

It is sometimes associated with cystocoele.

Pelvic floor exercises help and a number of operations to help support the bladder neck have been devised.

URGE INCONTINENCE:

Means "when you've gotta go, you've gotta go." In other words, the desire to micturate, when it occurs, is immediate and unstoppable.

Although some cases relate to cystitis, stroke, or dementia, for most patients a cause isn't found and the condition is put down to a "hyperkinetic" or "unstable" bladder.

Urge incontinence is hard to treat in orthodox practice and depends on drugs to reduce bladder sensitivity and "bladder training" regimes in which the patient is encouraged to slowly increase the amount of urine held in the bladder before emptying.

TRUE INCONTINENCE:

Means a gross disturbance of sphincter control. It may be **active** (eg bedwetting in children) or **passive** (eg leaking fistula, neurological disorder, surgical damage, etc)

Treatment is of the underlying cause.

NOTE:

Overflow incontinence is a paradoxical phenomenon seen in patients with longstanding urinary retention. The overfull bladder "overflows" and leaks urine.

CONTRACEPTION

| **METHOD** | | | **DRAWBACKS** |

Pregnancies per 100 women–years:

	Best result	Worst	
Coitus interruptus	20	>20(!)	Drawing back .....
Natural fertility awareness	1	30	Labour intensive
Barrier:			
Condoms	0.4	4	Need conscientious application of
Caps/diaphragms	1.9	7	correct procedures. The use of spermicidal creams or foams is always recommended with barrier methods.
Intra-uterine devices	0.5	4	Cause dysmenorrhoea and heavy periods. Can predispose to pelvic infection. Usually only suitable for parous women. They require skilled insertion to ensure proper placement and avoid perforation of uterus.
Hormones:			
Oestrogen/progesterone combined oral contraceptives	0.1	–	Nausea, breast tenderness/enlargement, intermenstrual spotting, weight gain and mood disturbance are common "minor" side effects. Jaundice, hypertension and the risk of **DVT** are major possible complications. May also predispose to migraine, cervical erosions, thrush and chloasma (deepening of facial pigmentation).
Progesterone only pills	1	4	Irregular bleeding, weight gain, acne.
Morning after pills	–	–	Same as combined pills – especially nausea.
Depot progesterone	1	4	As progesterone only pills.
Sterilization	–	0.1	Tends to be irreversible. Anaesthetic risk in female. Recovery from vasectomy often takes longer than generally admitted.

For a more detailed discussion of these methods, refer to a standard textbook of gynaecology.

INFERTILITY

May be **primary** (couple have never been pregnant) or **secondary** (have had children but now can't become pregnant).

If several months of regular intercourse have passed without contraception, the following may be investigated:

Male:

? Normal penis + testes

? Frequency of intercourse

? Enough normal, motile sperm

? Normal seminal fluid

? Sperm able to penetrate cervical mucus

Female:

? Normal pelvic anatomy

? Regular ovulation + normal cyclical endometrial changes

? Blocked Fallopian tubes

? Appropriate changes in cervical mucus at ovulation

Management:

The management is to treat the cause (if possible).

Drugs are available to stimulate sperm and ovum production.

Blocked Fallopian tubes can be bypassed by in vitro* fertilization followed by re-implantation of the fertilized egg directly in the uterus.

Lack of sperm production leads some couples to seek artificial insemination by a donor (but remember that a large number of the anonymous donors are medical students .....).

*   In test tube.

IMPORTANT GYNAECOLOGICAL SYMPTOMS

and their differential diagnosis —

PAIN

ACUTE LOWER ABDOMINAL PAIN:

Non-pregnant:

> Fibroids
> Salpingitis
> Ovarian tumours (? torsion, bleeding or rupture)
> Endometriosis
> Appendicitis

Early pregnancy:

> Abortion
> Degeneration of fibroids
> Impaction of retroverted uterus
> Ectopic pregnancy
> Corpus luteum haemorrhage
> Stretching of round ligaments
> Pyelonephritis
> Appendicitis

Late pregnancy:

> Labour
> Placental abruption*
> Ruptured uterus
> Pyelonephritis
> Appendicitis
> Rectus muscle haematoma

---

*   See chapter 27.

CHRONIC LOWER ABDOMINAL PAIN:

Endometriosis
Uterine tumours (eg fibroids)
Uterine displacements
Chronic salpingitis
Ovarian tumours
Peritoneal adhesions

BACKACHE:

Dysmenorrhoea
Malposition of uterus
Pelvic infection
Endometriosis
Pelvic tumours
Pregnancy

BLEEDING

PRE-PUBERTAL BLEEDING:

Vaginal trauma or foreign body
Precocious puberty
Bleeding disorder (purpura, acute leukaemia)
Various other rare conditions

BLEEDING DURING REPRODUCTIVE PERIOD:

Abortion
Ectopic pregnancy
Bleeding endometrium: PID
Uterine neoplasms
Oestrogen secreting ovarian tumours
DUB (dysfunctional uterine bleeding)
Systemic bleeding disorder
Cervical bleeding: Erosions
Polyps
Carcinomas
Vaginal bleeding: Trauma
Retained foreign body (eg tampon)
Urethral caruncle
Carcinoma

POST-MENOPAUSAL BLEEDING:

Uterus:

Atrophic endometritis
Neoplasms (including fibroids and oestrogenic ovarian tumours)
Hormone therapy

Cervix:

Erosion
Polyps
Carcinoma

Vagina:

Retained foreign body
Atrophic vaginitis
Urethral caruncle
Carcinoma

VAGINAL DISCHARGE

White, non-infected:

Normal
Pregnancy
Cervical erosion* or polyp
Fibroids or endometrial polyps
IUDs
General ill health

Cottage cheese:

Candida

Purulent:

Cervical erosion
Cervicitis

---

*   Remember, "the pill" predisposes to cervical erosions.

Cervical polyps
Trichomoniasis
Neglected tampon
Atrophic vaginitis/endometritis
Bacterial vaginitis (children)

Watery:

Uterine cancer
Urine from a fistula
Leaking amniotic fluid in pregnancy

Blood stained:

Cervical erosion
Polyp or carcinoma
Senile endometritis or vaginitis
Abortion
Retained foreign body

URINARY SYMPTOMS

FREQUENCY AND DYSURIA:

Urethra:

NSU
Gonorrhoea
Traumatic urethritis
Urethral caruncle
Urethral diverticulum

Bladder:

Pelvic operations
Pelvic radiotherapy
Pregnant uterus pressing on bladder
Pelvic tumour pressing on bladder
UTI

INCONTINENCE:

True incontinence
Stress   "
Urge   "
Overflow   "

PAINFUL INTERCOURSE (dyspareunia*)

Lower genital tract:

Anatomical abnormality of vagina
Rigid hymen
Local infection/inflammation
Post operative scarring
Post episiotomy
Post radiotherapy
Atrophic vaginitis
Spasm of perivaginal muscles ("vaginismus")

Upper genital tract:

PID
Endometriosis
Cervicitis
Retroverted uterus
Ovarian cyst
Degenerating fibroid
Ca cervix or uterus
Psychosexual disturbance

*   pronounced dis-par-oonee--ah.

27. Introduction to Obstetrics

'You ask me about my
future, and I tell you
about my children.'

Susan Griffin

INTRODUCTION TO OBSTETRICS

OVERVIEW

Complications of Pregnancy

> Vomiting
> Spontaneous abortion
> Hypertension
> Ante-partum haemorrhage
> Abnormalities in the volume of amniotic fluid

Ectopic Pregnancy

The diabetic Pregnancy

Therapeutic Abortion

This chapter contains a brief review of some common complications of pregnancy that may occur in the months leading up to labour, together with a consideration of ectopic pregnancy, the diabetic pregnancy and therapeutic abortion.

The mechanisms of labour and the complications that may arise during the different stages of a birth are only properly understood through practical experience and are thus not discussed here. (Much useful information can, however, be found in orthodox texts on midwifery.)

COMPLICATIONS OF PREGNANCY

There are several conditions complicating pregnancy that arise **as a result of the pregnancy itself** but you should remember that a pregnant woman can also suffer from **all** the conditions that may afflict a **non**-pregnant woman.

Perhaps the most important complications of pregnancy are –

› Vomiting
› Hypertensive disorders (pre-eclampsia, eclampsia and essential hypertension)
› Spontaneous abortion
› Ante-partum haemorrhage (abruptio placentae and placenta praevia)
› Abnormalities in the volume of amniotic fluid (poly and oligohydramnios)
› Rhesus incompatibility (see chapter 4)

VOMITING

Nausea (± vomiting) occurs in about 1/3rd of normal pregnancies during the first trimester. It usually stops around 14 weeks, but may occur at any stage.

It is sometimes due to intercurrent illness and is more severe with twins and "hydatidiform mole."*

If vomiting persists and starts to affect the mother's general health, it is called "hyperemesis gravidarum."** This is generally thought to be psychogenic and often gets better on admission to hospital. Serious cases may require IV fluid replacement.

Anti-histamine drugs are used in orthodox medicine to alleviate morning sickness and are thought to be safe. However, most practitioners feel that it is best to avoid ANY medication in pregnancy.

---

*   A peculiar neoplasm of trophoblastic tissue.
** A great deal of throwing up by a pregnant person .....

SPONTANEOUS ABORTION

Abortion is defined as "expulsion of the conceptus" before the twenty eighth week of pregnancy. At least 10% of pregnancies end in abortion. The majority occur in first 12 weeks.

Common causes include –

› Foetal abnormality
› Uterine abnormality
› Severe maternal illness
› Drugs

Trauma rarely causes spontaneous abortion (unless there is instrumental interference with the uterine cavity).

THREATENED ABORTION:

A "threatened abortion" presents as slight bleeding which resolves spontaneously, with continuation of the pregnancy.

Management is bedrest until fresh bleeding stops. Ultrasound is used to confirm the presence of an intact gestation sac in the uterus.

INEVITABLE ABORTION:

Severe bleeding, pain, dilatation of the cervix and expulsion of any part of the uterine contents is termed "inevitable abortion".

Unfortunately, an inevitable abortion may be **complete or incomplete** (and may even be **missed** altogether). Incomplete and missed abortions carry a risk of continued bleeding and infection.

Management involves surgical evacuation of material from the uterus (+ antibiotics if necessary).

Note that some people have a predisposition to repeated abortion with no evident cause.

HYPERTENSION

Hypertension in pregnancy may be due to pre-existing "essential" hypertension or to kidney disease. However, hypertension and proteinuria may appear in pregnancy in women with *no* past history of high blood pressure. When this occurs, the condition is termed **pre-eclampsia**.

Rarely, pre-eclampsia may progress more or less rapidly to **eclampsia** with grossly elevated blood pressure, fits, coma and possibly death.

A whole book could be written (and probably has been) on the theories of causation of pregnancy induced hypertension but, so far, no theory has led to successful prevention of the condition.

Clinical features:

The disease is more common in teenage primigravidae,* in women over thirty five and in twin pregnancies.

Any rise in BP greater than 20mmHg systolic or 10mmHg diastolic above the average BP of early pregnancy is suggestive of pre-eclampsia. Signs of fluid retention and proteinuria may also be present.

Headache with vomiting and epigastric pain** suggest the need for urgent intervention.

The longer pre-eclampsia continues, the more likely it is that the foetus will be underweight. Severe pre-eclampsia may result in death of the baby before birth. Eclampsia may result in the death of the mother and baby.

Management:

There is no satisfactory treatment or preventive strategy. All patients with a persistent or increasing rise in BP (and those with proteinuria and oedema) are admitted to hospital for rest and observation (of the foetus and the mother).

---

*   Primigravidae – "primip" for short – means a woman having her first pregnancy.

** From liver damage.

Since ending the pregnancy is the only actual "cure," any evidence of severe maternal or foetal compromise warrants either induction of labour (35 weeks+) or Caesarian section (less than 34 weeks).

Antihypertensive drugs (usually methyldopa or hydralazine) are used for the treatment of impending eclampsia. If progressive hypertension occurs before the foetus is big enough to survive delivery, these drugs may also be used to "buy time" and thus allow a normal labour.

Prognosis:

The foetal mortality in pre-eclampsia is 3% (30% in eclampsia). Pre-eclampsia in one pregnancy means a 50% chance of recurrence in the next.

ANTE-PARTUM HAEMORRHAGE

Bleeding from the placental site after 28 weeks but before birth of the child. It may arise from a normally situated placenta (**abruptio placentae**) or from a placenta situated partly or wholly in the lower uterine segment (**placenta praevia**).

ABRUPTIO PLACENTAE:

Seems to be related to poor nutritional/social background.
30% of cases are associated with eclampsia.
The bleeding may be **concealed** (retained within the uterus) or **revealed**. Slight **concealed** haemorrhage presents as pain and some uterine tenderness with a live foetus. Severe cases present with shock, severe continuous abdominal pain and a dead foetus. In cases of suspected slight concealed haemorrhage, admission to hospital for observation is crucial since any evidence of foetal distress will be taken as an indication for Caesarian section.

Severe cases require pain relief, treatment of shock and urgent delivery of the foetus.

Revealed haemorrhage may present as anything from slight bleeding to copious bleeding with uterine tenderness and a dead foetus. The rule is that **all cases of bleeding in pregnancy should be admitted to hospital for observation (without vaginal examination).**

Treatment depends on confirmation of the diagnosis, the degree of blood loss and the health of the foetus.

PLACENTA PRAEVIA:

This means that the placenta is situated in the lower part of the uterus. It presents as painless, often recurrent bleeding.

Because the placenta occupies the lower uterine segment the foetal head cannot "engage."* If labour starts, catastrophic bleeding may occur.

Management involves admission to hospital for ultrasound examination to determine the exact position of the placenta. If placenta praevia is found then a Caesarian will be performed at about 38 weeks (in most cases).

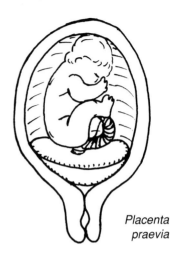

Placenta praevia

ABNORMALITIES IN THE VOLUME OF AMNIOTIC FLUID

POLYHYDRAMNIOS:

Means excess "liquor"** and usually appears after about the 30th week. The mother complains of discomfort and breathlessness and the uterus appears bigger than expected. The cause is unknown but it is associated with twins, foetal abnormalities, placental abnormalities, diabetes and rhesus incompatibility.

The condition may be complicated by pre-eclampsia, malpresentations of the foetus, premature labour or prolapse of the umbilical cord and thus the associated foetal mortality is quite high. Before 36 weeks, it is sometimes worth drawing off some of the excess fluid through a fine needle. Beyond 36 weeks, labour may be artificially induced to avoid the problem getting worse.

OLIGOHYDRAMNIOS:

Means too little liquor and is frequently associated with foetal abnormality.

---

*   Fit properly into the pelvis.

**   Old fashioned (but still current) name for amniotic fluid.

ECTOPIC PREGNANCY

Any pregnancy not in the uterine cavity is ectopic. Most ectopic pregnancies are in the Fallopian tubes.

Previous mild pelvic infection may predispose to ectopic pregnancy by causing partial tubal blockage. IUDs are also associated with ectopics, presumably for the same reason.

An ectopic pregnancy at the lateral end of the tube will present later than a more medial one since it has more room to expand.

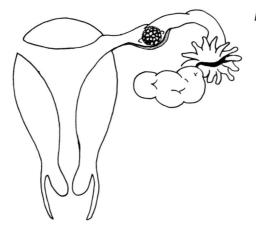

Ectopic pregnancy

Either way, since the tube cannot expand to accommodate the ever growing ovum, the "gestational sac" will eventually burst out of the tube into the peritoneum or rupture into the tubal lumen causing blood to leak out of the lateral end of the tube and into the pouch of Douglas,* behind the uterus.

Once the sac has ruptured, the "decidua"** that has grown within the empty uterus breaks down and uterine bleeding occurs.

---

*   James Douglas, 1675-1742, Scottish anatomist and royal physician.
**   Vascular proliferation of endometrial tissue lining the inside of the womb.

Clinical features:

The commonest presentation is that associated with slow leakage of blood from a not yet completely ruptured ectopic ie one or two missed periods, attacks of moderate to severe lower abdo pain and perhaps some vaginal bleeding. The patient will be pale, maybe with increased pulse rate and raised temperature. Lower abdominal tenderness ± guarding may be found on examination.

Complete rupture with severe intraperitoneal haemorrhage causes sudden severe abdominal pain (as if kicked in the guts) with possible collapse, unconsciousness and shock. The patient will have a rigid abdominal wall and severe tenderness on vaginal examination.

The differential diagnosis of ectopic pregnancy includes:

> Uterine abortion (more profuse bleeding that *precedes* pain)
> Salpingitis (vaginal discharge, high fever)
> Appendicitis
> Torsion of ovarian cyst (well defined abdominal tumour palpable, no evidence of pregnancy)

Management:

Management for **any** case of suspected ectopic pregnancy is **immediate** hospitalization and (almost certainly) urgent surgery.

THE DIABETIC PREGNANCY

The basic rule about the diabetic pregnancy is that nearly all the possible complications of pregnancy become both more likely and potentially more serious when compounded by this metabolic condition.

Pregnancy sometimes provokes diabetes (gestational diabetes) in a mother previously well, or may accelerate the eye, kidney and nerve complications affecting an established diabetic.

Pre-eclampsia, polyhydramnios, early labour, intra-uterine death, thrush and urinary tract infections are all relatively common complications of the diabetic pregnancy and the tendency for the babies of diabetic mothers to grow rather large often complicates labour.

The practice in most of Britain is to "induce" diabetic pregnancies at about 38 weeks (since most intra-uterine deaths occur late).

A diabetic labour needs careful and sophisticated management, not only to maintain normal blood sugar in the mother but to deal with the possibility of hypoglycaemia or respiratory distress in the baby.

THERAPEUTIC ABORTION

Abortion simply means expulsion of the "products of conception" before 28 weeks of pregnancy (as currently defined in English law). Most abortions are spontaneous.

Therapeutic abortion (termination of pregnancy) is performed for about 1/5th of the recognized pregnancies in Britain.

Termination of pregnancy may be performed before **24 weeks** if two medical practitioners agree that one or more of 4 indications exist ie:

> Risk to mother's life if pregnancy continues (renal disease, hypertension, heart disease; about 5% of total).
> Risk to physical or **mental** health of woman (87% of total).
> Risk to health of existing children (physical or mental; less than 2% of total).
> Risk of congenital abnormality (commonest cause rubella; 0.7% of total).

A single practitioner is permitted to perform an abortion in an emergency if s/he suspects that a woman is in immediate danger of death or serious injury (0.4% of total).

The remaining cases involve a combination of indications.

About 200,000 abortions are performed each year in the UK, the majority between 9 and 12 weeks. More abortions are carried out privately than on the NHS.

Methods of abortion include:

> Vaginal evacuation through a catheter (plus the use of "polyp forceps" and curettage to remove harder foetal parts if between 10 and 12 weeks); vaginal evacuation is not possible after the 12th week and needs general anaesthesia after 8 weeks.
> Intravenous prostaglandins may be used after 12 weeks to induce a 12-18 hour "mini-labour." May need evacuation of remnants.
> Intra-uterine injections of irritant substances or prostaglandins to kill the foetus and produce spontaneous contractions.
> Mini Caesarian (rarely done).

The risks of termination include:

> haemorrhage
> infection (may lead to infertility)
> damage to cervix or uterus
> psychic trauma

28. Emergencies

It is not so important to be

serious

as it is to be

serious about

what's important.

Laroff

EMERGENCIES

OVERVIEW

Introduction

Myocardial Infarction

Acute Left Ventricular Failure

Status Asthmaticus

Diabetic Emergencies

Status Epilepticus

Bacterial Meningitis

Temporal Arteritis

Fractured Neck of Femur

Heroin Overdose

INTRODUCTION

In these days of high tech intensive care and skilled reconstructive surgery, it is hard to deny that orthodox medicine is pre-eminent in the management of many acute, life threatening conditions. However, to develop skills in emergency medicine you need to be allowed to get things wrong occasionally, to learn from your mistakes and to stretch the boundaries of your experience without fear of censure.

I believe that society has given orthodox doctors a licence to fail (and sometimes to kill) in return for the promise of help with *any* condition at *any* time of the day or night. It could even be argued that this basic "contract" is crucial to the maintenance of orthodox supremacy in **other** areas of healthcare, despite growing public dissatisfaction with the day to day management of common, non-life threatening conditions. It certainly underpins much of the cynicism of orthodox doctors towards alternative therapies when, at three o'clock on a wintery Sunday morning dealing with an elderly patient with a massive GI bleed, they wonder where the acupuncturists, herbalists, homeopaths and osteopaths are.

The commitment by orthodox doctors to take on all-comers, 24 hours a day, has produced a team approach to acute illness that utilizes many different disciplines and levels of skill. The orthodox practitioner nearly always has the back up of other people with more experience of the particular presenting problem.

Moreover, the tacit agreement that doctors are allowed to fail without much public criticism (as long as they try their best) allows the orthodox profession to **publish** details of their experiences and methods, and thus to analyse their successes and failures. This produces great cohesion within the orthodox system.

A gynaecologist, orthopaedic surgeon, cardiologist and anaesthetist are, to all intents and purposes, as different from each other as an acupuncturist, homeopath, herbalist and osteopath and yet, in the management of, say, severe trauma, all these orthodox practitioners may need to work together to help the patient over the worst of the illness.

• • •

24 HOUR ACCESSIBILITY

TEAMWORK

SHARED EXPERIENCE AND SKILL

WILLINGNESS TO HAVE A GO AT ANY PROBLEM

OPEN DISCUSSION OF SUCCESS AND FAILURE

Since these are rarely seen in alternative medicine as yet, we must ask:

› In what sense are we *alternative* therapists if we can't offer immediate and continuing care for *any* medical problem that may present to us and
In what sense are we *complementary* if we have no routine way of referring our patients to the doctors we are "complementary" to.

Patients surely have the right to expect that they will be offered the **best** available treatment for their illnesses and this necessarily involves the ability of practitioners to recognize those conditions best dealt with by **other** disciplines. The following pages outline a brief **selection** of conditions for which orthodox medicine may be the most appropriate therapy currently available.

NOTE:

It could be argued that there are really *three* classes of medical "emergency" likely to face the *alternative* practitioner, ie –

1) Conditions where orthodox skills in plumbing, carpentry and physiological support are unequivocally necessary to preserve life and function.

2) Conditions where orthodox nursing and 24 hour resources are necessary for the patient to recover (although orthodox *therapy* is not necessarily crucial).

3) Conditions that are so "serious" that everyone *assumes* they should be dealt with by "the doctors" despite the fact that analysis of treatment outcome would suggest that the patient may be better off at home or under the care of an alternative discipline.

It is up to you to decide which conditions fall into which category ....

MYOCARDIAL INFARCTION*

Necrosis of heart muscle due to lack of oxygen resulting from compromised blood supply.
5 people per thousand have MIs each year in UK.

Aetiology:

> SMOKING
> Hypertension
> High serum cholesterol
> Being male and post-menopausal female
> Getting older
> Family history of heart disease
> Western diet
> Emotional stress
> Lack of exercise
> Social deprivation
> Gross obesity
> Diabetes
> Gout
> The contraceptive pill

Pathology:

Most heart attacks are caused by **coronary artery atherosclerosis/thrombosis.**

Clinical features:

Severe crushing central chest pain radiating up into the throat and down the arms. Unlike angina, the pain of MI may well last for longer than 30 minutes. Breathlessness, fear and nausea ± vomiting are common. There may be a past history of angina.

Heart attack victims look ill and frightened with cold, clammy hands and feet. The pulse rate will be raised and the blood pressure is often abnormal. The temperature may go up in the hours following the MI but rarely higher than 38.5°C.

---

*   This is a summary of information outlined in chapter 6 and chapter 11.

Severe chest pain may be caused by many conditions other than is-chaemic heart disease, eg oesophagitis, pericarditis, pleurisy, nerve root and rib lesions, pneumonia and pulmonary embolus.

Investigations:

ECG, chest X-ray and various blood tests are crucial to the orthodox assessment of the extent of heart muscle damage.

Orthodox management:

There is no specific treatment for myocardial infarction but appropriate management of the many possible complications (arrhythmias, heart failure, shock, cardiac arrest etc) can save life. Moreover a calm, "safe" atmosphere, pain relief (morphine), oxygen, vasodilator drugs, anticoagulation and bed rest will all help reduce the incidence of complications and improve prognosis in the acute phase. MI survivors are gently mobilized and are often able to return home after 2 weeks for a 2-3 month break from work. Certain patients will be offered investigations to assess their suitability for coronary artery bypass surgery.

Prognosis:

Of 100 patients having an MI, 25 will die immediately and 75 will reach hospital alive.

1 of these will die in A+E.
8 will die in the first week and
4 will die before discharge.
62 will leave hospital (2 having had CPR*) of whom **55 will still be alive 1 year later.**

The number of coronary arteries blocked and the age of the patient affect the ultimate prognosis. There is no clear strategy to prevent future attacks, but avoiding known risk factors makes sense.
Some physicians recommend prophylactic β-blocker therapy.

NOTES:

The elderly and diabetics sometimes have clinically "silent" MIs.

---

*   Cardio-pulmonary resuscitation

ACUTE LEFT VENTRICULAR FAILURE

Acute inability of the left ventricle to maintain an output sufficient to meet the body's circulatory demand. It is the commonest cause of acute pulmonary oedema.

Who gets it:

Anyone. Past history of cardiovascular disease is common.

Aetiology:

Valvular heart disease, ischaemic heart disease (including MI), hypertension, intrinsic heart muscle disease and drugs which decrease the rate and strength of ventricular contraction. "Constrictive" pericarditis may produce LVF by restricting left ventricular filling.

Pathology:

The symptoms and signs of acute LVF result from an excess of extracellular fluid in the lungs secondary to pulmonary venous congestion; when the left ventricle fails, pulmonary venous congestion must follow because of the back pressure transmitted via the left atrium to the pulmonary veins and thence to the lung capillaries from which fluid leaks out.
Fluid retention , if present, will exacerbate the situation.

Clinical features:

> Severe breathlessness (worse for lying down = orthopnoea)
> Wheeze
> Cough with frothy pink sputum
> Great distress and anxiety
> Tachypnoea
> Tachycardia
> Alternate strong and weak pulse beats
> Gallop rhythm of heart on auscultation
> Fine "crackles" heard in chest (especially at lung bases)
> Cyanosis if deteriorating
> May be signs of right ventricular failure as well

Investigations:

The orthodox approach requires immediate chest X-ray and ECG (? MI) together with "baseline" blood tests.

Orthodox management:

Sit patient up, *massive* reassurance, give oxygen (if no history of lung disease), drip, heroin IV (if no lung disease) to relieve distress, strong diuretic IV, fluid restriction and frequent monitoring of vital functions.

Prognosis:

Hard to generalize.

Poor general health, severe heart damage and co-existent lung disease all worsen prognosis. Orthodox treatment can nevertheless be dramatically effective and has saved many lives.

Sometimes the condition worsens despite treatment. Falling blood pressure may herald the onset of cardiogenic shock (90% fatal). This requires intensive life support.

NOTE:

In an absolute emergency, in the middle of a desert (and sometimes in A+E), bleeding off up to 500 ml of blood may just off-load the heart enough to preserve life .....

STATUS ASTHMATICUS

Acute severe asthma, not responsive to usual treatment. Unrelieved, it may lead to respiratory failure, dehydration, cardiac arrest and death.

Who gets it:

> **Anyone,** but usually a patient known to have asthma. There may have been a **recent deterioration** of respiratory function and a history of admission to hospital during acute attacks.

>> There may also be a history of recent respiratory tract infection or exposure to a known allergic precipitant.

Pathology:

Generalized bronchial muscle spasm causing airway obstruction complicated by inflammation of the bronchial mucous membranes with production of thick, sticky mucus.

Clinical features:

Asthma attacks cause dyspnoea, cough, wheeze (especially in expiration, which is prolonged), hyperinflation of chest, tachycardia and (often) the use of the accessory muscles of respiration.

Danger signs:

> › No response to normal treatment
> › Inability to talk or drink
> › Continuing distress with decreasing wheeze
> › Pulse rate >130, or (worse) bradycardia
> › Pulsus paradoxus (an exaggeration of the normal decrease in systolic BP during inspiration felt as diminished pulse volume during inspiration)
> › As the situation becomes absolutely critical, diminished breath sounds, confusion and cyanosis may occur

Differential diagnosis:

> › Acute airway obstruction (foreign body, tumour)
> › Tension pneumothorax
> › Severe respiratory tract infection
> › Acute pulmonary oedema

Investigations:

Chest X-ray, assessment of "peak flow", **blood gases** to assess if there is respiratory failure.

Orthodox management:

Sit patient up, salbutamol nebulizer, oxygen, intravenous aminophylline (if patient not already on theophylline), intravenous steroids, IV mainten-ance of fluid/electrolyte balance, consider antibiotics if evidence of chest infection, continuous close monitoring of general condition, pulse, blood gases and urine output.

Patient may need artificial ventilation if exhausted or has cardiac arrest.

May also require a period of "maintenance" steroid therapy after dis-charge.

Complications:

› Drug sensitivity reaction
› Spontaneous pneumothorax
› Ventilatory failure

Prognosis:

There are **1000 asthma deaths per year in the UK;** deaths in hospital are more likely to occur early in the morning.

» Once again, early treatment by an experienced team carries a good prognosis for recovery from the acute situation.

DIABETIC EMERGENCIES*

The two common **life threatening** metabolic disturbances affecting diabetics are:

HYPOGLYCAEMIA and HYPERGLYCAEMIC KETOACIDOSIS.

> Diabetes may be primary (idiopathic) or secondary to pancreatic disorders, drug therapy (eg thiazide diuretics and steroids) or other disease (eg acromegaly).
>
> Secondary diabetes is relatively rare but there are over **500,000 cases** of primary diabetes diagnosed in the UK at the present time.
>
> Clinically, diabetes may be classified as **insulin dependent (IDD) or non-insulin dependent (NIDD).***

Clinical features:

HYPOGLYCAEMIA:

> Usually the result of excess antidiabetic medication combined with exercise, ↓ food intake or ↑ alcohol intake. Symptoms come on rapidly and may be relieved by eating a couple of sugar lumps.
> Before having a fit or going into a coma, the patient becomes agitated, sweaty, confused and aggressive. The pulse will be fast. If not treated rapidly (oral or intravenous glucose), irreversible brain damage → death may occur.

HYPERGLYCAEMIC KETOACIDOSIS:

> Caused by insulin lack and progressively increasing blood glucose. Slow onset, often precipitated by infection or cessation of insulin therapy. Patient bone dry, overbreathing, breath smelling of acetone, vomiting, confused, ↓BP and, eventually, coma.
> Management requires much experience and involves IV insulin, fluid replacement, correction of electrolyte and acid/base imbalance and treatment of precipitating infection (if present).
> Untreated, patients may develop secondary infection, GI bleeding, cerebral oedema, clotting disorders and shock → death.

---

*   See also chapter 15.

STATUS EPILEPTICUS

Epileptic fits should not be allowed to go on for longer than about 20 minutes because of the danger of brain swelling, brain damage or death from cardiorespiratory depression. Prolonged fitting without recovering consciousness is called **status epilepticus.**

Who gets it:

Anyone. At least 6% of the population have had a (non-febrile) convulsion at some time in their lives. **900 people per 100,000 have "established" epilepsy in the UK.**

People with primary (idiopathic) **grand mal** epilepsy are always at risk of status epilepticus, especially when they alter, forget, give up or change the dosage of their orthodox medication. Symptomatic epilepsy (see chapter 16) may also produce status epilepticus.

Pathology:

Persistent abnormal neuronal discharge.

Clinical features:

Prolonged fitting.
Easy to recognize if tonic-clonic; harder with partial seizures.

Orthodox management:

Keep the airway clear. Keep the patient breathing.
Intravenous or rectal Valium usually brings the situation under control. Otherwise, a drip is set up to maintain fluid/electrolyte/acid-base balance and a continuous infusion of Valium is given. If this doesn't work, a variety of other drugs can be tried. Last resort is general anaesthesia (+ intubation and artificial ventilation).

» It is also important to treat any precipitating underlying pathology (eg meningitis).

Prognosis:

Prompt action by a well co-ordinated and experienced team should produce a good outcome (depending on the nature of the precipitating pathology).
Children are particularly prone to permanent brain damage after "recovery" from status epilepticus.

BACTERIAL MENINGITIS

Infection of the arachnoid and pia mater. It can be caused by a variety of micro-organisms.

Incidence:

Difficult to assess but causes about 300 deaths per year in England and Wales.

Causative organisms:

The commonest **bacteria** causing meningitis are:

Meningococcus (aka Neisseria meningitidis)
Pneumococcus (aka Streptococcus pneumoniae)
Haemophilus influenza (more common in small children)
E. coli (more common in neonates)

The **TB bacillus** and some **viruses** also cause meningitis.

Aetiological factors:

› Skull fracture
› Severe middle ear or sinus infections
› Pneumonia and other severe infections
› Overcrowding (for meningococcal meningitis)

Tuberculous meningitis is commoner in Asian communities.

Pathogenesis:

Having reached the meninges via the bloodstream or by direct spread from a nearby focus of infection, micro-organisms spread through the sub-arachnoid space and provoke a gross **inflammatory reaction**.

The pus in the CSF creates a good "culture medium" for the further multiplication of bacteria or viruses.

Untreated, this can lead to thrombosis of cerebral veins, infarction of brain tissue, hydrocephalus, circulatory collapse and death. Patients that survive may be left with permanent brain damage.

Transmission:

Meningococcal meningitis sometimes causes epidemics in closed communities since the organism lives in the **nasopharynx** and can be spread by **droplet infection**.

Pathology:

Exudate accumulates within the **sulci** of the brain and around the **optic chiasma**. The CSF looks cloudy. Under the microscope, infected tissue shows intense inflammatory reaction (particularly around blood vessels) with numerous organisms present. In severe **meningococcal** meningitis, the heart, joints, adrenal glands and skin may also become involved.

Clinical features:

> › Increasingly severe bursting **headache** with **photophobia**.
> › Patient lies curled up and has **fever**.
> › Signs of **meningeal irritation**, ie neck rigidity and pain on passive extension of knee with hips flexed.

As the condition gets worse, drowsiness, confusion, fits and cranial nerve palsies may develop. In **meningococcal meningitis**, a characteristic **haemorrhagic rash** is seen particularly on the lower limbs.

Management:

If meningitis is suspected, a diagnostic **lumbar puncture** is always performed and a sample of CSF is sent for "culture". Treatment then depends on the type of organism found, but a combination of **benzyl penicillin** and **chloramphenicol** will deal with most bacterial causes. There is no treatment for **viral** meningitis (which is usually less severe). **Tuberculous** meningitis (which often has an *insidious* onset with signs developing *late*) requires prolonged, specialist treatment.

Prognosis:

Overall mortality (despite treatment) for bacterial meningitis is 10% (80% in newborn infants). The complications of epilepsy, deafness and mental retardation are much more likely to occur in children. Most patients with viral ("aseptic") meningitis make a complete and uncomplicated recovery but tuberculous meningitis has a 15-20% mortality and high risk of post-infective complications.

TEMPORAL ARTERITIS

An uncommon inflammatory condition affecting arteries of the head, especially temporal arteries. Also known as giant cell arteritis or cranial arteritis.

Who gets it:

Old people of both sexes, F>M; **rare under 60 years.**

Aetiology:

Unknown. Sometimes appears in association with **polymyalgia rheumatica** (see chapter 19).

Pathology:

Inflammation of the whole thickness and circumference of lengths of affected arteries.

The inflammatory reaction is characterized by the appearance of multinuclear "giant cells"– hence the name. The process may affect the **temporal** arteries, ophthalmic*/retinal arteries, cerebral arteries and sometimes the coronary and other arteries.

Clinical features:

Severe headache with burning and tenderness (and sometimes redness) over temporal arteries.
There may also be visual blurring plus face, jaw and mouth pain.
Systemic manifestations are common and include fever, malaise, depression, weight loss, sore joints and sore muscles.

Investigations:

ESR (can be high)
Haemoglobin (often low)

Biopsy of temporal artery under local anaesthetic shows characteristic inflammatory changes.

---

*   The ophthalmic arteries are branches of the temporal arteries.

Orthodox management:

> High dose prednisolone (steroids), up to 60 mg/day, to suppress the symptoms and prevent blindness. The dose is gradually reduced over 2 years, using the ESR as an indicator of disease activity.

Side effects:

> The side effects of **steroids** (see chapter 8).

Prognosis:

> **Blindness occurs in one or both eyes in 1/3rd of untreated patients.** A small number will develop blindness **despite** steroid therapy. Early steroid therapy may very occasionally lead to recovery of vision *after* blindness occurs.

FRACTURED NECK OF FEMUR

A common fracture of the proximal femur which, untreated, may lead to avascular necrosis of the femoral head.

Who gets it:

The elderly, (especially old women*). Young adults engaged in strenuous activity (eg soldiers on forced marches carrying heavy packs) may occasionally suffer femoral neck "stress" #'s.** Severe trauma to the hip (eg car accident) may also cause #NOF (often combined with dislocation).

Pathology:

Since the head of the femur receives its main blood supply through the femoral neck, with some additional supply through the capsular retinaculum and down the ligamentum teres, the danger of avascular necrosis of the femoral head after fractured neck of femur increases:

1)   the more proximal the fracture
2)   the more displaced the fracture (capsular retinaculum torn)
3)   the older the patient

Avascular necrosis causes the head of the femur to collapse. Although usually associated with #NOF, it also occurs in alcoholics, patients on steroids, after radiotherapy and even spontaneously. It causes pain and continuing disability.

Apart from the risk of avascular necrosis, NOF fractures are difficult to deal with because the proximal fragment of bone can't be immobilized or manipulated from the outside.

Clinical features:

›   The affected leg appears shortened and externally rotated
›   There is tenderness in groin over fracture site
›   Any attempt to move the hip is painful
›   The patient cannot raise the affected leg from the bed

---

*   Even minor trauma can cause #NOF in old people.
**   # is short hand for fracture.

Occasionally, more proximal #'s become "impacted."* In such cases, there is still pain in the groin but there may be no other abnormal physical signs. Impacted fractures are easily missed.

NOTE: In posterior **dislocation** of the hip – eg after a car accident where the knee contacts the dashboard at speed – the affected leg is flexed, adducted and internally rotated (the sole of foot rests on the opposite instep). Pain is referred along the distribution of the sciatic nerve.

Investigations:

X-rays.

Orthodox management:

Surgery, eg **"internal fixation"** (younger patients and impacted fractures in older patients) or replacement of the femoral head and neck with a **prosthesis**** (older patients with unimpacted fractures in whom the risk of avascular necrosis and poor fracture healing is greater).

If the fracture fails to unite after internal fixation, total hip replacement (with a new ball and socket) may be necessary.

Patients are mobilized as soon as possible.

Side effects:

As with all major surgery, complications include infection, bed sores, pneumonia, venous thrombosis, pulmonary embolus and death.

Prognosis:

By and large, the surgical treatment of hip fracture, dislocation and degeneration is very satisfactory (particularly from the patient's point of view). Unfortunately, many old people return home to exactly the same circumstances in which they had their original fall.........

---

*   jammed.
**   Artificial replacement part.

HEROIN OVERDOSE

Self administered drug poisoning accounts for 10% of acute "medical" hospital admissions in the UK.

Overdose with heroin, morphine or other "narcotic" pain killers represents a relatively small proportion of the overall problem. The following brief description of the features of the narcotic overdose is simply a way of introducing the problems associated with the management of suspected overdose/poisoning which:

1) Requires a team approach and a degree of specialist knowledge;
2) May be complicated by an inaccurate or incoherent "history" from the patient;
3) May rapidly turn into the management of an unconscious patient.

Priorities:

In any case of suspected overdose, the immediate priorities are:

› MAINTAIN THE AIRWAY

› CONSIDER THE NEED FOR ARTIFICIAL RESPIRATION
  (+ external cardiac compression)

› IF THE PATIENT IS UNCONSCIOUS,
  USE THE RECOVERY (semi-prone) POSITION

Clinical features suggesting narcotic overdose are:

› Injection marks
› ↓ rate of respiration
› ↓ BP
› Pinpoint pupils
› Sweating

The patient may go on to develop fits, arrhythmias, hypothermia, renal failure and, of course, coma.

Management:

A drug called **naloxone** (Narcan) can reverse the effects of opiates and alter the problem into that of opiate withdrawal (characterized by anxiety, perspiration, tremors, goosebumps, vomiting, diarrhoea, and if severe, ↑ BP and tachycardia).

Methadone may be used to ease the withdrawal period.

THE BASIC HOSPITAL MANAGEMENT OF ANY SUSPECTED OVERDOSE IS

1) Maintain airway and ventilation.

2) Try to ascertain the nature of the overdose (examine pills, look at bottles, examine blood and urine samples).

3) If a poison is swallowed, empty the stomach if the patient is conscious and the substance ingested was not corrosive or petroleum based.

4) General nursing care and maintenance of homeostasis.

5) Seek advice from poison centre.

6) Consider the need for "forced diuresis" (aspirin o/d) or dialysis (paracetamol, paraquat).

NOTE 1:

The London poison information service is on **071-955-5000** (also regional centres).
If you are with someone suspected of o/d or poisoning, **keep any vomit** for later chemical analysis (first aid measures take precedence of course).

NOTE 2:

The hospital method of emptying the stomach is called "gastric lavage" and requires the passing of a lubricated tube into the stomach via the mouth. Apart from aspirin and antidepressant overdose, it is rarely worthwhile emptying the stomach more than 4 hours after ingestion of the poison.

Inducing vomiting (eg with ipecacuanha) is effective in children and adults, but should never be attempted unless the patient is **fully conscious** with a cough and a gag reflex. Salt or mustard solutions should **never** be used.

Vomiting must never be induced after ingestion of petrol, paraffin, corrosives or caustics because of the risk of aspiration into the lungs.

Oral adsorbents such as activated charcoal are sometimes useful to prevent further gastric absorption of substances known to be toxic in small amounts (eg antidepressants).

29. The Principles of First Aid

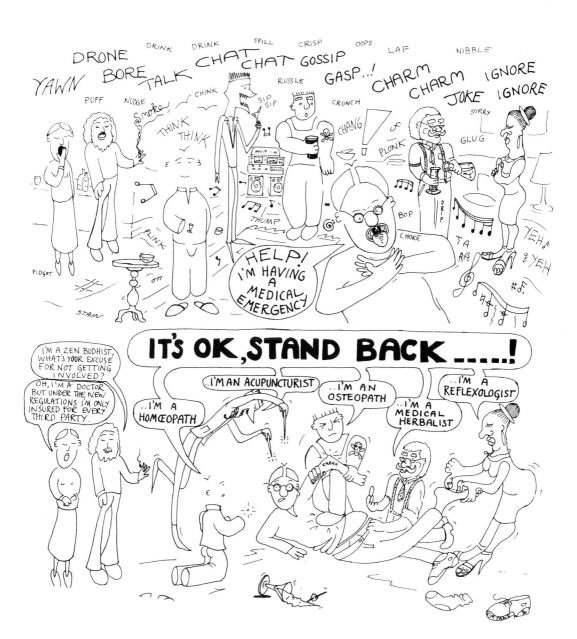

THE PRINCIPLES OF FIRST AID

OVERVIEW

Introduction

> The aims of first aid
> General approach
> Priorities
> Diagnosis
> Treatment
> Disposal
> Report
> Summary

Resuscitation

> Priorities
> Algorithm

Common Conditions Requiring First Aid

> Burns
> Choking
> Drowning
> Fainting
> Fits
> Heart attack
> Overdose
> Shock
> Stroke
> Unconsciousness

INTRODUCTION

This chapter is merely a brief aide-memoire and must be read in conjunction with an approved first aid training manual (eg Red Cross/St. John's). **No amount of reading is a substitute for a full, practical first aid training.**

THE AIMS OF FIRST AID

PRESERVE LIFE

PREVENT FURTHER DETERIORATION

PROMOTE RECOVERY

GENERAL APPROACH

Don't panic.
Don't put yourself in danger when approaching the casualty.
If appropriate, take charge calmly but firmly.
Note the time.

PRIORITIES

Do whatever is necessary to **minimize danger** to yourself, the casualty and any bystanders – further casualties will just make things worse.
Organize the bystanders.
Call for assistance.

Assess casualty (or casualties) for life threatening conditions and take immediate action as follows:

› If blocked airway → clear airway

› If absent breathing → mouth to mouth

› If absent pulse → ECC (External Cardiac Compression)

› If major bleeding → direct pressure to control it

› If unconsciousness → recovery position

› If shock → reasonable warmth, quiet, raise legs* if appropriate.
   Keeping a patient with shock too warm will make things worse.

*　(the casualty's)

DIAGNOSIS

If there is no immediate threat to life and help is on the way, take a brief **history** (from bystanders as well) and then perform a brief **general examination**. Start at the head and work down. Look for Medic-alert etc. Assess level of consciousness every 10 minutes. Keep an eye on respiration rate and pulse.

TREATMENT

Preserve life by maintaining open airway, correct positioning of patient, resuscitation techniques as appropriate and control of major bleeding.

Prevent deterioration by dressing wounds, immobilizing large wounds and fractures, keeping the patient as comfortable as possible (consistent with appropriate treatment).

Promote recovery by massive reassurance, attempting to relieve discomfort, handling the casualty gently and protecting the casualty from wet and cold.

DISPOSAL

Depends on nature and severity of condition.

Anyone who has been unconscious or who is in shock should be assessed in hospital.

REPORT

For serious cases transferred to an A+E department, try and provide a brief **report** giving estimated time of accident, description of injuries, changes in levels of consciousness, skin colour changes, estimate of blood loss, unusual behaviour by casualty, any treatment given.

SUMMARY

☐ DON'T MAKE THINGS WORSE

☐ GET HELP

☐ KEEP CASUALTIES ALIVE

☐ DON'T GIVE UP

- ☐ DON'T MOVE CASUALTIES MORE THAN ABSOLUTELY NECESSARY
- ☐ DO NOT REMOVE CLOTHING UNNECESSARILY
- ☐ DO NOT GIVE ANYTHING BY MOUTH IF CASUALTY UNCONSCIOUS OR IF THERE IS ANY POSSIBILITY OF INTERNAL INJURY OR NEED FOR OPERATION
- ☐ DON'T TRY TO DO TOO MUCH
- ☐ DON'T LET BYSTANDERS CROWD ROUND
- ☐ BE AS GENTLE AND REASSURING AS YOU POSSIBLY CAN
- ☐ DON'T KEEP ASKING THE CASUALTY QUESTIONS

and remember

- ☐ THE CASUALTY MAKING THE MOST NOISE IS UNLIKELY TO BE IN THE MOST IMMEDIATE DANGER

RESUSCITATION

PRIORITIES:

- ☐ OPEN AIRWAY
- ☐ BREATHE FOR THE CASUALTY
- ☐ CIRCULATE THE BLOOD
- ☐ NEVER GIVE UP

ALGORITHM:

› Check breathing

› Open airway and clear out foreign matter (including dentures)

› Four swift inflations if no contraindications

› Check **carotid** pulse

› If *definitely* no pulse, start combined mouth to mouth and external cardiac compression with patient on hard surface (check for return of pulse after first minute and then every three minutes)

› Make sure that you are performing both techniques effectively

› For adult casualty and one first aider, 15 compressions at 80 bpm followed by 2 full ventilations and repeat ad lib

› If heart beat present, 16 ventilations per minute

› If spontaneous breathing and heartbeat, **recovery position**

› If two first aiders, 5 compressions @ 60 bpm to one inflation

› If child, mouth to mouth around lips *and* nose @ 20 breaths per minute ECC with **one hand** @ 100 bpm

› If infant, as for children but ECC with **two fingers**

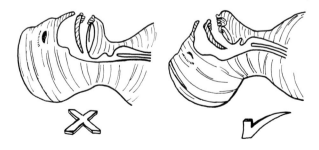

COMMON CONDITIONS REQUIRING FIRST AID

BURNS

IF CLOTHES ON FIRE, RESTRAIN CASUALTY FROM RUNNING OUT-
SIDE, WRAP IN HEAVY FABRIC (non-nylon) SHROUD (damp if possible)
AND LAY DOWN AS SOON AS POSSIBLE.

DO NOT ROLL PATIENT ALONG GROUND.

IF MINOR

PLACE UNDER SLOWLY RUNNING COLD WATER UNTIL PAIN SUB-
SIDES.

REMOVE RINGS ETC BEFORE SWELLING ENSUES.

DO NOT APPLY OINTMENTS OR BURST BLISTERS.

ONLY USE A DRESSING IF ABSOLUTELY NECESSARY AND THEN
ONLY NON-ADHESIVE, NON-FLUFFY AND ABSOLUTELY STERILE.

IF SEVERE

LAY CASUALTY DOWN, MAKE COMFORTABLE AND PROTECT BURNT
AREA FROM CONTACT WITH GROUND IF POSSIBLE.

REMOVE RINGS, WATCHES, BELTS, OTHER CONSTRICTING CLOTH-
ING.

DON'T REMOVE ANYTHING STICKING TO BURN.

IF EXTENSIVE, LIGHTLY COVER WITH MOST STERILE NON-FLUFFY
MATERIAL TO HAND.

IF CASUALTY CONSCIOUS, GIVE FREQUENT SIPS OF COLD WATER.

CHOKING

REMOVE DEBRIS, FALSE TEETH, ETC FROM MOUTH.

ENCOURAGE COUGHING.

BEND PATIENT OVER AND SLAP BETWEEN SHOULDER BLADES (up to 4 times).

CHECK MOUTH AGAIN FOR DISLODGED OBSTRUCTION.

IF CHOKING NOT RELIEVED, TRY ABDOMINAL THRUST.

IF PATIENT BECOMES UNCONSCIOUS YOU MUST IMMEDIATELY AT-TEMPT ARTIFICIAL VENTILATION.

IF THIS PROVES IMPOSSIBLE, REPEAT BACK SLAPPING AND ABDOMI-NAL THRUST (if necessary).

DROWNING

CLEAR AIRWAY AND START RESUSCITATION ASAP (in water if possible).

PLACE IN RECOVERY POSITION AS SOON AS NORMAL BREATHING ESTABLISHED.

KEEP CASUALTY WARM.

FAINTING

POSITION CASUALTY SO THAT GRAVITY HELPS RESTORE BLOOD FLOW TO BRAIN.

MAINTAIN OPEN AIRWAY.

LOOSEN TIGHT CLOTHING + FAN AIR ON FACE.

BEWARE INJURIES SUSTAINED DURING FALL.

FIRMLY RESIST OTHERS' ATTEMPTS TO SIT PATIENT UP OR GIVE ALCOHOL.

NIL BY MOUTH UNTIL FULLY CONSCIOUS.

FITS

BE ABLE TO DESCRIBE EXACTLY WHAT HAPPENS.

CLEAR A SPACE AROUND CASUALTY AND DO YOUR BEST TO PRO-TECT FROM INJURY (carefully loosen clothing at neck if possible) AND DISCOURAGE A CROWD FROM FORMING.

DON'T RESTRAIN CASUALTY.

DO NOT TRY TO PUT ANYTHING IN MOUTH.

WHEN CONVULSIONS FINISHED, PLACE IN RECOVERY POSITION AND ALLOW CASUALTY TO WAKE IN OWN TIME.

DON'T CALL AMBULANCE UNLESS CASUALTY CONTINUES TO HAVE FITS, REMAINS UNCONSCIOUS FOR MORE THAN FIFTEEN MINUTES OR SUSTAINS INJURY DURING FALL.

HEART ATTACK

BE PREPARED TO RESUSCITATE.

IF PATIENT CONSCIOUS, SUPPORT IN HALF SITTING POSITION WITH KNEES BENT.

ENCOURAGE PATIENT TO REST QUIETLY UNTIL AMBULANCE ARRIVES.

IF UNCONSCIOUS, BUT BREATHING NORMALLY, PLACE IN RECOVERY POSITION AND WAIT.

BE PREPARED FOR PULSE AND BREATHING TO CEASE.

OVERDOSE

IF STILL CONSCIOUS, ASK WHAT HAS BEEN TAKEN — REMEMBER, MAY LOSE CONSCIOUSNESS AT ANY MOMENT.

DO NOT ATTEMPT TO INDUCE VOMITING.

BE PREPARED TO RESUSCITATE.

RECOVERY POSITION IF UNCONSCIOUS.

TRY AND SEND SAMPLE OF VOMIT PLUS ANY PILLS, BOTTLES ETC TO HOSPITAL WITH PATIENT.

SHOCK

REASSURE AND COMFORT.

LAY CASUALTY ON BACK ON BLANKET WITH HEAD TURNED ON ONE SIDE.

IF CONDITION ALLOWS, RAISE LEGS.

KEEP CASUALTY REASONABLY WARM.

LOOSEN TIGHT CLOTHING.

NIL BY MOUTH.

MONITOR BREATHING, PULSE AND CONSCIOUSNESS.

BE PREPARED TO RESUSCITATE IF NECESSARY.

STROKE

THERE IS VERY LITTLE YOU CAN DO EXCEPT LOOSEN CONSTRICTING CLOTHING, LAY CASUALTY DOWN WITH HEAD AND SHOULDERS SLIGHTLY RAISED AND HEAD TO THE SIDE.

GIVE MASSIVE REASSURANCE.

BE PREPARED FOR UNCONSCIOUSNESS, SHOCK AND CARDIO-RESPIRATORY ARREST.

UNCONSCIOUSNESS

DO NOT LEAVE CASUALTY UNATTENDED IF POSSIBLE.

ENSURE CLEAR AIRWAY.

BE PREPARED TO RESUSCITATE.

PERFORM REGULAR CHECKS OF CONSCIOUSNESS LEVEL.

IF BREATHING NORMALLY, PLACE IN RECOVERY POSITION AND COVER WITH BLANKET.

IF YOU SUSPECT SPINAL INJURY, NO MOVING UNLESS VITAL TO SUSTAIN LIFE.

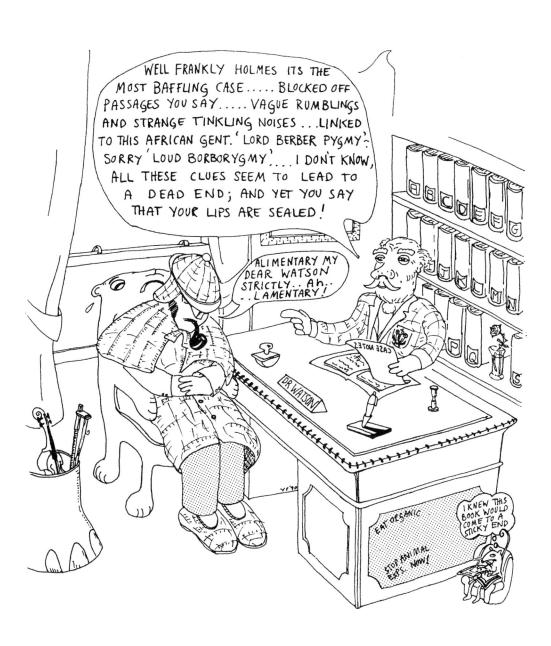

DICTIONARY OF DIFFERENTIAL DIAGNOSIS

OVERVIEW

The Nervous System

Blackouts
Brain death
Confusion
Convulsions/fits
Facial pain
Fatigue
Funny turns

Headache
Pins and needles
Tremor
Unconsciousness
Vertigo
Weakness
Walking difficulty

The Cardiovascular and the Respiratory System

Breathlessness
Chest pain
Clubbing
Cough

Cyanosis
Haemoptysis
Palpitations
Wheeze

The Gastro-intestinal System

Constipation
Diarrhoea
Dysphagia
Indigestion

Nausea and vomiting
Rectal bleeding
Weight loss

Urinary Tract

Dysuria and frequency
Haematuria
Polyuria

Psychiatry

Anxiety
Depression
Suicidal behaviour

ENT

Hoarseness
Sore throat
(see also chapter 25)

Fevers

Acute fever
Pyrexia of unknown origin
Fever plus rash

Miscellaneous

Hypothermia

Gynaecology

See chapter 26

NERVOUS SYSTEM

BLACKOUTS

Blackouts – recurring episodes of sudden loss of consciousness – frequently cause diagnostic difficulty.

It is important to take a detailed history of events leading up to an attack and also to find out as much as possible about the blackout itself.

Causes include:

› "Drop attacks" (patient falls to ground and immediately gets up again. Seen in Parkinson's disease, epilepsy and vertebrobasilar insufficiency)
› Epilepsy
› Fainting
› Hypoglycaemia
› "Stokes-Adams attacks"* – episodes of complete heart block causing the heart to stop for a short time. More likely to occur in older patients
› Vertebrobasilar "insufficiency" (may be accompanied by dizziness and visual disturbance)

BRAIN DEATH

There are 3 criteria essential to the medico-legal diagnosis of death:

› A KNOWN UNTREATABLE CAUSE

› DEEP COMA WITH NO RESPONSE (except spinal reflexes) TO ANY STIMULUS

› ABSENT BRAIN STEM FUNCTIONS ie: no corneal, cough or gag reflexes; absent eye movements and no "doll's eye" movement; fixed, dilated pupils; no "caloric" reflexes; no spontaneous respiration

» The diagnosis must be made by a "consultant" in association with one other doctor.

---

* William Stokes, 1806-1878, Irish physician and art lover.
   Robert Adams, 1791-1875, Irish professor of surgery and surgeon to Queen Victoria.

CONFUSION

Confusion is defined as clouding of consciousness with loss of contact between the patient and his/her environment. Other features include failure of recent memory, disorientation and "emotional lability". It is seen more frequently in the elderly.

Causes:

> "Small" strokes
> Cardiac, respiratory, renal or liver "failure"
> Any severe acute infection, especially if high fever (eg meningitis, pneumonia, malaria)
> Drug overdose (almost any type)
> Hypo- or hyperglycaemia or other metabolic disturbance
> Thyroid disorders
> Steroid overdose
> High blood calcium (eg from multiple secondary tumours in bone)
> Alcohol
> Vitamin deficiencies

CONVULSIONS/FITS

Causes:

IDIOPATHIC EPILEPSY: (see chapter 16)

FOCAL CEREBRAL LESIONS: Birth injury
Congenital malformations
Tumours
Trauma
Vascular accidents (eg stroke)
Hypertension
Infections (meningitis etc)
Degenerative diseases
(eg pre-senile dementia)

METABOLIC DISTURBANCE: Pyrexia (especially children)
Low **oxygen**
Low **sugar**
Low **calcium**
Low **magnesium**
Electrolyte imbalance
Kidney failure

Liver failure

Drugs + poisons (eg lead poisoning, alcohol withdrawal, anti-depressant overdose)

FACIAL PAIN

A patient complaining of "pain in the face" may have pathology in almost any structure above the neck (eg eyes, sinuses, teeth etc). The pain may be acute or chronic.

Common causes include:

Acute: Eye disease
Sinusitis

Chronic: Trigeminal neuralgia
Cluster headaches
Migraine
Dental problems
TMJ syndrome
Post-herpetic neuralgia

FATIGUE

Physical:

Endocrine/metabolic: Diabetes
Hypoglycaemia
Thyroid disease (especially myxoedema)
Cushing's syndrome
Addison's disease

Multi-system: Rheumatoid arthritis
Connective tissue disorders
Sarcoid

Infective/inflammatory: TB
Infectious mononucleosis
Post viral syndromes (including ME)
Chronic pyelonephritis

Neoplasia

Nutritional imbalance
provoked by:

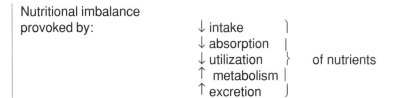

$\left.\begin{array}{l} \downarrow \text{intake} \\ \downarrow \text{absorption} \\ \downarrow \text{utilization} \\ \uparrow \text{ metabolism} \\ \uparrow \text{excretion} \end{array}\right\}$ of nutrients

Psychic:

Fatigue may be related to anxiety and depression. If so, it tends to have a long history and relate to stress. It might be worse in the morning and fluctuate in intensity over the day or the week. Pleasurable activity is less tiring.

For many people, the emotional and intellectual demands of work, relationships and surviving in modern society are profoundly stressful and fatiguing.

Environmental:

› Alcohol overuse and abuse
› Lack of exercise
› Workaholism
› Family stresses (young children can be very tiring)
› Occupational factors (noise, dust, lighting, etc)

Drug induced:

› Sedatives and tranquillizers
› Anti-convulsants
› Analgesics
› Tetracycline
› Steroids
› Oral contraceptives
› Digoxin
› β-blockers
› Ergotamine
› Vitamin A and D

(The message is, "whatever the complaint, ask what drugs are being taken." Fatigue may be a symptom of impending toxicity – see chapter 8.)

FUNNY TURNS

Sometimes patients complain of attacks of unwellness which appear to defy conventional diagnostic classification. These come under the heading of "funny turns".

Common causes:

› More or less straightforward conditions obscured by language or communication difficulties between practitioner and patient
› Hypoglycaemia
› Temporal lobe epilepsy
› Panic attacks
› Hyperventilation

HEADACHE

Headache is one of the commonest presentations in primary care. Beware the following patterns:

› Recent onset with increasing frequency, severity and duration
› Onset over 40 years of age
› Evidence of vascular disease
› Signs of meningeal irritation
› History of trauma

Don't forget that drugs, low blood sugar and simple colds and 'flu can cause headache.

Severe acute headache:

Acute meningitis
↑ ICP
Temporal arteritis
Subarachnoid haemorrhage

Chronic headache:

Tension
Migraine
Cervical spine lesions
Past head injury

PINS AND NEEDLES

The sensation of pins and needles may arise from:

Peripheral nerves:	Peripheral neuropathies
	Trauma
	Compression (eg carpal tunnel)
Nerve roots:	Prolapsed IV disc
Spinal cord compression:	Tumours
	Prolapsed IV disc
Medical conditions affecting spinal tracts:	Syphilis
	MS
	Vitamin B12 deficiency
General:	Hyperventilation

TREMOR

> Normal "physiological" tremor
> Benign familial tremor
> Thyrotoxicosis
> Parkinson's disease (resting tremor)
> Cerebellar disease (intention "tremor" – actually more of a jerking movement)

UNCONSCIOUSNESS

Think –

DRUGS (? pinpoint pupils of heroin overdose, ? alcohol on breath)

EPILEPSY (? incontinence, bitten tongue, Medic-alert bracelet)

DIABETES (acetone on breath in ketoacidosis, sweating in hypoglycaemia, ? sugar in pocket, Medic-alert etc)

HEAD INJURY

HYPOTHERMIA

NOTE:

Simple observations and some anatomical knowledge often point to the underlying pathology, eg:

› Hemiplegia → suggests STROKE.
› Stiff neck → implies meningitis.
› Irregular, non-reactive pupils and a squint ("strabismus") → imply increasing intracranial pressure affecting **brainstem** structure. This is an **extremely** dangerous situation.
› Problems in maintaining "vital" functions → implies serious damage to brainstem and, possibly, imminent demise.

In general terms, the rules are:

☐ KEEP THE PATIENT ALIVE (see chapter 29).

☐ GET HELP.

☐ TRY AND GET SOME SORT OF "HISTORY" FROM FRIENDS, RELATIVES, BYSTANDERS.

☐ ASSESS THE LEVEL OF COMA AND NOTE ANY CHANGES THAT OCCUR WHILST WAITING FOR HELP TO ARRIVE.

The following is a more complete list of causes of coma:

COMMON

Drugs and poisons

CNS causes:	Stroke
	Sub-arachnoid haemorrhage
	Subdural or extradural haematoma
	Brainstem tumour
	Concussion
	Post-epileptic fit
Metabolic:	Hypoxia
	Hypoglycaemia
	Hyperglycaemia
Vital organ or system failure:	Liver failure
	Renal failure
	Respiratory failure
	Hypothermia

LESS COMMON

Infection:	Meningitis
	Encephalitis
	Cerebral malaria
Vascular:	Severe hypertension
	Disseminated intravascular coagulation (DIC)
	Fat embolism
Endocrine:	Addisonian crisis
	Hypothyroidism
	Hypopituitarism
Metabolic:	Thiamine deficiency
	Porphyria

VERTIGO

With deafness and tinnitus → Menière's.

With history of chronic otitis media → labyrinthitis.

With double vision and problems speaking → brainstem lesion.

Related to neck movements → vertebrobasilar insufficiency (often associated with cervical spondylosis).

Only felt on lying down → Benign postural vertigo.

Only felt on standing up → Postural hypotension.

NOTE:

The appearance of progressive deafness, with tinnitus, mild vertigo and 7th, 6th and 5th cranial nerve palsies suggests the possibility of a neurofibroma of the 8th nerve, called an **acoustic neuroma.** This condition is potentially treatable but disastrous if ignored.

WEAKNESS

Post-infection neuropathy (the Guillain-Barré syndrome*)
Motor neurone disease

Myasthenia gravis

Muscular dystrophy

Endocrine + metabolic disease (eg Cushing's syndrome, alcohol abuse, thyrotoxicosis, abnormal blood calcium)

Cancer "myopathy"

Peripheral neuropathy

WALKING DIFFICULTY

Cerebellar lesions (eg MS, stroke)

Spastic paralysis (eg stroke)

Motor neurone disease

Dorsal column sensory loss (syphilis, diabetes, B12 deficiency)

Parkinson's disease

Hysteria

Arthritis

Peripheral vascular disease

* Georges Guillain, 1876-1961, French professor of neurology.
  Jean Barré, 1880-1967, eminent neurologist and professor at the University of Strassbourg.

CARDIOVASCULAR/RESPIRATORY SYSTEM

BREATHLESSNESS

Breathlessness that is appropriate is not abnormal. Pathological breathlessness is the recognition by the patient of an inappropriate relationship between activity and respiratory effort eg:

› Lung disease (COAD, asthma, pulmonary embolus and infection)
› Cardiac disease (IHD, heart failure)
› Anaemia
› Metabolic disturbance (eg diabetic ketoacidosis)
› Obesity
› Fever
› "Psychogenic" hyperventilation

CHEST PAIN

Chest pain is a common clinical problem but it is often difficult to pin down the cause. Disorders of different systems – any of which may cause chest pain – often co-exist in the same patient and obvious physical abnormalities may only be present when the patient is actually experiencing chest pain. Things get even more complex when you remember that the heart, the great vessels, the oesophagus, the pleura, the chest musculature and the structures around the hila of the lungs all share afferent pain fibres.

The following anatomical classification of the differential diagnosis of chest pain provides a starting point in the diagnostic maze –

THE HEART

Myocardium:	Ischaemia
	Infarction
	Myocarditis
Pericardium:	Pericarditis

INTRATHORACIC STRUCTURES

Bronchial tree and pleura:	Pneumonia
	Pleurisy
	Tumours
	Pneumothorax

Oesophagus:	Reflux
	Hiatus hernia
	Tumours
	Spasm
	Strictures
Aorta:	Aneurysm
Miscellaneous mediastinal structures:	Tumours of lymph nodes
Diaphragm:	Inflammation
	Tumours

NECK AND CHEST WALL

Skin and breasts:	Herpes zoster
	Mastitis
Muscles:	Intercostal myalgia
Bones:	Trauma
	Cancer secondaries
	Arthritis
	Fractures
	Costochondral joint injury or inflammation
Spinal cord:	Inflammation
	Compression of nerve roots

ABDOMINAL STRUCTURES

Stomach and duodenum:	Ulcers
	Gastric cancer
Liver + biliary tract:	Cholecystitis
Pancreas:	Pancreatitis
Peritoneum:	Peritonitis
Spleen:	Splenomegaly
Kidneys:	Various
Large bowel:	Various

NOTE:

☐ Ischaemic pain is often described as crushing, constricting, heavy, pressing, squeezing, wind or indigestion.

☐ Pleural pain is sharp and localized and made worse by deep inspiration and coughing.

☐ Pericardial pain consists of a dull retrosternal ache with a sharper left sided component exacerbated by respiration, coughing and posture change.

☐ Oesophageal pain is deep, retrosternal, burning or boring.

☐ The pain of a "dissecting" aneurysm of the aorta is similar to MI pain but more abrupt and sharp. The patient will rapidly go into shock.

☐ Pain associated with structural disease of the upper vertebrae can be reproduced exactly by pressure over the affected area. It may wake the patient at night.

☐ Peptic ulcer pain bears some relationship to eating and is relieved by antacids.

The following algorithm may also prove useful:

CHEST PAIN

Continuous, consider:	MI
	Pneumothorax
	Tumour
	Dissecting aneurysm
Intermittent, consider:	On exertion = Angina
	On breathing = Pleuritic
	On movement = Spinal nerve root irritation
	On eating = GI tract

CLUBBING

Respiratory:	Bronchiectasis
	Lung abscess
	Lung cancer
	TB
	Cystic fibrosis
	Fibrosing alveolitis

Cardiac:	Congenital heart disease
	Bacterial endocarditis
Gut:	Inflammatory bowel disease
	Primary biliary cirrhosis
	Malabsorption syndromes
General:	Familial

COUGH

The cough reflex is one of the defence mechanisms of the respiratory tract.

Cough may be due to **airway irritation** – in which case it will be **dry** – or it may be due to **excessive bronchial secretion** – in which case it will be **"productive"**.

Drugs, head injury and anaesthesia may all depress the cough reflex and cause secretions to collect in the large airways. This may lead to infection.

Coughs that persist for more than 6 weeks should be taken particularly seriously.

NON-PRODUCTIVE:

› Anxiety
› Foreign body in pharynx, larynx, trachea or bronchi
› Habit
› Interstitial lung disease
› Lower respiratory tract irritation (fumes, dust etc)
› Upper respiratory tract infection

PRODUCTIVE:

› Asthma
› Bronchial neoplasm
› Bronchiectasis
› Chronic bronchitis
› Foreign body
› Lung abscess
› Pneumonia
› Pulmonary venous congestion

HAEMOPTYSIS:

> Acute or chronic bronchitis
> Bronchiectasis
> Foreign body
> Left ventricular failure/mitral stenosis (pink and frothy)
> Lung neoplasm (primary or secondary)
> Pulmonary infarction
> TB

If someone complains of a productive cough, EXAMINE A SPUTUM SAMPLE:

> Asthma → Very sticky sputum of varying colours
> Bronchiectasis → Large volume of purulent sputum
> Chronic bronchitis → Variable amount of mucous or purulent sputum
> Lung abscess → Purulent, foul smelling sputum
> Pneumonia → Little sputum at first followed by purulent sputum until recovery

A significant proportion of patients who cough up blood turn out NOT to have a serious pulmonary lesion.

CYANOSIS

Cyanosis means blue discoloration of the skin.

It is most easily seen in the lips, the tongue, the mucous membranes of the mouth and the nail beds.

It suggests diminished haemoglobin oxygen saturation.

PERIPHERAL CYANOSIS:

Blueness confined to the nail beds of the fingers and toes. It suggests abnormally high oxygen in areas where blood flow is restricted.

Thus peripheral cyanosis may be caused by:

> Peripheral vasoconstriction due to cold or vascular disease.
> Sluggish peripheral blood flow due to "hyperviscosity" of the blood.
> Decreased cardiac output may produce a state in which the hands, feet, tips of ears, tip of nose etc are not receiving sufficient blood flow (although the tongue and mucous membranes may still be pink).

CENTRAL CYANOSIS:

This suggests that desaturated blood is being pumped from the left ventricle into the systemic circulation.

Causes:

› Abnormal haemoglobin
› High altitude
› Gross hypoventilation (head injury, chest injury, drug induced respiratory depression, etc).
› "Shunting" of venous blood from the right side of the heart to the left. This occurs in a variety of congenital heart defects.
› When pulmonary blood flows through diseased or collapsed areas of lung which are receiving no air, a **ventilation/perfusion imbalance** is created. Ventilation/perfusion imbalance due to chronic obstructive pulmonary disease is probably the commonest cause of central cyanosis.

HAEMOPTYSIS

Bronchitis and bronchiectasis are the commonest causes of haemoptysis.

Other causes include:

› Inhaled foreign body
› Lung carcinoma (1° or 2°)
› Pulmonary hypertension (eg LVF, mitral stenosis)
› Pulmonary infarction (eg after pulmonary embolus)
› TB

PALPITATIONS*

NON-CARDIAC:

> Stress/strong emotion
> Alcohol, tea, coffee, tobacco
> Thyrotoxicosis
> Electrolyte imbalance (too much or too little potassium, acid-base imbalance, etc)
> ↓ oxygen and ↑ carbon dioxide in the blood in respiratory disease
> Hypotension
> Drugs

CARDIAC:

> MI
> Hypertension
> Atrial fibrillation
> Mitral valve prolapse
> Connective tissue disorders affecting heart
> Inflammation or degeneration of myocardium

WHEEZE

Wheezing suggests airflow obstruction. The obstruction causing wheeze may be localized or generalized. Not all patients with asthma wheeze and not all wheezing patients have asthma.

Local causes:

> Impacted foreign body
> Impacted lumps of mucus
> Localized compression or narrowing of the airways

General causes:

> Asthma
> Bronchitis
> Emphysema

---

* A complaint of palpitations may relate to changes in the rate, rhythm or force of the heart beat.

GASTRO-INTESTINAL SYSTEM

CHRONIC CONSTIPATION

Painful anal disease:	Fissure
	Fistula
	Haemorrhoids
Neoplastic	Large bowel cancer
Endocrine/metabolic:	Hypercalcaemia
	Hypothyroidism
Neurological:	Hirschsprung's disease*
	Spinal cord damage
Iatrogenic:	Anticholinergic drugs
	(eg some antidepressants)
	Opiates (eg codeine)
Psychogenic:	Depression
Various:	Irritable bowel syndrome
	Low fibre intake
	Old age
	Pregnancy
	Prolonged immobility or ill health

DIARRHOEA

Infective:	Amoebae
	Salmonellae
	Shigellae
	Staphylococci
	Vibrio
Inflammatory:	Crohn's
	Ulcerative colitis
Malabsorption syndromes	(producing steatorrhoea)
Endocrine + metabolic:	Diabetes (due to autonomic neuropathy)
	Thyrotoxicosis

*   Harald Hirschsprung, 1830-1916, Danish physician, professor of paediatrics, Copenhagen.

Neoplastic:	Large bowel carcinoma
Iatrogenic:	Following antibiotic therapy or bowel resection
Psychogenic:	Anxiety
General:	Food sensitivity "Irritable bowel"

DYSPHAGIA*

Mechanical:

Affecting the lumen of the oesophagus:	Foreign bodies
Affecting the wall of the oesophagus:	Tumours Strictures Webs
Pressing on the oesophagus from the outside:	Tumours Goitre Aortic aneurism

Neurological:

Stroke affecting brainstem
Demyelinating disease
Polyneuropathy
Achalasia of the oesophagus
Chagas disease
Polio

Muscular:

Systemic sclerosis
Myasthenia gravis
Oesophageal spasm

---

*   Difficulty swallowing.

INDIGESTION

- › Anticholinergic drugs (eg some antidepressants)
- › Anxiety/emotion
- › Diabetic neuropathy
- › Gastric neoplasm
- › Inflammatory disorders of gallbladder, liver or pancreas
- › Iatrogenic (eg after "vagotomy" for stomach ulcer)
- › Migraine
- › Peptic ulcer disease

NOTE:

Ischaemic heart disease sometimes presents as a complaint of "indigestion."

NAUSEA AND VOMITING

Any "acute abdomen"	(see chapter 13)
"Gastroenteritis"	
Stomach diseases:	Ulcers
	Carcinoma
	Pyloric stenosis
Toxic:	Alcohol
	Chemicals
	Many drugs (eg morphine)
Metabolic:	Chronic renal failure
	Hypercalcaemia
	Diabetic ketoacidosis
	Liver disease
Hormonal:	Pregnancy (first 3 months)
Severe pain or anxiety	
Neurological:	$\uparrow$ ICP
	Meningitis
	Menière's
	Migraine

RECTAL BLEEDING

- › Haemorrhoids
- › Anal fissures
- › Tumours (malignant and benign) of colon/rectum
- › Crohn's disease/ulcerative colitis
- › Amoebic + bacillary dysentery

WEIGHT LOSS

GI tract:	Malabsorption
	Gastric ulcer
Endocrine:	Hyperthyroidism
	Diabetes mellitus
Neoplasia:	All, but particularly stomach + oesophagus
Chronic infection or inflammation	
Psychiatric:	Depression
	Anorexia nervosa
General:	Any serious illness
	Dietary restriction

URINARY TRACT

DYSURIA AND FREQUENCY

› Urinary tract infection (urethritis and cystitis)
› Prostatic disease
› Urinary tract stones
› Bladder tumours

HAEMATURIA

Prostatic disease

Urethral trauma

Bladder disease: Tumours
                    Stones
                    Trauma

Kidney disease: Glomerulonephritis
                    Polycystic disease
                    Stones
                    Carcinoma
                    Analgesic "nephropathy"
                    Acute pyelonephritis
                    Trauma

Bleeding disorders (eg sickle cell disease – see chapter 23) and bacterial endocarditis occasionally present as haematuria

» **Painless haematuria should always raise the suspicion of urinary tract malignancy.**

POLYURIA

› Increased fluid intake
› Diuretics
› Diabetes (mellitus + insipidus)
› Renal failure
› Hypercalcaemia

PSYCHIATRY

ANXIETY

? NORMAL OR "PATHOLOGICAL"

Does patient have a personality predisposed to anxiety?
Can the anxiety be explained by the patient's general situation?

If pathological –

? Known anxiety "syndrome" (agoraphobia, claustrophobia, etc)
? Symptom of another psychiatric illness (eg depression)
? Associated with a medical condition (eg thyrotoxicosis)

If anxiety syndrome – which one?

› Phobic disorder
› Agoraphobia
› Panic disorder
› Post-traumatic stress

ANXIETY SYNDROMES:

Phobic disorders:

Irrational fear of specific objects – becomes pathological when the fear starts to play a large part in the person's life.

Agoraphobia:

Marked fear of being in public places or of being alone.

Panic disorders:

Apprehension and fear accompanied by autonomic symptoms (palpitations, butterflies in stomach).

Post-traumatic syndrome:

The development of various anxiety symptoms following a traumatic event. The onset is often delayed. Nightmares and feelings of guilt are common.

DEPRESSION

Depression has been discussed in chapter 17. The formal classification of depression is a complex subject beyond the scope of this book. However, the following diagnostic scheme may prove useful.

"Medical" disorders that may present as depression:

› Myxoedema
› Parkinson's disease
› Myasthenia gravis
› Addison's disease (generalized adrenocortical hormone deficiency)
› Rheumatoid arthritis
› Dementia
› Schizophrenia

The following drugs are also known to cause depression in some people:

› Methyldopa (for hypertension)
› Oral contraceptive (up to 6% of users)
› Steroids
› Anticonvulsants (eg phenytoin)
› Levodopa (for Parkinsonism)
› Appetite suppressants
› Digoxin (for heart failure)
› Indomethacin (for joint disease)
› Griseofulvin (for treatment of persistent fungal infections)

Depression is often associated with anxiety disorders such as agoraphobia and may accompany any severe illness (eg post myocardial infarction).

SUICIDAL BEHAVIOUR

Potential suicide is regarded as a medical emergency. **Threats of suicide should always be taken seriously.** Most suicides give several warnings before committing the act.

Associated disorders:

Depression:	The risk is often greater as the patient starts to recover.
Schizophrenia:	Paranoid or Messianic delusions and post-psychotic depression may precipitate a suicide attempt. "Voices" may direct actions.
Personality disorders:	May be manipulative, attention seeking or a means of escape from a difficult situation. There is often a history of multiple attempts.
Confusional states:	Organic brain damage; drug/alcohol abuse; hallucinated psychosis.

Incurable disease

Assessment of risk:

A person who has carefully worked out the method is at greater risk.

Previous attempts:	Each attempt has a better chance of succeeding.
Method:	Does the person have the available means to kill themselves
Mental state:	The more depressed, anxious and agitated a person is, the greater the risk of suicide. Hallucinatory voices of compelling nature are particularly dangerous.
Age + sex:	Most attempting = females from mid-teens to early twenties. Most succeeding = middle aged or old men.

Marital status:	Single, divorced, separated or widowed = higher risk.
Family history:	A person with a family history of suicide is at higher risk.
Impulsive personality:	Higher risk
Drugs/alcohol:	History of abuse = higher risk.
Culture/religion:	May diminish or increase risk.

ENT

HOARSENESS

Acute + chronic laryngitis

Laryngeal tumours

Pharyngeal tumours

Hypothyroidism

Recurrent laryngeal nerve palsy (eg after thyroid surgery)

SORE THROAT

Viral pharyngitis

Streptococcal pharyngitis

Quinsy

Infectious mononucleosis

Vincent's angina*

Diphtheria

* Jean Hyacinthe Vincent, 1862-1950, French professor of bacteriology.

FEVERS

ACUTE FEVER

Raised temperature may relate to altered physiological states (pregnancy, menstrual cycle, exercise etc) but is usually a sign of organic
disease eg:

› ANY INFECTION

› AUTO-IMMUNE DISEASE

› MI, PULMONARY INFARCTION, CEREBRAL HAEMORRHAGE

› CANCER (especially renal cell carcinoma and lymphoma)

› CRUSH INJURIES

› HAEMATOLOGICAL DISORDERS (such as acute haemolysis)

› DRUG REACTIONS

› METABOLIC DISORDERS (eg gout)

NOTE:

Fever in the very young, the very old, the immunocompromised and
overseas travellers may imply serious illness.

Most simple "viral" fevers resolve within four days.

The following are some common causes of fever lasting up to two weeks:

› Influenza

› Infectious mononucleosis

› Zoonoses (such as brucellosis)

› "Travellers" diseases (eg malaria, typhoid, amoebiasis)

› Endocarditis

› Abscesses

› Drug fevers

› Septicaemia

Continuing fever defying diagnosis despite basic conventional testing is
referred to as **pyrexia of unknown origin** and is considered below.

PYREXIA OF UNKNOWN ORIGIN (PUO)

50% INFECTIONS
20% NEOPLASMS
15% AUTO-IMMUNE
15% MISCELLANEOUS

About 10% of cases of PUO are never "given" a firm diagnosis.

Infections include:

> TB
> Brucellosis
> Cytomegalovirus
> Endocarditis
> Infectious mononucleosis
> Malaria
> Amoebiasis
> Psittacosis
> Toxoplasmosis
> Q fever
> Deep seated abscesses

Neoplasms include:

> Lymphomas
> Kidney
> Lung and liver cancers
> Disseminated cancer

Auto-immune includes:

> Polymyalgia rheumatica
> Rheumatoid arthritis
> SLE

Miscellaneous includes:

> Drug fevers
> Inflammatory bowel disease
> Cirrhosis of liver
> "Factitious" fevers

FEVER PLUS RASH

☐ ANYONE WITH AN HAEMORRHAGIC RASH SHOULD BE AD-
MITTED TO HOSPITAL IMMEDIATELY.

☐ SEVERELY ILL PATIENTS WITH HIGH FEVER AND A MACULO-
PAPULAR RASH (± SHIVERING, SWEATING AND JOINT PAIN)
MAY ALSO REQUIRE HOSPITALIZATION.

☐ MANY LIFE THREATENING INFECTIOUS DISEASES ARE
TREATABLE BY ORTHODOX THERAPY.

Important and common causes of fever + maculopapular rash:

Bacterial:

› Meningococcal meningitis (though the rash is *usually* haemorrhagic)
› Scarlet fever
› Staphylococcal infection
› Syphilis

Viral:

› Measles
› Rubella
› Infectious mononucleosis
› Typhus

and just about any other virus you can think of ......

Various:

› Any drug
› Erythema multiforme
› Juvenile rheumatoid arthritis
› SLE

MISCELLANEOUS

HYPOTHERMIA

Hypothermia is defined as a fall of body temperature to below 35°C (95°F) as measured by a low reading thermometer in the rectum.

Severe hypothermia leads to coma.

The condition is likely to occur in three groups of people:

1) Healthy adults subjected to external cold, especially when under the influence of alcohol or vasodilator drugs.

2) The elderly or infirm in poorly heated accommodation, especially following an accident or stroke.

3) People with endocrine disorders particularly thyroid, pituitary or adrenal failure.

Urgent removal to hospital for gradual rewarming and monitoring is essential since there is imminent danger of a cardiac arrhythmia. Bronchopneumonia is a common complication of hypothermia.

FURTHER READING

Students and practitioners of complementary medicine have little time to to devote to background reading in orthodox medicine but it is sometimes useful to be able to study a topic of particular interest in greater detail.

The following selection of books may be worth looking at.

Expensive but detailed; quite heavy going:

The Oxford Textbook of Medicine: Oxford University Press.
Bailey and Love's Short Practice of Surgery: Harding, Rains and Ritchie; Lewis.
Muir's Textbook of Pathology: J. R. Andersen; Arnold.
A Guide to Physical Examination: Barbara Bates; J.B. Lippincott Company.

Middle price range; concise but readable:

Modern Medicine: Read et al; Pitman.
Scott: An Aid to Clinical Surgery; H.A.F. Dudley; Churchill Livingstone.
Lecture Notes on Pathology: Blackwell.
or
Pathology Illustrated: Govan et al; Churchill Livingstone.
Clinical Skills: Bouchier and Morris; W.B. Saunders.

Relatively cheap; austere but detailed enough for most purposes:

Medicine, the Bare Bones: Friedman and Moshy; Wiley (covers all medical and surgical disciplines).
Short Textbook of Pathology: Unibooks (or any low price general pathology text).
Lecture Notes in History Taking and Clinical Examination: Blackwell.

Whichever textbooks you choose, it is essential that you also purchase the following:

The British National Formulary (listing uses, doses, side effects and contraindications for all drugs available in the UK).
The Red Cross/St John Ambulance First Aid Manual.
A medical dictionary, eg *Black's Medical Dictionary,* ed. C.W.H. Havard.

You might also find the following useful as background reading:

Health and Disease, a Reader: Black et al; Open University Press.
Nursing Practice and Health Care: Hinchliff et al; Arnold.
Long Cases in General Medicine: R.E. Pounder; Blackwell.

Index

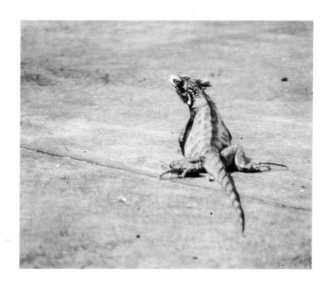

Index

A

α-1-antitrypsin deficiency
  emphysema 269
abortion
  spontaneous 45, 631
  syphilis 153
  therapeutic 638
abruptio placentae 633
abscess 20
  appendicitis 316
  Crohn's disease 311
  peritonitis 298
  pneumonia 279
acanthosis nigricans
  malignancy 552
acholuric jaundice 320
acid alcohol fast bact. 112
acidosis
  diabetes 365
acne rosacea 538
acne vulgaris 537–538
acoustic neuroma 686
acromegaly 350
  carpal tunnel syndrome 451
  pituitary tumour 348
  skin manifestations 552
ACTH secretion
  medullary carcinoma 346
  pituitary tumour 347
actinomyces 113
acute arterial obstruction 260
acute bronchitis 282
Addison's disease 355
  auto-immune 62
  hypoparathyroidism 359
  skin manifestations 552
adenocarcinoma 81
adenoiditis 581
adenoma 81
ADH secretion
  diabetes insipidus 352
adhesions

bowel obstruction 298
  diverticulitis 314
adverse drug reactions 170–174
agoraphobia 422, 710
AIDS 145
AIDS related complex 146
albumin, lowered
  nephrotic syndrome 481
alcohol
  acute pancreatitis 327
  Ca-oesophagus 330
  chronic pancreatitis 329
  cirrhosis 322
  Cushing's disease 353
  diabetic coma 369
  hepatitis 321
  hyperlipidaemia 370
aldosterone secretion
  Conn's syndrome 356
alleles 39
allergic oedema 96
allergic rhinitis 578
allergy 60–61
alopecia 62
Alport's syndrome 482
alveolitis
  hypersensitivity 61
Alzheimer's disease 406
amniocentesis 48
amniotic fluid
  abnormalities 634
amyloidosis
  nephrotic syndrome 481
  primary 25
  secondary 25
anaemia
  AIDS 146
  arthritis 439
  auto-immune haemolytic 61, 516
  β-Thalassaemia Major 516
  B12 and folic acid 513
  Ca-bronchus 274

Ca-colon/rectum 332
Ca-oesophagus 330
Ca-stomach 330
chronic disease 517
clinical features 510
congenital 514
definition 510
HF 240
hypothyroidism 517
impaired red cell formation 520–526
infective endocarditis 249
introduction 510
iron deficiency 512
leukaemia 523
liver disease 517
malabsorption 314
malignant malaria 155
neoplasia 83
pathological consequences 510
pernicious 62
polymyalgia rheumatica 458
porphyrias 372
red cell destruction/loss 514–516
sickle cell 41, 515
thalassaemia 516
uraemia 517
anaphylaxis 60
  chemical reaction 60
  shock 99
aneurysm
  arteriosclerosis 91
  atheroma 91–92
  definition 92
  aortic 152
  dissecting
angina
  "prinzmetal's" 243
  "unstable" 243
  congenital HD 256
  definition 242
  reflux 308

stroke 386
anginose glandular fever 135
angioneurotic oedema 97
angiosarcoma 81
angular stomatitis 304
animal experiments 165
ankylosing spondylitis 445
anorexia
    Addison's disease 355
    bowel obstruction 299
    Ca-bronchus 274
    gout 449
    hepatitis 321
    hypercalcaemia 358
    nervosa 427
ante-partum haemorrhage 633
anti-nuclear factor
    arthritis 439
antibodies 54, 56
    anaphylaxis 60
    arthritis 439
    auto-immune conditions 456
    blood groups 67
    IgE 60
    IgG 61
    IgM 61
    immunization 64
    neutralization 56
    organ specific 62
    phagocytosis 56
    production 59
    secretion 57
    SLE 457
anticholinesterases
    myasthenia gravis 399
anticoagulant therapy 179,
    386, 388
antigens 54
    antigen/antibody complex 61
    blood groups 67
    on RBC: A, B + Rhesus 67
    Rhesus 68
    tissue reactivity 60
anxiety 422
    asthma 271
    depression 701
    differential diagnosis 700
    hyperthyroidism 341
    neurotic depression 422

phaeochromocytoma 357
    syndromes 700
aphthous stomatitis 302
aplasia 72
apoptosis 23
appendicitis, acute 316
    peritonitis 297
aqueous humour
    See water jokes
arrhythmia
    malabsorption 315
    myocardial infarction 645
    overdose 658
arteriosclerosis 91
arteritis
    temporal 63, 654–655
arthritis
    bacillary dysentery 142
    carpal tunnel syndrome 451
    classification 438
    drug therapy 442
    gonorrhoea 148
    gout 448
    inflammatory bowel disease
    312, 447
    introduction 439
    psoriasis 534
    psoriatic 447
    reactive campylobacter 139
    Reiter's disease 446
    rheumatoid 21, 25, 62, 440–
    442
    seronegative 445–447
    Sjögren's syndrome 307
    Still's disease 447
arthrosis 439
asbestos
    carcinogenesis 75
ascites
    Ca-colon/rectum 332
    Ca-liver 334
    Ca-stomach 331
    cirrhosis 323
    oedema 96
    portal hypertension 323
    RVF 241
aspergillosis
    asthma 271
aspiration pneumonia 280

Ca-oesophagus 330
asthma 60, 271–272
    acute severe 648
    sputum 692
    wheeze 694
    juvenile 61
    status asthmaticus 648
atheroma 91
    diabetes 367
    hyperlipidaemia 370
    intermittent claudication 259
atherosclerosis 91, 239
    coronary 242
    coronary artery 644
    hyperlipidaemia 371
athlete's foot 542
atrial fibrillation 253
    Ca-bronchus 274
    hyperthyroidism 340
    stroke 388
atrial septal defect
    congenital HD 256
atrophy 72
atypical pneumonia 279
Australia antigen test
    hepatitis B 322
auto-immune disorders 62, 63,
456
    classification 62
    connective tissue 63
    multisystem 62
    organ specific 62
autolysis 23
autosomes 44

B

B-lymphocytes 56, 57, 59
β-Thalassaemia Major 516
bacillary dysentery 141
bacteraemia 111
bacteria 110, 113–114
bacterial classification 111
bacterial endocarditis
    streptococci 137
bacterial infection
    immune response 57

basic clinical science

shock 99
bacterial meningitis 124, 380, 653
bacteriuria
    asymptomatic 486
bacteroides 114
balance disorders 395–396
bamboo spine 445
basal cell carcinoma 544
basophils
    anaphylaxis 60
    description 59
BCG vaccination 277
Behcet's syndrome
    stomatitis 302
Bell's palsy 402
berry aneurysm 384
biliary colic 327
    gallstones 326
bioavailability 168
bipolar disorder 421
black outs 679
bladder cancer 494
bladder stones 490
bleeding disorders 518–519
    Christmas disease 519
    classification 94
    Factor IX deficiency 519
    Factor VIII deficiency 519
    haemophilia 519
    Henoch Schönlein purpura 518
    idiopathic thrombocytopenic purpura 518
    leukaemia 523
    von Willebrand's disease 519
blepharitis 22, 538, 565
blindness
    temporal arteritis 655
    Paget's disease 466
    temporal arteritis 458
blood groups 67–68
    group A 67, 330
    group AB 67
    group B 67
    group O 67, 309
    Rhesus factor 68
blood pressure

measurement 232–233
blood transfusion 67
    HDN 68
    incompatible 61
blurred vision 563
bone cancer
    osteogenic sarcoma 471
    Paget's disease 466
bordetella pertussis
    whooping cough 290
borrelia vincentii
    Vincent's angina 303
bowel obstruction 298
    acute abdomen 296
    Ca-colon/rectum 332
    Ca-stomach 331
    Crohn's disease 311
    diverticulitis 314
    hernia 318
bowel perforation
    Crohn's disease 312
    ulcerative colitis 311
bradyarrhythmias 255, 648
brain abscess 380
    epilepsy 409
    stroke 386
brain atrophy
    dementia 406
brain damage
    hypoglycaemia 650
    meningitis 125
    status epilepticus 651
brain death 679
brain scan 380
brain tumour 408
    epilepsy 409
    trigeminal neuralgia 392
breast examination 230–231
breathlessness
    differential diagnosis 688
bronchiectasis 285
    cystic fibrosis 291
    sputum 692
    whooping cough 290
bronchiolitis 288
bronchitis
    acute 282
    bronchopneumonia 277, 278
    chronic 268

influenza 283
    sputum 692
bronchopneumonia 277, 278
brucella 114
Buerger's disease
    thrombophlebitis 262
bulimia 427
bulla 553
Burkitt's lymphoma 77, 135
burns 30
    first aid 668
    shock 99
butterfly rash 457

C

cachexia 83
caesarian section
    ante-partum haemorrhage 633
    pre-eclampsia 633
calcitonin 468
    medullary carcinoma 346
    Paget's disease 466
calcium
    deficiency, renal failure 485
    high 469
    low 468
    renal osteodystrophy 467
    urolithiasis 490
campylobacter 114, 139
    gastroenteritis 300
cancer
    grading 81
    staging 81
    theories of cause 79
candida 303, 541
    angular stomatitis 304
    diabetic pregnancy 637
carcinogenesis
    definition 75–78
    multifactorial 75, 77
    summary 77
carcinogenic agents
    endogenous 76
    exogenous 75
    initiators 76

promoters 76
viruses 76
carcinoma 81
  bowel obstruction 298
  bronchus 273–274
  brain 407–408
  breast 76
  cervical 77
  cervix, genital herpes 149
  cheek 304
  cirrhosis 324
  colon, inflam. bowel disease 312
  colon/rectum 332
  Cushing's disease 353
  gastroenteritis 300
  hernia 317
  liver 334
  liver cell 77
  lung 273
  nasopharyngeal 77
  oesophagus 330
  pancreas 333
  stomach 330
  thrombophlebitis 262
  tongue 305
cardiac arrest
  myocardial infarction 645
  status asthmaticus 648–649
cardiac oedema 97
cardiac rhythm disturbances 252–255
cardiac tamponade 251
cardiogenic shock 99, 647
  LVF 647
cardiomyopathy 258
cardioversion 254
carpal tunnel syndrome 451
case control/cohort studies 191
caseating granulomata
  TB 275
cataract 562, 570
  hypoparathyroidism 359
catarrh 585
  bronchiolitis 288
  whooping cough 290
cell degeneration and death 23
  mechanisms 23
  nuclear changes 23

cellulitis 540
central cyanosis 693
cerebellar signs
  Ca-bronchus 274
  multiple sclerosis 403
cerebral embolus
  infective endocarditis 249
cestodes 118
chalazion 565
chancre
  syphilis 152
chemosis 340
chest pain 213
  angina 242
  Ca-bronchus 274
  differential diagnosis 688
  hypertension 246
  pericarditis 251
  pneumonia 279
  pneumothorax 286
  TB 276
chickenpox 127
  encephalitis 380
  oral ulceration 303
  shingles 136
  virus 115
childhood diseases 288–291
chlamydia trachomatis 118
  NSU 151
cholangitis 326
cholecystectomy 326
cholecystitis 22
  acute 326
  chronic 327
  gallstones 326
  peritonitis 297
  typhoid 144
cholelithiasis 325
cholera 140
  acute abdomen 296
cholestatic jaundice 320
cholesteatoma 573
cholesterol
  hyperlipidaemia 370
  IHD 239
  stones 325
Christmas disease 94, 519
chromosomal abnormalities 44–45

autosomal 46
cri du chat 46
Down's syndrome 46
Edwards' syndrome 46
mosaicism 45
numerical 45
Patau's syndrome 46
spontaneous abortions 45
structural 45
syndromes 47
translocation 45
chronic obstructive airway disease 268–270
circinate balanitis
  Reiter's disease 446
circulatory disorders 87
cirrhosis 322
  ascites 96
  hepatoma 334
  intraheptic cholestasis 320
claustrophobia 422
cleft lip
  multifactorial inheritance 47
clinical examination 207
  blood pressure measurement 232–233
  breast 230–231
  cardiovascular system 213–216
  dermatomes and myotomes 225–226
  endocrine disease 229
  gastrointestinal system 220–222
  heart sounds 234
  integrated approach 209
  joint movement 228
  nervous system 223–224
  orthodox approach 208
  quick "screening" 210–212
  respiratory system 217–219
  system by system 213
  tendon reflexes 227
clinical genetics 35
clinical trials 192
  controlled 192
  cross over 193
  design 193
  double blind 192

basic clinical science

phase I-IV 165
placebo effect 192
randomized 192
type 1 errors 194
type 2 errors 194
clostridia 112–113
clotting disorders 93–95
club foot 47
clubbing 215, 217
    Ca-bronchus 274
    cirrhosis 324
    COAD 270
    congenital HD 256
    cystic fibrosis 291
    differential diagnosis 690
    infective endocarditis 249
    malabsorption 315
cluster headaches 391
coagulative necrosis 24
coarctation of the aorta 256
coeliac disease 314, 549
cold sores 303, 540
colic 296
coliform bacteria 112
colitis 22
collagen 27, 30
colliquative necrosis 24
coma
    causes 685
    eclampsia 632
    ketoacidosis 650
    mid-brain infarction 387
    overdose 658
    pontine infarction 387
    subarachnoid haemorrhage
    385
    typhoid 144
commensals 119
Committee on Safety of
Medicines 163
Committee on the Review of
Medicines 163
complement system 19, 61
condylomata lata 152, 153
    syphilis 152
confusion
    asthma 272
    diabetic coma 369
    differential diagnosis 680

porphyrias 372
    suicidal behaviour 702
congenital heart disease 239,
    256–257
congenital rubella syndrome
    129
congestive cardiac failure 241
conjugation 320
conjunctivitis 566
    acne rosacea 538
    Reiter's disease 446
Conn's syndrome 356
connective tissue disorders
63, 452, 456
constipation
    antidepressants 428
    bowel obstruction 299
    differential diagnosis 695
    hernia 317
    high calcium 469
    hypercalcaemia 358
    hypothyroidism 344
    irritable bowel 314
    porphyrias 372
    typhoid 143
contraceptive pill 239, 619
contractures 30
conversion hysteria 423
cor pulmonale 269
corneal arcus senilis 370
corneal ulcer 561
coronary artery bypass 242,
    645
corticosteroids 353
corynebacterium acnes 113,
    537
Costen's syndrome 392
cough 217
    acute bronchitis 282
    asthma 271
    bronchiolitis 288
    Ca-bronchus 274
    chronic bronchitis 268
    croup 289
    differential diagnosis 691
    hernia 317
    influenza 283
    LVF 240
    pneumonia 279

TB 275
    whooping 290
cough headache 392
coxsackie virus 115, 117
crabs 150, 543
cradle cap 532
cranial arteritis 654
cranial nerve palsy
    extradural haemorrhage 382
    meningitis 125, 379, 653
    pituitary tumour 347
    subarachnoid haemorrhage
    385
craniopharyngioma 348
cretinism 343
cri du chat 46
Crohn's disease 311, 325,
    332, 447
    Ca-colon/rectum 332
    gallstones 325
croup 289
crystal deposition 448–449
Cushing's disease 353
Cushing's syndrome 83, 229,
    347, 552
cutaneous drug reactions 551
cutaneous malignancy 544–
    547
CVS disease 237ff
cyanosis
    acute LVF 646
    arterial obstruction 260
    asthma 272
    bronchiolitis 288
    central 215
    COAD 270
    congenital HD 256
    croup 289
    deep vein thrombosis 261
    differential diagnosis 692
    HF 240
    intermittent claudication 259
    ischaemic foot 260
    pneumothorax 286
    status asthmaticus 648
cystic fibrosis 41, 291
cystitis 477, 486, 503
cystoscopy 505
cytomegalovirus infection

117, 134

D

dandruff
  seborrhoeic eczema 532
deafness 584
  congenital syphilis 153
  Meniere's disease 395
  meningitis 380, 653
  Paget's disease 466
  TIA 389
deep vein thrombosis 261
  Ca-pancreas 333
  oedema 96
  venous ulcers 263
dehydration
  fever 108
  shock 99
  status asthmaticus 648
  ulcerative colitis 311
delerium 417
  acute brain syndromes 426
  typhoid 143
delusion 417
delusions 406, 417
dementia 406
  brain ischaemia 92
  Ca-bronchus 274
  hypothyroidism 344
  Parkinson's disease 397
  syphilis 152
demyelinating diseases 403–
  405
dendritic ulcer 561
dental caries 137
depersonalization 418
depression 568
  anorexia nervosa 427
  bipolar disorder 421
  dementia 407
  differential diagnosis 711
  high calcium 469
  hyperparathyroidism 358
  hypothyroidism 344
  low calcium 469
  neurotic 422

polymyalgia rheumatica 458
  psychotic 421
  suicidal behaviour 702
derealization 418
dermatitis 532–533
  allergic contact 533
  direct irritant 532
  varicose veins 262
  See also eczema
dermatitis herpetiformis 315,
  549, 552
dermatomes and myotomes
  225–226
dermatomyositis 63, 460
dermatophyte infections 541
Dermodex folliculorum 538
dermoid cyst 81
diabetes 364–369
  acromegaly 350
  acute abdomen 296
  arterial disease 92
  Ca-pancreas 333
  chronic pancreatitis 329
  coma 369, 684
  complications 366
  Cushing's disease 354
  diabetic amyotrophy 368
  diet 366
  emergencies 650
  gallstones 325
  gastroenteritis 300
  hyperlipidaemia 370
  IHD 239
  intermittent claudication 259
  ischaemic foot 260
  ketoacidosis 365, 369, 650
  myocardial infarction 644
  nephrotic syndrome 481
  polyhydramnios 634
  pregnancy 637
  proteinuria 479
  retinopathy 367
  silent MI 645
  skin 552
  stroke 386
  Type 1 (IDD) 364, 650
  Type 2 (NIDD) 364, 650
diabetes insipidus 352
  pituitary tumour 347

diabetes mellitus 364–369
  See chapter 15
diarrhoea 283, 300
  AIDS 146
  anaphylactic shock 99
  Ca-stomach 331
  campylobacter 139
  cholera 140
  Crohn's disease 311
  diabetes 368
  differential diagnosis 695
  diverticulitis 313
  dysentery 141
  gastroenteritis 300
  hyperthyroidism 340
  irritable bowel 314
  malignant malaria 155
  medullary carcinoma 346
  Reiter's disease 446
  shock 99
  typhoid 143
  ulcerative colitis 311
diplopia
  myasthenia gravis 399
  SLE 457
disorders of lipid metabolism
  370–371
disseminated intravascular
coagulation 94
diverticular disease 313
  bowel obstruction 298
  gastroenteritis 300
  peritonitis 297
DNA virus 76
dominant genes 40,43
double vision 563
Down's syndrome 46, 48, 256
drop attacks 679
droplet spread
  chickenpox 127
  measles 131
  meningitis 379, 653
  rubella 129
drowning 669
drug classes 177–185
  anti-emetics 179
  anti-epileptics 179
  antibacterials 177
  anticholinergic 178

anticoagulants 179
antidepressants 179
antihistamines 179
antipsychotics 179
anxiolytics 180
β-blockers 180
barbiturates 180
biguanides 185
bronchodilators 180
cardiac glycosides 180
cytotoxics 181
demulcents 181
diuretics, loop 182
diuretics, potassium sparing 182
diuretics, thiazide 185
dopadecarboxylase inhibitors 181
dopaminergic 181
expectorants 181
hypnotics 181
immunosuppressants 181
lithium salts 181
loop diuretics 182
mast cell stabilizers 182
NSAIAs 182
oxytocics 182
potassium sparing diuretics 182
prostaglandins 182
salicylates 182
sedatives 181
steroids 183
sulphonylureas 185
sympathomimetics 185
thiazide diuretics 185
vasodilators 185
drug interactions 175–176
drug poisoning 658
drug withdrawal 160
Duchenne muscular dystrophy 42, 401
duodenal ulcer 309
Dupuytren's contracture 324
dysentery 141
    amoebic 141
    gastroenteritis 300
    Reiter's disease 446
dysphagia 220, 586

Ca-oesophagus 330
Ca-stomach 331
differential diagnosis 696
dysphasia 387
dyspnoea 214–215
    acute bronchitis 282
    angina 242
    asthma 271
    Ca-bronchus 274
    COAD 270
    hyperthyroidism 340
    LVF 241
    pleurisy 281
    pneumonia 279
    pneumothorax 286
    status asthmaticus 648
dysuria
    gonorrhoea 147
    NSU 151

E

E. coli
    meningitis 124, 378, 652
    prostatitis 499
ear 572
    glue ear 574
    mastoiditis 575
    otitis externa 572
    otitis media, acute 572
    otitis media, chronic 573
    otitis media, complications 575
    otitis media, secretory 574
    otosclerosis 576
earache 583
eardrum injury 575
eating disorders 427
ecchymosis 95
echovirus 117
eclampsia 632–633
ectopic pregnancy 635–636
ectropion 565
eczema 532–533, 552
    See also dermatitis
Edwards' syndrome 46
Eisenmenger's syndrome 256

electroconvulsive disorders 409–411
elephant 531
embolism
    arterial obstruction 260
    atrial fibrillation 254
    infective endocarditis 249
    stroke 386
emphysema 268
empyema 326
encephalitis 22, 380
    chickenpox 127
    epilepsy 409
    genital herpes 149
    measles 131
    Parkinson's disease 397
encephalomyelitis
    influenza 284
    mumps 132
encephalopathy
    hepatic 324
    malignant malaria 155
    pertussis vaccine 133
endocarditis 22, 249
    valvular heart disease 247
endogenous pyrogens 108
endotoxins 111
enteric fever 300
enterobacteria 114
enterovirus 115
entropion 565
enzyme induction 175
eosinophils,description 59
epidemiological methods 191
    analytic studies 191
    case control/cohort studies 191
    clinical trials 192
    descriptive studies/surveys 191
    intervention studies 192
epidemiology, common terms
    cohort 196
    cost benefit analysis 196
    cost effectiveness 196
    cross-sectional 195
    false negatives 195
    false positives 195
    incidence 195
    inference of causality 196

marginal analysis 196
prevalence 195
prospective 196
retrospective 195
secular trends 196
sensitivity 195
specificity 195
epididymal cyst 500
epididymitis 503
epigenetic theory 79
epiglottitis, acute 289
epilepsy 409, 651
blackouts 679
cerebral tumour 408
differential diagnosis 680
eclampsia 632
first aid 670
funny turns 683
hypoparathyroidism 359
malignant malaria 155
meningitis 125, 379, 380, 653
narcotic overdose 658
neoplasia 83
osteomalacia 465
porphyrias 372
SLE 457
TIA 388
unconsciousness 684
vertigo 396
epistaxis 585
Epstein-Barr virus 117, 135
erysipelas 128
erythema multiforme 550
erythema nodosum 137
inflam. bowel disease 312
TB 275
erythrodermic psoriasis 534
erythropoietin 511
ESR 439
infection 109
polymyalgia rheumatica 458
exophthalmos 340
exotoxins 111
extracerebral haemorrhage 382
extradural haemorrhage 382
extrahepatic cholestasis 320
extrasystoles 253

extrinsic asthma 271
exudate
constituents of 19
eye disease 559–561, 566–570
acute conjunctivitis 566
acute iritis 566
acute keratitis 561
assessment 560
blurring 563
cataract 562, 570
corneal ulcer 561
diabetic retinopathy 563
double vision 563
floaters 564
glaucoma, acute 568
glaucoma, simple 563
headache 564
introduction 559
nystagmus 564
painful eyes 564
red eye 561
retinal detachment 562
sight, gradual loss 562
sight, sudden loss 562
sore eyelids 565
vitreous haemorrhage 562
watering 564

F

facial nerve palsy
Bell's palsy 402
parotid tumour 306
facial pain
differential diagnosis 681
Factor IX deficiency
haemophilia 519
Factor VIII deficiency
haemophilia 519
fainting 99, 214
blackouts 679
congenital HD 256
epilepsy 410
first aid 670
SVT 254
Fallot's tetralogy

congenital HD 256
famine oedema 98
fasciculation
motor neurone disease 405
fat necrosis 24
fatigue
Ca-bronchus 274
congenital HD 256
differential diagnosis 681
hyperthyroidism 340
LVF 240
TB 276
fatty degeneration 23
febrile convulsions 410
femoral hernia 318
femur, fractured neck of 656–657
fever
acute 705
acute bronchitis 282
acute cholecystitis 326
acute pyelonephritis 477
appendicitis 316
arthritis 441
chickenpox 127
Crohn's disease 311
deep vein thrombosis 261
differential diagnosis 705–707
erysipelas 128
German measles 129
gingivostomatitis 303
gout 449
hepatitis 321
infection 108
infective endocarditis 249
influenza 283
lobar pneumonia 278
measles 131
meningitis 125, 379, 653
neoplasia 83
osteomyelitis 470
plus rash 707
pneumonia 279
polyarteritis nodosa 459
polymyalgia rheumatica 458
PUO 706
rheumatic fever 248
Still's disease 447

basic clinical science

TB 275
thyrotoxic crisis 342
ulcerative colitis 311
Vincent's angina 303
viraemia 116
fibrin 31, 93
fibrinogen 93
fibrinoid necrosis 24
fibrinolytic system 93, 94
fibroblast 20, 27, 30
fibrocytes 27
fibroma 81
fibrosarcoma 81
fibrosis 27, 31
liver 322
pneumonia 279
TB 277
filariasis
asthma 271
first aid 663
aims 664
approach 664
diagnosis 665
disposal 665
introduction 664–666
priorities 664
report 665
resuscitation 667
summary 665
treatment 665
fistula 21, 314
Ca-colon/rectum 332
Crohn's disease 311
fits
See epilepsy
flight of ideas 418
hypomania 421
floaters 564
fluid overload
LVF 241, 646
pre-eclampsia 632
focal seizures 410
foetal abnormalities
oligohydramnios 634
polyhydramnios 634
spontaneous abortion 631
therapeutic abortion 638
foetal distress
abruptio placentae 633

foetal mortality
hypertension 633
polyhydramnios 634
folic acid deficiency
anaemia 513
stomatitis 302
food poisoning
clostridium 113
gastroenteritis 300
irritable bowel 314
salmonella 143
funny turns
differential diagnosis 683
Fusiformis fusiformis
Vincent's angina 303

G

galactorrhoea
hyperprolactinaemia 349
gallstone ileus 326
gallstones 325
acute pancreatitis 327
extrahepatic cholestasis 320
gangrene 24
arterial obstruction 260
bowel obstruction 298
intermittent claudication 259
gastric erosion
GI haemorrhage 299
gastric polyps
Ca-stomach 330
gastric ulcer 309
gastritis 22
Ca-stomach 330
gastroenteritis 300
acute abdomen 296
campylobacter 139
gastrointestinal haemorrhage
299
gastrointestinal neoplasm 330–
334
genes 37, 40
definition 43
dominant 43
recessive 43
the genetic code

DNA 36
genes 37
nucleotides 36
sequence 37
triplets 37
genetic counselling 48–49
genetic defects
incomplete penetrance 40
variable expression 40
transmission of 39–43
genetic disorders
dominant 41
recessive 41
sex linked 42
genital herpes 149
genital infestations 150
germ theory 106
German measles 129
giant cell arteritis 654
polymyalgia rheumatica 458
giardiasis 300
gingivostomatitis 303
glandular fever
CMV-infection 134
EBV-infection 135
hepatitis 321
glaucoma
acute 568
closed angle 568
secondary 568
simple 563
glomerulonephritis 477
acute 482
chronic renal failure 484
hypersensitivity 61
nephrotic syndrome 481
proteinuria 479
streptococcal 137
glucocorticoids 353
gluten enteropathy 314, 549
glycosuria
diabetes 365
goitre 339
acromegaly 350
Graves' disease 340
hyperthyroidism 340
hypothyroidism 343
gonorrhoea 112, 147, 499
gout 448

carpal tunnel syndrome 451
hyperlipidaemia 370
IHD 239
leukaemia 523
neoplasia 83
Gram negative 112, 114
Gram positive 112
grand mal epilepsy 410
granulation 28
diagram 29
Graves' disease 339, 341
growth hormone secretion 350
pituitary tumour 348
guanine 36
Guillain-Barré syndrome
weakness 687
gumma
congenital syphilis 153
syphilis 152
gynaecomastia 349
cirrhosis 324
hyperthyroidism 341

H

haem production 372
haemarthrosis
haemophilia 519
haematemesis
Ca-stomach 331
cirrhosis 323
peptic ulcer 310
haematological malignancy
leukaemias 520, 522
lymphoma 524
lymphomas 520
myelomatosis 525
myeloproliferative disorders
520–521
plasma cell tumours 520
haematuria 480
acute nephritis 482
bladder cancer 494
differential diagnosis 699
prostatic hypertrophy 497
renal carcinoma 493
haemoglobin 320

haemolysis
gallstones 325
malignant malaria 155
haemolytic disease of the newborn (HDN) 68
haemophilia 42, 519
clotting disorders 94
Haemophilus influenza
croup 289
meningitis 124, 378, 652
pneumonia 279
haemopoiesis 511
haemoptysis 217
Ca-bronchus 274
differential diagnosis 692–
693
LVF 240
TB 276
half life 167
hallucination 418
acute brain syndromes 426
schizophrenia 420
hand,foot & mouth disease 303
Hashimoto's disease 62, 343
hayfever 60, 61, 578
HBsAG test 322
headache 283, 390–394
acromegaly 350
chickenpox 127
Costen's syndrome 392
cough 392
depression 392
differential diagnosis 683
erysipelas 128
hypertension 246
malignant malaria 155
meningitis 124, 379, 653
migraine 390
migrainous neuralgia 391
phaeochromocytoma 357
pituitary tumour 347
post-herpetic neuralgia 394
pre-eclampsia 632
subarachnoid haemorrhage
385
subdural haemorrhage 384
temporal arteritis 391, 458,
568
tension 392

Tic Douloureux 392
TMJ syndrome 392
trigeminal neuralgia 392
typhoid 143
Heaf test 277
heart defects
Down's syndrome 46
Edwards' syndrome 46
multifactorial inheritance 47
Patau's syndrome 46
XO 47
heart failure 240–241
acromegaly 350
atrial fibrillation 253
COAD 270
common causes 239
congenital HD 256
congestive 241, 251
diagram 238
drugs 241
extrasystoles 253
high calcium 469
hyperthyroidism 340
infective endocarditis 249
LVF 240
management 241
myocardial infarction 645
Paget's disease 466
pleurisy 281
proteinuria 479
rheumatic fever 248
RVF 241
thyrotoxic crisis 342
heartburn 308
helper cells 56
hemianopia 387
hemiplegia
meningitis 125
stroke 387
subarachnoid haemorrhage
385
Henoch-Schönlein purpura
acute nephritis 482
streptococci 137
vasculitis 94
hepatic encephalopathy 324
hepatitis 22, 321
amoebic dysentery 141
cirrhosis 322

hepatoma 334
  inflam. bowel disease 312
  intrahepatic cholestasis 320
hepatoma 334
hernia 317
  bowel obstruction 298
  hiatus 308
heroin overdose 658–659
herpes labialis 303
herpes simplex 540
  corneal ulcer 561
  encephalitis 380
  erythema multiforme 550
  stomatitis 303
  virus 117
herpes zoster 136, 540
  oral ulceration 303
  post-herpetic neuralgia 394
heterolysis 23
heterozygous 40
hiatus hernia 308
hip dislocation 657
  congenital 47
hip replacement 657
hirsutism
  hyperprolactinaemia 349
histamine 19, 59, 271
  anaphylaxis 60
histogenesis 80
histrionic 424
HIV infection 146
hoarseness 586
  croup 289
  differential diagnosis 704
Hodgkin's lymphoma 520, 524
homozygous 39
hordeolum 565
Huntington's chorea 41
hydatidiform mole 630
hydrocephalus
  dementia 407
  meningitis 125
hydrocoele 500
  epididymitis 503
  testicular malignancy 496
hypercalcaemia
  hyperparathyroidism 358
  renal failure 483
hypercalcuria 491

hypercapnia 217
hypercholesterolaemia 370
  nephrotic syndrome 481
hyperemesis gravidarum 630
hyperglycaemia
  coma 369
  diabetes 364–365
  ketoacidosis 650
hyperkalaemia 483
hyperlipidaemia 370–371
hypernephroma 493
hyperparathyroidism 229, 358
  chronic pancreatitis 329
  high calcium 469
  peptic ulcer 309
hyperpigmentation
  Addison's disease 355
hyperplasia 73
hyperprolactinaemia 349
  pituitary tumour 348
hyperpyrexia 108
hypersensitivity 60
  anaphylactic shock 99
  blood transfusions 61
  complement system 61
  cytolytic 61
  delayed, cell mediated 61
  immune complex 61
  Type 1 60
  Type 2 61
  Type 3 61
  Type 4 61
hypertension 239, 481
  acromegaly 350
  acute nephritis 482
  Alport's syndrome 482
  arterial disease 92
  atrial fibrillation 253
  Conn's syndrome 356
  Cushing's disease 354
  definition 245–246
  diabetes 368
  gout 449
  hyperlipidaemia 370
  IHD 239
  intermittent claudication 259
  LVF 241, 646
  myocardial infarction 644
  phaeochromocytoma 357

polyarteritis nodosa 459
porphyrias 372
pregnancy 632
proteinuria 479
SLE 457
stroke 386
TIA 389
valvular heart disease 247
hyperthyroidism 339–341
  heart failure 240
  keratitis 561
  osteoporosis 464
hypertrophy 73
hyperuricaemia 449
hyperventilation 683
hypocalcaemia 410
hypoglycaemia 650
  blackouts 679
  coma 369
  diabetes 650
  diabetic labour 637
  epilepsy 410
  funny turns 683
  TIA 388
hypomania 421
hypoparathyroidism 62, 359
  low calcium 468
  thyroid surgery 342
hypopituitarism 351
  pituitary tumour 347
hypoplasia 72
hypopyon 567
hypostatic pneumonia 278
hypotension
  Addison's disease 355
  adrenal crisis 355
  antidepressants 428
  asthma 272
  diabetes 368
  diabetic coma 369
  extrasystoles 253
  malabsorption 315
hypothermia
  differential diagnosis 708
  overdose 658
hypothyroidism 229, 343
  anaemia 517
  carpal tunnel syndrome 451
  dementia 407

hyperlipidaemia 370
hypopituitarism 351
hypoventilation 693
hypovolaemic shock 99
hypoxia 217
hysteria 423

I

idiopathic thrombocytopenic
purpura 518
illusion 418
immune response
   allergy 60
   cell mediated 55
   humoral 55
   sequence 57
   simplified description 56–57
immune system 54
   effector cells 54, 56
immunization 64
   active 64
   current policy in UK 65
   passive 64
immunoglobulins 19, 56
   response modes 55
   self recognition 55, 57, 62
   surface markers 55
   tolerance 54
immunosuppression 181, 302
impetigo 130
impotence
   multiple sclerosis 404
incontinence 616–618
   multiple sclerosis 404
   syphilis 152
indigestion
   differential diagnosis 697
infection
   bacterial 108
   course and outcome 121
   diabetes 368
   general effects 108–109
   human defences 119
   immunity 64
   metabolic changes 109
   opportunistic 117

   routes of entry 119
   viral 116
   virulence 120
infectious mononucleosis
   EBV-infection 135
infective agents
   types 110–118
infertility
   gonorrhoea 147
   hyperprolactinaemia 349
   hyperthyroidism 341
infiltrations 25
inflammation
   abscess 20
   acute 16
   chemical 18
   chemical mediators 19
   chronic 21
   effects 19
   exudate 19
   fistula 21
   Lewis' triple response 17
   oedema 96
   organization 20
   resolution 20
   sequence of events 18
   sinus 21
   suppuration 20
inflammatory bowel disease
311
   campylobacter 139
   gastroenteritis 300
influenza 283–284
   bronchopneumonia 278
   encephalitis 380
inheritance
   auto-immune diseases 62
   blood group 67
   dominant 40
   hypersensitivity 61
   incomplete penetrance 40
   multifactorial 47
   recessive 41
   sex linked 42
   variable expression 40
insomnia 429
insulin
   diabetes 364
   diabetic coma 369

interferon 120
intermittent claudication 214,
259
   atheroma 92
intracranial pressure
   cerebral tumour 408
   extradural haemorrhage 382
   raised 380, 685
   stroke 388
   subdural haemorrhage 384
intrahepatic cholestasis 320
intrinsic asthma 271
iodine insufficiency 343
iridectomy 569
iritis
   acute 566
   ankylosing spondylitis 445
   inflam. bowel disease 312
   Reiter's disease 446
iron deficiency
   anaemia 512
   stomatitis 302
irritable bowel syndrome 314
   gastroenteritis 300
ischaemia 91, 92, 690
ischaemic foot 260
ischaemic heart disease 242–
244, 645
   acute LVF 646
   angina 242
   atrial fibrillation 253
   common causes 239
   diabetes 367
   hyperlipidaemia 370
   hypothyroidism 344
   indigestion 697
   risk factors 239
IUD 635
IVU 505

J

jaundice 220, 320
   biliary colic 327
   Ca-colon/rectum 332
   Ca-liver 334
   Ca-pancreas 333

Ca-stomach 331
cirrhosis 324
gallstones 326
hepatitis 321
hyperlipidaemia 370
malignant malaria 155
neoplasia 83
primary biliary cirrhosis 325
joint movement
  normal ranges 228
joint pain 437ff
  acromegaly 350
  hepatitis 321
  infective endocarditis 249
  rheumatic fever 248
JVP 241, 251

K

Kaposi's sarcoma 146
karyolysis 23
karyorrhexis 23
keloid 31
keratinocytes 545
keratitis 561
  congenital syphilis 153
keratoderma blenorrhagica
  Reiter's disease 446
ketoacidosis 365, 369, 650
ketone bodies 365
ketosis
  fever 109
kidney disease
  common presentations
  479–485
  See also renal medicine
kidney stones 490
  complications 492
  Cushing's disease 354
  gout 449
  high calcium 469
  hyperparathyroidism 358
killer cells 56
kinins 19
klebsiella 114, 279
Klinefelter's syndrome 47
Koebner's phenomenon 535

Korsakoff's psychosis 426
kuru 117

L

labyrinthitis 686
lactobacillus 113
laryngeal nerve palsy
  thyroid surgery 342
laryngitis 581
  croup 289
LD50 test 165
left ventricular failure 240
  pulmonary oedema 97
legionnaire's disease 279
legionella pneumophila 114
leptospira 114, 321
leucoplakia 304
leukaemia 520
  acute lymphoblastic 522
  acute myeloid 522
  chronic lymphatic 522
  chronic myeloid 522
Lewis' triple response 17
lice 543
lichen planus 535
lichenification 553
lipoma 81
liposarcoma 81
listeria 113
lithium salts 181
liver
  anaemia 517
  carcinoma 334
  clotting disorders 94
  enlarged 146, 153, 249, 334,
  350
  liver abscess 141
  liver failure 155, 221, 323
  malignant malaria 155
  porphyrias 372
  RVF 241
lobar pneumonia 278
low back pain
  classification 450
lumbar puncture 125, 379, 653
lung abscess

sputum 692
lung cancer 251, 273, 353
lupus erythematosus, systemic
  auto-immune 63
  skin manifestations 552
lymphadenopathy 447
  AIDS 146
  CMV-infection 134
  congenital syphilis 153
  EBV-infection 135
  genital herpes 149
  German measles 129
  neoplastic 83
  syphilis 152
lymphocytes 54–55, 58–59
lymphoid tissues 58–59
lymphoma 520, 524
  Hodgkin's 524

M

macrophage 57, 59, 61
macule 553
malabsorption 314
  chronic pancreatitis 329
  Crohn's disease 312
  gastroenteritis 300
malar flush 215
malaria 154, 155, 296
malignant disease
  aetiology 82
  clinical features 82–83
  clinical manifestations 83
  danger signals 82
  mortality league table 82
  pathological features 80
malignant melanoma 546
Mallory-Weiss syndrome 299
manic depression 421
Mantoux test 275, 277
mast cells 60
mastoidectomy 574
mastoiditis 575
measles 131
  bronchopneumonia 278
  croup 289
  risk groups 65

virus 115, 117
the medical model 6–10
Medicines Act 163
Medicines Commision 163
medullary carcinoma
    thyroid 346
melaena
    GI-haemorrhage 299
    peptic ulcer 310
memory
    dementia 406
    Korsakoff's psychosis 426
memory cells 56
Meniere's disease 395, 686
meningeal irritation 125, 379, 385, 653
meningitis 22, 124, 378
    bacterial 380, 652–653
    complications 380, 653
    epilepsy 409
    faecal streptococci 137
    genital herpes 149
    headache 683
    meningococcus 112, 124, 378, 652
    mumps 132
    TB 277
    tuberculous 380, 653
    unconsciousness 685
    viral 379, 653
menstrual disturbance
    Addison's disease 355
    anorexia nervosa 427
    hyperprolactinaemia 349
    hyperthyroidism 341
    hypopituitarism 351
mental retardation
    CMV-infection 134
    cri du chat 46
    Down's syndrome 46
    meningitis 125, 380, 653
    non-specific 41
    stereotypies 419
mental state
    assessment 432–433
merozoites 154
metabolic bone diseases 464–467
metabolic disorders 363

metaplasia 73
metastasis 80
micturating cystogram 506
mid-brain infarction 387
migraine 390, 396
migrainous neuralgia 391
Mikulicz disease 307
miliary tuberculosis 277
mineralocorticoids 353
Minister of Health 163
mitral valve disease
    atrial fibrillation 253
    mitral regurgitation 241
molluscum contagiosum 541
monocytes, description 59
mononeuritis multiplex
    diabetes 368
morning sickness 630
mosaicism 45
motor neurone disease 405, 451
mountains 456
mouth, dry
    Mikulicz disease 307
    Sjögren's syndrome 307
movement disorders 397–398
multiple myeloma 520
multiple sclerosis 403
    trigeminal neuralgia 392
    vertigo 396
mumps 132
    encephalitis 380
    salivary glands 306
    virus 115, 117
Murphy's sign 326
muscle spasm
    hypoparathyroidism 359
    malabsorption 315
muscle weakness
    Duchenne muscular dystrophy 401
    myasthenia gravis 399
    osteomalacia 465
muscular dystrophy 400
mutations 38, 40
    epigenetic theory 79
myalgic encephalomyelitis 381
myasthenia gravis 399
    hyperthyroidism 341

mycobacteria 112, 113, 275
mycoplasma 114, 279
myelofibrosis 521
myeloma 25, 520, 525
    high calcium 469
    nephrotic syndrome 481
myeloproliferative disorders 520–521
    gout 448
myocardial infarction 243, 644–
    acute abdomen 296
    atrial fibrillation 253
    bradycardia 255
    cardiac rhythm disturbance 252
    extrasystoles 253
    fever 108
    LVF 241
    pericarditis 251
    shock 99
    valvular heart disease 247
    ventricular fibrillation 254
myocarditis 22
    typhoid 144
myringotomy 574
myxoedema 343

N

nasal polyps 579
nausea
    angina 242
    appendicitis 316
    bowel obstruction 299
    Ca-stomach 331
    differential diagnosis 697
    hepatitis 321
    hypercalcaemia 358
neck stiffness
    See meningeal irritation
necrobiosis lipoidica diabeticorum 368, 552
necrosis 24, 26
    caseous 24
    coagulative 24
    colliquative 24

fat- 24
fibrinoid 24
gangrene 24
neisseria 114
nematodes 118
neoplasia 71
    autonomous growth 74
    local effects 83
    malignant versus benign 80
    metastatic effects 83
    systemic effects 83
nephritis
    acute 482
    Alport's syndrome 482
    haematuria 480
    renal oedema 98, 482
nephrocalcinosis 492
nephrotic syndrome 482
    diabetes 368
    hyperlipidaemia 370
    oedema 98, 482
    proteinuria 479
nervous system 377
    differential diagnosis 679–687
nettle rash 539
neuralgia
    post herpetic 136
neurofibromatosis 41, 686
neuropathy
    Ca-bronchus 274
    diabetes 368
    polyarteritis nodosa 459
    porphyrias 372
neurosis 422–423
    hysterical 423
    obsessive/compulsive 423
neurotic depression 422
neutrophil 59
the NHS 197–204
the NHS Act 197
night sweats 276
nits 150, 543
nodules
    arthritis 440
    gout 448
nose 577–579
    allergic rhinitis 578
    hayfever 578

nasal polyps 579
nosebleed 585
sinusitis 577
NSU 151
    Reiter's disease 446
nucleotides 36, 43
    mutations 38
nystagmus 564
    multiple sclerosis 404

O

obesity
    arterial disease 92
    diabetes 365
    IHD 239
    intermittent claudication 259
    myocardial infarction 644
obstetrics 629
oedema 96
    acute pulmonary 646
    allergic 96
    anaphylaxis 60
    angioneurotic 97
    cardiac 97
    croup 289
    deep vein thrombosis 261
    definition 96–98
    famine 98
    generalized 97
    in LVF 240
    in RVF 241
    local 96
    malabsorption 314
    nephrotic syndrome 481
    pulmonary 97, 240
    renal 98
    SLE 457
    venous ulcers 263
oesophageal varices 299
oligohydramnios 634
oliguria 482
    See renal failure
oncogenic theory 77
oncogenic viruses 79
oophoritis 132
ophthalmic herpes 136

ophthalmoplegia 340
opiate withdrawal 658
optic neuritis
    multiple sclerosis 403
oral contraceptives
    carpal tunnel syndrome 451
    myocardial infarction 644
    Raynaud's phenomenon 452
    stroke 386
oral herpes simplex infection 303
oral thrush 303
orchidectomy 496
orchitis 132, 502
organic brain syndromes 426
organization 20
orthopnoea 214
osmotic diuresis 365
osteoarthritis 443
osteogenic sarcoma 471
osteomalacia 465
    hyperparathyroidism 358
    low calcium 468
osteomyelitis 470
osteoporosis 464
    Cushing's disease 354
otitis externa 22, 572
otitis media 22
    acute 572
    chronic 573
    complications 575
    secretory 574
otosclerosis 576
ovarian failure, premature
    auto-immune 62
overdose 658–659
    first aid 671
    London poison information centre 659
overhydration 483

P

pacemaker 252
Paget's disease 466
pain

acute cholecystitis 326
appendicitis 316
arterial obstruction 260
biliary colic 327
bowel obstruction 299
Ca-tongue 305
chronic cholecystitis 327
deep vein thrombosis 261
diverticulitis 313
gastroenteritis 300
irritable bowel 314
peptic ulcer 310
peritonitis 297
pleuritic 281
pulmonary embolus 287
salivary tumour 306
ulcerative colitis 311
varicose veins 262
Vincent's angina 303
palpitations 214
antidepressants 428
atrial fibrillation 253
differential diagnosis 694
hyperthyroidism 340
phaeochromocytoma 357
pancreatic insufficiency
cystic fibrosis 291
pancreatitis
acute 296, 327
acute abdomen 296
Ca-pancreas 333
campylobacter 139
chronic 329
hyperlipidaemia 370
low calcium 468
mumps 132
peritonitis 297
panic disorders 422, 683, 700
pannus 440
papilloedema 245, 347
papilloma 81
papule 553
para-influenza
virus 117
paralysis agitans 398
paralytic ileus 297
paranoia 418
parasites 118
parathyroid adenoma

hyperparathyroidism 358
phaeochromocytoma 357
parathyroidectomy 358
paratyphoid 144
Parkinson's disease 397, 428,
568, 679
paronychia 541
parotid gland 306
mumps 132
Sjögren's syndrome 307
paroxysmal supraventricular
tachycardia 254
paroxysmal ventricular
tachycardia 254
Patau's syndrome 46
patent ductus arteriosus 256
pediculosis 150, 543
pelvic inflammatory disease
22, 147, 151, 297, 609, 611,
635
pemphigoid 549
pemphigus vulgaris 548
peptic ulcer 309
GI-haemorrhage 299
hyperparathyroidism 358
pain 690
peritonitis 297
reflux 308
perforated bowel
acute abdomen 296
appendicitis 316
Ca-colon/rectum 332
diverticulitis 314
pericardial pain 700
pericarditis 251
acute LVF 646
Ca-bronchus 274
chronic constrictive 251
SLE 457
TB 277
peripheral cyanosis 692
peripheral vascular disease
259–263
peritonitis 297
acute abdomen 296
acute cholecystitis 326
diverticulitis 314
peritonsillar abscess 580
perleche 304

personality disorders 424–
425, 702
pertussis 133, 290
pertussis vaccine 65
Peter Pan dwarfism 351
petit mal epilepsy 410
PGL 146
phaeochromocytoma 346, 357
phagocytosis 19, 121
by macrophages 59
by neutrophils 59
pharmacodynamics 167
pharmacokinetics 167
pharmacology 159
pharyngeal pouch 586
phenylketonuria 41
phobic disorders 700
photophobia
meningitis 379, 653
migraine 390
pigment stones 325
pins and needles
differential diagnosis 684
pituitary problems 343, 347–
353
pityriasis rosea 536
pityriasis versicolor 542
Pityrosporum ovale 542
placebo effect 192
placenta praevia 633
placental abnormalities
polyhydramnios 634
plaque 553
plasma cell tumours 520
plasma cells 56, 59
plasmodium
malaria 154
pleural effusion 279
pleurisy 281
RVF 241
pleural pain 690
pleurisy 22, 281
pneumonia 279
SLE 457
pneumococci
meningitis 124, 378, 652
pneumonia 279
pneumocystis carinii
AIDS 146

pneumonia 22, 278–280
acute abdomen 296
AIDS 146
aspiration 308
bronchopneumonia 278
faecal streptococci 137
femur, fractured neck of 657
influenza 283
lobar 20
pulmonary oedema 97
sputum 692
typhoid 144
whooping cough 133, 290
pneumonitis
chickenpox 127
measles 131
pneumothorax 286, 649
point mutations 38, 43
polio virus 115, 117
polyarteritis nodosa 459
acute nephritis 482
asthma 271
auto-immunity 63
polycystic disease of the
kidneys 41
polycythaemia
neoplasia 83
thrombophlebitis 262
polycythaemia rubra vera 521
polydipsia
Conn's syndrome 356
diabetes 365
diabetes insipidus 352
hypercalcaemia 358
polyhydramnios 634
diabetic pregnancy 637
polymyalgia rheumatica 458
auto-immunity 63
temporal arteritis 654
polymyositis
auto-immunity 63
polyneuropathy
Bell's palsy 402
polyposis coli 41
polyuria
Conn's syndrome 356
diabetes insipidus 352
differential diagnosis 699
hypercalcaemia 358, 469

porphyrias 372–373
portal venous obstruction 323
porto-systemic connection 323
post-herpetic neuralgia 394
post-primary TB 276
post-renal failure 484
post-traumatic syndrome 700
post-viral syndrome 381
postural hypotension 686
postural proteinuria 479
potassium loss
Conn's syndrome 356
Cushing's disease 354
potency 169
potentiation 169
pre-eclampsia 632
diabetic pregnancy 637
polyhydramnios 634
pre-renal failure 483
pregnancy
abruptio placentae 633
diabetic pregnancy 637
placenta praevia 634
polyhydramnios 634
pre-eclampsia 633
amniotic fluid 634
ante-partum haemorrhage
633
carpal tunnel syndrome 451
complications 630–634
deep vein thrombosis 261
diabetic 637
ectopic 297, 635–636
German measles 129
HDN 68
hernia 317
HF 240
hypertension 632
risk of HDN 68
spontaneous abortion 631
vomiting 630
pretibial myxoedema
hyperthyroidism 341
primary biliary cirrhosis 325
primary hyperaldosteronism
356
primary hyperparathyroidism
358
primary TB 275

primigravidae 632
proctitis
gonorrhoea 147
prokaryotic organisms 110
prolactin secretion
drugs 349
hyperprolactinaemia 349
physiological causes 349
pituitary tumour 348
prolactinoma 348
prophylaxis 162
prostaglandins E2 108
medullary carcinoma 346
therapeutic abortion 638
prostatic disease
cancer 495
epididymitis 503
hypertrophy 497–498
prostatitis 499
gonorrhoea 147
NSU 151
prosthesis 657
proteinuria 479
acute nephritis 482
diabetes 366
hypertension 245
nephrotic syndrome 481
pregnancy 632
SLE 457
proteus 114
protozoa 118
proud flesh 31
pruritus vulvae 365, 599–600
pseudomonas 114
psittacosis 279
psoriasis 534
erythrodermic 534
psoriatic arthritis 447, 534
psychopath 424
psychosis 420–421
porphyrias 372
SLE 457
psychosomatic 419
pubic lice 150
pulmonary embolism 287
asthma 271
deep vein thrombosis 261
femur, fractured neck of 657
pulmonary hypertension 269

pulmonary oedema 97, 240
  congenital HD 256
  malignant malaria 155
pulmonary stenosis
  congenital HD 256
pulmonary TB 275
pulmonary venous congestion
  acute LVF 646
pulsus paradoxus
  asthma 272
  pericardial effusion 251
  status asthmaticus 648
pupillary abnormalities
  extradural haemorrhage 382
  mid-brain infarction 387
purpura 553
  idiopathic thrombocytopenic
  518
  SLE 457
pyaemia 111
pyelogram, retrograde 506
pyelonephritis
  acute 477
  chronic 477
  chronic renal failure 484
  diabetes 368
  typhoid 144
pyknosis 23
pyloric obstruction 309
pyogenic bacteria 112
pyrexia 108
pyrexia of unknown origin 706
pyrogens
  endogenous 108

Q

q-fever 279
quinsy 580

R

rabies virus 117
rash
  antidepressants 429

fever 707
  meningitis 379, 653
  SLE 457
  Still's disease 447
Raynaud's phenomenon 259,
452
  scleroderma 460
  SLE 457
recessive genes 40
  expression 43
rectal bleeding 301, 313
  Ca-colon/rectum 332
  differential diagnosis 698
reflux nephropathy 477
reflux oesophagitis 308
regurgitation
  congenital HD 256
Reiter's disease 446
Reiter's syndrome
  NSU 151
  stomatitis 302
renal artery stenosis
  hypertension 481
renal cancer
  varicocoele 501
renal carcinoma 493
renal failure
  acute 483
  acute pancreatitis 328
  Alport's syndrome 482
  cholera 140
  chronic 484
  epilepsy 410
  glomerulonephritis 477
  gout 448
  hypercalcaemia 469
  hyperlipidaemia 370
  hyperparathyroidism 358
  hypocalcaemia 468
  malignant malaria 155
  overdose 658
  pericarditis 251
  renal osteodystrophy 467
  SLE 457
renal medicine 476
  See also kidney disease
renal oedema 98
renal osteodystrophy 467
renal TB 277

resolution
  acute inflammation 20
respiratory failure 217, 272,
648
  COAD 269–270
respiratory syncytial virus
  (RSV) 117
  bronchiolitis 288
  viral pneumonia 280
respiratory system 267
  differential diagnosis 688–
  694
  observations 217
  points in history 217
  recording findings 219
  sequence of examination
  218
rest
  heart rate 252
resuscitation 667
retarded growth
  congenital HD 256
retinal detachment 562
rhesus factor 68
rhesus incompatibility
  polyhydramnios 634
rheumatic fever 248
  infective endocarditis 249
  streptococci 137
  valvular heart disease 247
rheumatoid arthritis 440–442
  osteoporosis 464
  pericarditis 251
  rheumatoid factor 439
  valvular heart disease 247
  vasculitis 94
rhinitis 22
rhinophyma 538
rhinorrhoea 578
rhinovirus 117
rickets 465
rickettsiae 118
rickety rosary
  osteomalacia 465
right ventricular failure 241
rigors 108
  malaria 155
  pneumonia 279
ringworm 541

basic clinical science

RNA-virus 76
rodent ulcer 544
rose spots
    typhoid 143
rotavirus 117
rubella 129
    congenital HD 256
    encephalitis 380
    virus 115
rubor 16

S

sacro-iliitis
    Reiter's disease 446
salivary gland disease 306
    Mikulicz disease 307
    stones 306
    tumour 306
salmonella 112, 114
    gastroenteritis 300
    paratyphoid 144
    typhoid 143
salpingitis 22, 147, 151, 297,
    604, 611, 635
sarcoidosis 469
sarcoptes scabei 150, 543
scabies 150, 543
scaly skin conditions 534–536
    lichen planus 535
    pityriasis rosea 536
    psoriasis 534
scarlet fever 137
schizophrenia 420
    hallucinations 418
    suicidal behaviour 702
scleroderma 63, 460
sclerosis
    osteoarthritis 443
    systemic 460
scurvy 94
secondary
    hyperparathyroidism 358
seminoma 496
septic infarction 111
septic shock 99
septicaemia 111

campylobacter 139
    meningitis 124
seronegative arthritides 439,
    445–447
sex chromosomes 44, 47
shigellae 112, 114
shingles 136, 540
shock 99–101
    acute pancreatitis 328
    anaphylactic 99
    cardiogenic 99
    cholera 140
    diagram 100
    ectopic pregnancy 636
    first aid 665, 672
    hypovolaemic 99
    ketoacidosis 650
    myocardial infarction 645
    outcome 101
    septic 99
shunts
    congenital HD 256
sialolithiasis 306
sickle cell anaemia 515
sinus formation 21
sinusitis 577
sinusoids 322
Sjögren's syndrome 63, 307
skin conditions, blistering
    548–550
    dermatitis herpetiformis 549
    erythema multiforme 550
    pemphigoid 549
    pemphigus vulgaris 548
skin conditions, infective 540–
    543
    bacterial 540
    candida 541
    cellulitis 540
    dermatophytes 541
    fungal 541
    herpes simplex 540
    herpes zoster 540
    molluscum contagiosum
    541
    pediculosis 543
    pityriasis versicolor 542
    scabies 543
    viral 540

    warts 540
skin conditions, malignant
    544–547
    basal cell carcinoma 544
    malignant melanoma 546
    squamous cell carcinoma
    545
skin manifestations
    of systemic disease 552
skin rash
    adverse drug reaction 174
    anaphylaxis 99
    chickenpox 127
    congenital syphilis 153
    erysipelas 128
    German measles 129
    hypersensitivity 61
    impetigo 130
    inflam. bowel disease 312
    measles 131
    meningitis 125
    porphyrias 372
    pubic lice 150
    shingles 136
    strep throat 137
    syphilis 152
    typhoid 143
SLE 457
    acute nephritis 482
    nephrotic syndrome 481
    pericarditis 251
    thromocytopenia 519
    vasculitis 94
smallpox 117
smoking
    arterial disease 92
    Ca-bronchus 273
    Ca-cheek 304
    Ca-oesophagus 330
    Ca-pancreas 333
    carcinogenesis 75
    COAD 269
    IHD 239
    intermittent claudication 259
    leukoplakia 304
    metaplasia 73
    myocardial infarction 644
    peptic ulcer 309
    stroke 386

social services 202
sodium retention
    Conn's syndrome 356
    Cushing's disease 354
spermatocoele 500
spina bifida 47
spirochaetes 114
spleen, enlarged
    AIDS 146
    CMV-infection 134
    congenital syphilis 153
    EBV-infection 135
    infective endocarditis 249
    malaria 155
spontaneous thrombophlebitis
    262
sporozoites 154
squamous cell carcinoma 545
stapedectomy 576
staphylococci 20, 112
    angular stomatitis 304
    impetigo 130
    infections 137
    osteomyelitis 470
    pneumonia 279
    prostatitis 499
staphylococci & streptococci
    infections 137–138
status asthmaticus 648–649
status epilepticus 651
steatorrhoea 329
stenosis
    congenital HD 256
stereotypies 419
steroid therapy 30
    adrenocortical atrophy 72
    Cushing's disease 353
    osteoporosis 464
    peptic ulcer 309
Stevens-Johnson syndrome
    550
Still's disease 447
Stokes-Adam's attacks 410,
    679
stoma 313
stomatitis 302
    angular 304
    aphthous 302
    malabsorption 315

Vincent's acute 303
viral infections 303
strangulation 298
strawberry tongue 138
strep throat 137, 248
streptococci 112
    α-haemolytic 137
    acute nephritis 482
    β-haemolytic 137
    cellulitis 540
    erysipelas 128
    faecal 137
    Henoch Schönlein purpura
        518
    impetigo 130
    prostatitis 499
    streptococcus pneumoniae
        278
    streptococcus pyogenes 112
stricture
    diverticulitis 314
    extrahepatic cholestasis 320
stridor 586
    croup 289
stroke 382
    atheroma 92
    epilepsy 410
    first aid 672
    stroke syndromes 386
    TIA 388
    unconsciousness 685
styes 565
subarachnoid haemorrhage
    384
    headache 683
subdural haemorrhage 383,
    407
submandibular gland
    stones 306
suicidal behaviour 702
sunlight 465
sunset 155
suppressor cells 56
suppuration 20
syncope 214
synechias 567
synovitis 440
syphilis 21, 152
    congenital 153

dementia 407
infective endocarditis 249
leukoplakia 304
valvular heart disease 247
systemic lupus erythematosus
    457
systemic sclerosis 552

T

T-lymphocytes 56–61
T4 339
tabes dorsalis 152
tachycardia
    acute LVF 646
    hyperthyroidism 340
    LVF 241
    overdose 658
    paroxysmal supraventricular
        254
    paroxysmal ventricular 254
    pericardial effusion 251
    porphyrias 372
    status asthmaticus 648
TB 21, 275–277
    acute abdomen 296
    Addison's disease 355
    carpal tunnel syndrome 451
    diabetes 368
    meningitis 378, 652
    pericarditis 251
telangiectasia
    definition 95
    hereditary haemorrhagic 94
telangiectasis 553
    acne rosacea 538
temporal arteritis 654–655
    headache 683
    polymyalgia rheumatica 458
temporal lobe epilepsy 411
tenosynovitis 441
teratoma 81, 496
tertiary hyperparathyroidism
    358
testicular atrophy 324
testicular malignancy 496
testicular torsion 504

basic clinical science

testicular tumours 500–501
tetanus 113
thalassaemia 516
therapeutic range 175
thought block
    schizophrenia 420
throat 580–582
    adenoiditis 581
    laryngitis 581
    malignant tumours 581
    quinsy 580
    tonsillitis 580
throat, sore
    differential diagnosis 704
thrombin 93
thrombocythaemia, essential
    521
thrombocytopenia 519
thrombocytopenic purpura 94
thrombophlebitis 261
    Ca-bronchus 274
    neoplasia 83
    spontaneous 262
    varicose veins 262
thrombophlebitis migrans 262
thrombosis 88
    arterial 90
    arterial obstruction 260
    atrial fibrillation 254
    coronary artery 644
    deep vein 96, 144, 261
    heart 90
    initiating factors 89
    meningitis 124
    stroke 386
    thrombophlebitis 261
    venous 90
thrombus 88
thrombus formation
    atrial fibrillation 254
thrush 541
    AIDS 146
    diabetes 368
    leucoplakia 304
    oral 303
thymine 36
thymus 58
    myasthenia gravis 399
thyroid disease 229, 339–346

skin manifestations 552
malignancy 339, 345
nodules 339
phaeochromocytoma 357
thyroidectomy 342
thyroiditis 345
thyrotoxic crisis 342
thyrotoxicosis 229, 339
    atrial fibrillation 253
    follicular carcinoma 346
    gastroenteritis 300
    high calcium 469
Tic Douloureux 392
tics 419
tinea capitis 542
tinea corporis 541
tinea cruris 542
tinea pedis 542
tinnitus 583
    Meniere's disease 395
tissue death 24
tissue healing 27–31
    by first intention 28
    by second intention 28
    complications 30
    delaying factors 30
    enzyme action 27
    fibrosis 27
    granulation 28–29
    regeneration 27
TMJ syndrome 392
tolerance 55
tonsillitis 580
tophi
    gout 448
transient ischaemic attack 388
traveller's diarrhoea 300
trematodes 118
tremor
    differential diagnosis 684
    multiple sclerosis 404
    Parkinson's disease 397
treponema 114, 152
trigeminal neuralgia 392, 564
triplets 37, 43
trisomy 46, 48
tropocollagen 27
TSH receptors 340
tubercle bacillus

discovery 106
    meningitis 124
tuberculin test 277
tuberculosis 275–277
tuberculous meningitis 380,
    653
tumour
    anaplastic 81
    classification 81
    histogenesis 80
    malignant 80
    nomenclature 81
Turner's syndrome 47, 256
TURP 497
twins
    polyhydramnios 634
    vomiting 630
tympanoplasty 574
typhoid 143
    acute abdomen 296

U

ulceration 26
    aphthous 302
    diabetes 368
    intermittent claudication 259
    ischaemic foot 260
    oral 303
    simple and malignant 26
    venous 263
    Vincent's angina 303
ulcerative colitis 311
    arthritis 447
    Ca-colon/rectum 332
ultrasound 506
    placenta praevia 634
    threatened abortion 631
uraemia 484
    acute nephritis 482
    anaemia 517
    bacillary dysentery 142
    renal failure 483
urethral stricture
    gonorrhoea 147
urethral syndrome 486
urethritis 486

ankylosing spondylitis 445
non-specific 151
post-gonococcal 148
uric acid 448
urinary retention 498
antidepressants 428
diabetes 368
genital herpes 149
See also prostatic disease
497ff
urinary tract infection 477, 486
diabetes 368
haematuria 480
proteinuria 479
urinary tract investigations
505–506
urinary tract malignancy 493–
496
bladder 494
kidney 493
prostate 495
testis 496
urinary tract stones 490–492
urobilinogen 320
urolithiasis 490–492
urology 489
urticaria 539
drug reactions 551

V

vaccination 65
contra-indications 64
principles 64–66
vaccine
BCG/TB 66
diphth./tetanus booster 65
diphtheria/tetanus/pertussis
65
measles, mumps, rubella 65
polio 65
polio booster 65–66
rubella 66
tetanus booster 66
vaccinia
virus 117
vaginal discharge 147, 623

Valsalva manoeuvre 254
valvular heart disease 245,
247
acute LVF 646
rheumatic fever 248
vampire 373
varicella-zoster 117
varicocoele 501
varicose veins 262
thrombophlebitis 261
venous ulcers 263
vasculitis 94
arthritis 440
Henoch Schönlein purpura
518
hypersensitivity 61
polyarteritis nodosa 459
SLE 457
stroke 386
vaso-vagal attack 99
venous ulcers 263
ventilation/perfusion imbalance
cyanosis 693
ventilatory failure
asthma 649
ventricular failure
240–241, 646–647
ventricular fibrillation 253–254
ventricular septal defect
congenital HD 256
vertebrobasilar insufficiency
blackouts 679
vertigo 686
vertigo 584
benign positional 686
brain stem ischaemia 396
differential diagnosis 686
labyrinth 396
Meniere's disease 395
multiple sclerosis 396, 403
postural 396
streptomycin 396
vestibular neuronitis 396
vesicle 553
vestibular neuronitis 396
vibrio cholerae 114, 140
Vincent's angina 303
viraemia 116
viral hepatitis 321

viral meningitis 379, 653
viral pneumonia 280
virion 115
virulence 120
viruses 76
Burkitt's lymphoma 77
cervical cancer 77
classification 117
definition 115
DNA 76
encephalitis 380
HIV 145
HSV-2 149
liver cell cancer 77
meningitis 378, 652
nasopharyngeal carcinoma
77
oncogenic 76, 79, 117
paramyxo 131
RNA 76
slow 117
varicella-zoster 127, 136
warts 77
visual field defects
pituitary tumour 347
vitamin B deficiency 302
vitamin C deficiency 30
vitamin D
calcium and phosphate
levels 468
osteomalacia 465
renal osteodystrophy 467
vitamin K
clotting disorders 94
vitiligo
Addison's disease 355
auto-immune disorders 62
vitreous haemorrhage 562
volvulus 298
vomiting 220
acute cholecystitis 326
anaphylactic shock 99
appendicitis 316
bowel obstruction 299
bulimia 427
Ca-stomach 331
diabetic coma 369
differential diagnosis 697
erysipelas 128

basic clinical science

extradural haemorrhage 382
gastroenteritis 300
GI-haemorrhage 299
hypercalcaemia 358
influenza 283
malignant malaria 155
Meniere's disease 395
meningitis 124
migraine 390
overdose 659
peptic ulcer 310
peritonitis 297
porphyrias 372
pre-eclampsia 632
pregnancy 630
shock 99
TIA 389
vestibular neuronitis 396
whooping cough 290
von Willebrand's disease
clotting disorders 94
haemophilia 519

W

warts 77, 117, 540
watering eye 564
weal 16, 553
weight loss
Addison's disease 355
ankylosing spondylitis 445
arthritis 441
Ca-bronchus 274
Ca-colon/rectum 332
Ca-oesophagus 330
Ca-pancreas 333
Ca-stomach 331
diabetes 365
differential diagnosis 698
high calcium 469
hyperthyroidism 340
malabsorption 314
neoplasm 83
peptic ulcer 310
polyarteritis nodosa 459
polymyalgia rheumatica 458
TB 276

ulcerative colitis 311
werewolf 418
wheeze
asthma 271
COAD 270
differential diagnosis 694
LVF 240
white blood cells 59
who am I 433
whooping cough 133, 278, 290
Wickham's striae 535
worms 118
wound healing
by first intention 28
by granulation 28–29
complications 30
delaying factors 30
keloid 31
proud flesh 31
by second intention 28
summary 30

X

x-chromosome 44, 47
x-linked 42
x-rays
carcinogenesis 75
xanthelasma 370
xanthomas 215, 370

Y

y-chromosome 44, 47
yeasts 118

Z

zinc deficiency 30

POSTSCRIPT

Now, at the end of three years' work, I would like to express my profound gratitude to family, friends, colleagues and students for their enthusiasm and support for this project. Hopefully, the next few years will see the publication of many new textbooks for students of natural medicine, reflecting a steady rise in standards of education and clinical training. It has been a privilege to have met so many talented, kind and committed people in the world of complementary/alternative medicine and I would like especially to thank the following –

Caroline Aldous
Nick Beak
Pia Birk
Nigel Bishop
Margery Bloomfield
Boss
Frances Büning
Suzi Chappell
Colin Croucher
Francesca Diebschlag
Peter Firebrace
Steve Gascoigne
Val Golden
Tim Goman
Holly Gothard
Paul Hambly
Richard James
Maurice Jennings
Lafayette
Ken Lunn
Kevin McSean
Cheryl Nicholson
Anna-Rosa Robertsdottir
Keith Robertson
Mike Robinson
Gordon Rowley
Mandy Smith
Helen Stapleton
Joyce Thomas
Linda Wilkinson
Hein Zeylstra

and also

Richard Adams
Shabaz Ahmad
Jane Aitchison
Elspeth Alexander
Trudi Allford
Gillian Allsop
Gil Alon
John Armstrong
Charlotte Arnold
Silvio Arnone
Polly Ashton
Mariana Aristidou
Chancal Atkinson
Dee Atkinson
Teresa Barlow
Jonathan Barnes
Sally Beazleigh
Nick Beak
Bendle
Lanny Benjamin
Ana Bennet
Lynn Bennet
Roisin Best
Ana Bie
Sue Birch
Pia Birk
Gillian Blacklock
Helen Bottomley
Mary Bove

Juliet Bowerman
Sandra Bradshaw
Paula Braga
Rex Brangwyn
Jade Britton
Nigel Brooke
Andrew Bryant
Frances Büning
Chris Bunkell
Jim Burgess
Greg Burke
Fiona Burns
Kerry Burrowes
Suely Camera
Amadis Cambell
Matthew Carratu
Peter Cavanaugh
Suzi Chappell
Despina Chrisofidou
Im Chuah
Wainwright Churchill
Beryl Churchman
Neil Clegg
Christopher Coker
Richard Collisson
Belinda Coppock
Paolo Coseschi
Alison Court
Atsuko Cowley
Carole Crowley
Freke De Graaf

Bob De La Warr
Jeremy De Souza
Anthony Deavin
Philip Delve
Timothy Dennis
Marc Deora
Anne Derby
Veronique Desjardins
Francesca Diebschlag
Clare Dobie
Oscar Donkor
Eva Duffin
Tilly Dunne
Charles Dunning
Richard Dyer
Ben Edwards
Martyn Edwards
Camilla Ewing
Louise Fenning
Geoffrey Fielding
Ingvild Flesland
Jennifer Fox
Helga Frank
Rhona Fraser
Karen Frivik
Enno Furste
Wolfgang Furste
Satyen Gadher
Jo Gardner
Rachel Gawen
Alison Geddes
Tony Ghazal
Edward Gilbert
Julie Gliese
Peter Gliese
Miguel Goni
Steve Guthrie
Andrew Graham
Jean Graham
Alison Grant
Carol Grealy
Nicki Green
Stuart Hale
Diane Hales

Rebecca Hallam
Paul Hambly
Afifah Hamilton
Jeff Hannaford
Teresa Harcourt
Marika Harding
Lesley Harris
Michael Harris
Catherine Harrison
Lindsay Hart
Vaughan Hedley
Ann-Christin Heltne
Diarmid Herlihy
Meredith Hernandez
Torben Hersborg
Hadassain Hilewitz
Alan Hoad
Steven Hoare
Philip Hochhauser
Jennifer Hodge
Amanda Holland
Philip Holmes
Catherine Horne
Stephanie Horton
Stephen Howard
Ruth Huddlestone
Diane Hunt
Penny Hutson
Elizabeth Huzzey
Alan Ibbitson
Sanjay Jayswal
Emma Jeffries
Kirsten Jensen
Linda Johansdottir
Timothy John
Diane Jones
Stephen Jones
Sue Kalicinska
Katherine Kavanagh
David Kellett
James Kemp
Cecile Kiener
Louise Kimber
Caroline King

Oran Kivity
Silvia Kon
Anna Konkurowich
Louise Krawchenko
Salia Krouri
Jacqueline Lambert
Jocelyn Lardy
Andrew Latter
Sheila Leet
Alison Ley
Karen Livesey
Judith Lloyd
Stephane Loiseau
Margarita di Lorenzo
Carole Louch
Christopher Low
Ian Low
Charlotte Lugg
Kenneth Lunn
Julia Lyndon
David McGinn
Sharon McLeod
Kevin McSean
John McTurk
Diana Mantripp
Nick Marcer
David Marriot
Janet Martin
David Matthews
Maire Mayne
Kalim Mehrabi
Karen Mejlaender
Amanda Milne
Jan Minnema
Kenneth Michie
Richard Moon
Bharti Moraiji
Alicia Morland
François Mounis
Jennifer Munro
Fiona Murray
Lene Mørch
James Moylan
Anthony Nevin

Andrew Newman
Brian Nicholls
Colin Nicholls
Stephen Noakes
Della Nock
Trudy Norris
Rosemary Norton
Steven O'Brien
Lip Ong
Ayokunnun Olarewaju
Peter Palmer
Simon Palmer
Annette Pantall
Gordon Parfett
Dawn Parkin
Jonathan Parsons
Alexi Pashourtides
Amanda Payne
John Pearson
Philip Pelham
Karen Pelling
William Penno
Matthew Peters
John Pichler
Birthe Pickwoad
Claire Piper
Diana Pitt
Ianto Powell
Marcelo Pragier
Simon Prideaux
Ceri Pritchard
Jeremy Pye
Caroline Quayle
Rachel Quickenden
Lou Radford
Anita Ralph
Sabine Raukamp
Philippa Rayne
Anna Reeve
Kyeth Ribbetson
Kay van Rietschoten
Robert Ritchie
Barbara Rivera
Anna Rosa Robertsdottir

Karen Robin
Tim Rofe
Carol Rogers
Jacqueline Rogers
Catherine Roguski
Martin Rose
Amaya Ross
Jackie Ross
Jason Rosser-Smith
Alan Rumsey
Ron Samra
Ninet Sapir
Roni Sapir
Delphine Sayre
Graham Scarr
Annette Schreiber
Sarah Sedgwick
Nicola Sell
Shahida Shuja
Barry Sibul
Karen Smallcorn
Amanda Smith
Gregory Smith
John Smith
Carmel Smythe
Peta Sneddon
Nicholas Snelling
Joanna Solan
Elizabeth Spiby
Pamela Stadlen
Helen Stapleton
Richard Starmer-Jones
Isobel Staynes
Keith Stelling
Tamsin Stewart
Tim Stillwell
Barrie Stone
Alison Strode
Heidi Stubbs
Anne Sullivan
Russel Sutton
Michael Talbot
Andrew Taylor
Heather Temple

Rhona Thomas
Charles Tisdall
Steena Todd
Jackie Townsend
Heidi Trondsen
Nicholas Tuckley
Alison Tyas
Jitendra Vara
Vangelis Vassalos
Piers Vigers
Pip Waller
Barbara Walsh
Richard Wegrzyk
Gillian Whybrow
David Wilson
Margaret Winton
Massih Yaghmaie
Dani Yakobson
Lise Zimmerman

If you cannot,

in the long run,

tell everyone

what you have been

doing,

your doing has been

worthless.

Erwin Schrodinger, "Science and Humanism"